Bleeding Edge

The Business of Health Care in the New Century

J.D. Kleinke

AN ASPEN PUBLICATION®
Aspen Publishers, Inc.
Gaithersburg, Maryland
1998

Library of Congress Cataloging-in-Publication Data

Kleinke, J.D.
Bleeding edge: the business of health care in the new century/
J.D. Kleinke
p. cm.
Includes bibliographical references and index.
ISBN 0-8342-1190-4
1. Medical care—United States.   2. Medical economics—United
States.   I. Title.
RA395.A3K57   1998
362.1'0973—dc21
98-20691
CIP

Cover art design by Mark Dangle.

Orders: (800) 638-8437
Customer Service: (800) 234-1660

About Aspen Publishers • For more than 35 years, Aspen has been a leading professional
publisher in a variety of disciplines. Aspen's vast information resources are available in both
print and electronic formats. We are committed to providing the highest quality information
available in the most appropriate format for our customers. Visit Aspen's Internet site for more
information resources, directories, articles, and a searchable version of Aspen's full catalog,
including the most recent publications: **http://www.aspenpublishers.com**
Aspen Publishers, Inc. • The hallmark of quality in publishing
Member of the worldwide Wolters Kluwer group.

Editorial Services: Denise H. Coursey
Library of Congress Catalog Card Number: 98-20691
ISBN: 0-8342-1190-4

Printed in the United States of America

1 2 3 4 5

*This book is dedicated to the memory of Merit Kimball,
health care journalist, teacher, and fellow believer
in the healing power of red rock canyons.
She would have disagreed with some of its conclusions,
shared others in the passionate defense of a cause,
and celebrated my right to draw them all.*

As water shapes its flow in accordance with the ground, so an army manages its victory in accordance with the situation of the enemy. And as water has no constant form, there are in war no constant conditions.

Sun Tzu, *The Art of War*

TABLE OF CONTENTS

FIGURES

PREFACE

This book could well carry the additional subtitle "as of this writing." Recurrence of this phrase throughout *Bleeding Edge* is *not* my attempt to hedge against some unforeseen legislative cataclysm destined to undo a decade of market-driven struggle by the U.S. health care system toward self-correction. Nor is it an attempt to spare myself from the next round of witchhunts by the popular media, which alternately embrace and condemn the contributions of hospitals, then drug companies, then HMOs, then back to hospitals. Rather, "as of this writing" acknowledges a pace of system change escalated to all-out battle royale, as today's health care industry transforms itself from sleepy, subsidized collegiality to bare-knuckles, zero-sum corporate organization.

The pervasiveness of this phrase reflects the use of what feels like a stylus and clay tablet to predict the outcome of a revolution best described in electronic pulses. Indeed, out at health care's bleeding edge is a collective disorientation, one created and sustained by the industry's intense, ceaseless market convulsions. As a result, many of the specific examples used to illustrate the principles developed and conclusions drawn throughout this book are daily superseded by more powerful examples, or modified by hard luck in their implementation, or occasionally repudiated by market resistance or government intervention.

Health system prognostication is made even more risky a business by the collective professional insecurities of those who crave it most. The conflicting values and growing anxiety that pervade today's health care organization render it especially vulnerable to the ever-changing management fashion designs of those who bill by the hour, and the musings of health care "futurists" informed more by anecdotes of failed experiments and false starts than rigorous strategic analysis. How far off the mark can even the most vigilant take us? Nothing less than the *Harvard Business Review* argued in 1992 that health care was "leaving the cycle of competition defined in the 1980s and entering a period in which public goals will be expressed."[1]

Whoops! Health care competition has accelerated so quickly since its "definition" in the 1980s that nearly 60 percent of the health care delivery system has changed ownership control, costs are falling relative to inflation, and the ranks of the uninsured—the beneficiaries of any expression of public goals—continue to grow. Real deflation in health care costs, inconceivable as recently as 1993 and driven less by managed care itself than by the systemic disciplines and behavior modifications it has imposed, is not an anomaly; rather, it is the beginning of a major restructuring of the entire health care delivery system.

But this good news may be far too little, too late: U.S. health care costs are still grossly out of proportion with the rest of the industrialized world and thus continue to act as a drag on U.S. business relative to foreign competitors. To complicate matters further, the fashionably contrarian talk among health care's *cognoscenti*, as of this writing, anticipates a renewal in health care inflation. The market-driven revolution in health care, it seems, proceeds two steps forward, one step back.

The vulnerability to faulty conjecture is understandable in health care: there is enormous uncertainty draped across its landscape at the close of the 20th century. The loudest voices you hear in today's health care enterprise tend to be the most shrill and the most confused. The typical health care executive is only now beginning to understand the system's diseases, inferred mostly from witnessing their subtle and not so subtle short-term curatives in the various forms of managed care. And it certainly does not help that the treatment of those underlying diseases proceeds while much of their symptoms rage on: the end result is a situation that could not be any more complex, bewildering or, at times, self-contradictory. The spectacular rise and just as spectacular crash and burn of Columbia/HCA Healthcare Corporation is only the most visible example. What is designed to work perfectly in the new century's health care system—unapologetic consolidation of inpatient capacity, the alignment of hospital and physician economic self-interests, aggressive assemblage of a complete continuum of care—may be a recipe for disaster in the remnants of the current century's system.

One of the few *benefits* of using what feels like a stylus and clay tablet to describe this revolution in progress is the enforced reliance for guidance on history books as much as the daily newspaper or Internet. Amidst all the confusion raging out at the bleeding edge of health care, the permanence of "writing a book" has forced me to find some lasting clarity, a few truisms cut from the time-tested templates of industrial history, and a more elastic sense of how things will work when the noise stops and the transformation of the U.S. health care system is complete. *Bleeding Edge* seizes upon the present, historic moment in health care. It applies various tools of traditional management theory—competitive strategic analysis, operations research, organizational design, and the like—to a $1 trillion business finally subject to the rules, traumas, and triumphs of any other industry. It proceeds on the principle that health care, despite its enormous share of the economy, is only now emerging as a full-fledged, modern industry. It also presupposes that, as health care gropes its way toward true industrial organization, management of the health care enterprise is undergoing a similar transformation: from folk art to industrial science; from reactive stewardship to strategic execution by its managers.

By analyzing the current churn in the context of a century's worth of system development, *Bleeding Edge* systematically cultivates a set of principles that will hold their shape, even as their most obvious embodiments inevitably change color faster than the daily media—

much less a full-blown book—can adequately track. The current and historic transformation of the health care system is very much a work in constant progress, and so too are the ideas generated within *Bleeding Edge*.

WHAT ABOUT THOSE 41 MILLION UNINSURED?

Reform of the system through marketplace principles is the best way to solve our most pressing and vexing health care policy issue: the uninsured. The Clintons had it exactly backwards. To serve the needs of a small, ever-shifting minority without private health insurance, they sought to tear down the entire system, a categorical fix for a line-item problem. It makes far more sense to let the health care community put its own house in order first; this will inevitably control costs and make insurance more affordable. This in turn will allow policy makers to leverage the successes of a self-reforming system when dealing with what is a labor-market pricing problem, rather than a failure of system performance. *As morally critical and intellectually compelling as this problem is, it unfortunately falls outside the scope of this book.*

My contribution is to find and articulate a better way to configure and manage the current health care system. I leave it to others—and hopefully myself at a later date—to figure out the financing of coverage for those 41 million and counting who have been priced out of the system. I will, however, drop one clue: the nation's uninsured are already receiving care, when their untreated illnesses rage out of hand, through the worst possible mechanism: uncompensated care provided by hospitals. The cost of this is already built into the system—in the tax breaks for not-for-profit hospitals and HMOs; in the bad debts written off by providers; and in the physician education funding provided by the federal government. The sources for financing the uninsured already exist within the system's current economic architecture. They simply need to be extracted, properly designed, and built onto the system like an extra wing.

YOUR TURN

Because everything this book seeks to describe is very much a constant work in progress, I will continue to adapt and amplify its analyses and examples in real-time, in response to the daily tumult of the health care marketplace. These explorations will be posted on the Internet at **http://www.hs-net.com** and will be linked back to the original text for reference. This activity will create ever newer material from a baseline of theory and understanding, and will yield a continuously "revised edition" of this book.

Best of all, this Web site will provide me with direct access to you, the reader, critic, and implementer of the ideas developed in this book. In the process, we will establish a forum for relating the abstractions and analyses of *Bleeding Edge* with the emerging realities of health care from readers in its trenches. I look forward to your joining me on this continuing adventure.

Denver, Colorado
April 1998

REFERENCE

1. R. Stevens, "The Hospital as an Organizational Chameleon: New-Fashioned for the 1990s," *Harvard Business Review*, November/December 1992, 91.

PART I

DIAGNOSIS

The history of medicine has been written as an epic of progress, but it is also a tale of social and economic conflict over the emergence of new hierarchies of power and authority, new markets, and new conditions of belief and experiences.

Paul Starr
The Social Transformation of American Medicine[1]

How much is a human life worth? In the United States, one heart attack patient's life is worth at least $200,000; in Europe, it is worth considerably less.

In 1993, biotech manufacturer Genentech finally proved the clinical superiority of its clot-busting drug, tissue Plasminogen Activator (t-PA), over streptokinase—a generic drug with similar clinical benefits but one-tenth the cost per patient—in a clinical trial involving 41,000 heart attack patients. The magnitude of that superiority? A 1 percent improvement in mortality.[2]

From a pure cost-effectiveness perspective, this puny improvement in mortality for an ultimately disabling condition does not justify t-PA's additional $1,850 cost per patient—unless the one extra person saved out of a hundred happens to be you. Or your father. Or your spouse.

Before and after the clinical trial, streptokinase continued to dominate the market in Europe. But within three months of the trial's results hitting the airwaves, t-PA's U.S. market share had risen from 50 to 66 percent.[3] This is particularly remarkable if you think back to 1993: the nation's demands for medical cost containment were reaching mob proportion; employers were herding millions of people into health maintenance organizations (HMOs) and preferred provider organizations (PPOs); and "managed care" was the cornerstone not only of plans to fix the economic woes of Medicare and Medicaid, but also of the Clintons' blueprint for reforming the entire system. Medicine cost too much, everyone agreed, and nearly everyone—except for those actually providing it—seemed to agree that managed care was the answer.

Meanwhile the nation's physicians were quietly going about the business of diagnosing and treating patients, which included increasing their relative use of t-PA at a cost of $185,000 ($1,850 per patient × 100 patients) to save one additional life.[4] Physicians willfully chose the leading-edge drug at more than 6 times the cost of its cheaper alternative—the efforts of managed care companies notwithstanding—because to do otherwise would be to practice clinically substandard medicine for individual patients. To do otherwise would chafe against the training, ethos, and self-determination of the nation's medical profession; it would ask physicians to ignore empirical truth and violate their Hippocratic oath; and it would place the rights of the individual behind the rights of the group, a cardinal sin in America. For committing this sin, the physician would be exposed to claims of medical malpractice. *Which would you have the jury believe, doctor: that you were not aware of a ground-breaking study on improved mortality for heart attack patients, published in the most prestigious medical journal in the world? Or that you simply chose to ignore it in the case of my client's husband, dead at the age of 52?*

Such is the culture of medicine in America. We demand the best, accept nothing less, and reward lawyers handsomely for making sure we get it. Even the imminence of certain death does not attenuate this cultural fact, as the clinical behaviors, costs, and outcomes of the typical intensive care unit (ICU) illustrate. Our national consciousness is steeped in optimism, hostile to all processes and manifestations of aging, and enraptured by a limitless faith in technology; as a people we have come to revile death as much a personal defeat as a personal loss. Death is an insult to the nation's proud heritage of scientific discovery and its well-financed infrastructure of miracle machinery. For an example of how thickly these beliefs run in our blood, one need look no further than the contrasting attitudes between Europe and the United States with regard to hospice versus ICU care for end-stage disease, heroic but ultimately futile battles against metastatic cancer, and physician-assisted suicide. In the United States, we fight to the end, regardless of what it costs.

That's the hard place.

Here's the rock: in the United States, health care costs too much. Health care consumes 13.6 percent of our economy—compared with 9.7 percent for Canada, 10.2 percent for the nations of Western Europe, and 8.3 percent for Japan.[5-7] Despite our appetite for leading edge drugs like t-PA, the additional $333 billion per year in economic share that we spend on health care in comparison to our trading partners buys the United States the highest infant mortality rate and lowest life expectancy in the industrialized world.[8] Meanwhile, half of the typical U.S. hospital sits empty, while the other half cannot push patients out the door fast enough. Many argue the nation has twice as many physicians as necessary, even though the average office-based physician attempts to diagnose and treat 19 patients in an average working day. And 41 million people live under the menace of no health insurance coverage.[9-12]

In an industry characterized by paradox, none is greater than the very stature of the industry itself: American medicine, with its prodigious research community, breathtaking technologies, and army of dedicated clinicians is a national treasure, net exporter, and creator of good jobs; the American system for financing, managing, and delivering that medicine is a national disgrace, a hodgepodge of conflicting interests, bureaucratic incoherence, and unworkable organizational designs. The United States is the best nation on earth when one has private health insurance and needs state-of-the-art medical care, but the "system" falls to pieces when it comes time to figure out how much that care really costs; exactly who should pay for it; and whether or not the care resulted in a good outcome, for a good price, and why.

Somebody should fix this!

This has been the clarion call from corporate America, consumers, the media, activists for the uninsured, and variously opportunistic politicians since the 1970s, when medical costs first started inching out of control. The call grew steadily louder through the 1980s, until it became a deafening roar in the early 1990s: the nation's inflationary monster had long since been slain and buried, but health care premiums were still increasing by double-digit figures every year.[13]

What is the source of the health care system's disconnect from all the progress made by the rest of the U.S. economy? There are two: bad economics and bad history.

YOU CALL THIS A MARKET?

The U.S. health care system is a mess because the economic behaviors driving it are not only irrational, but often perverse and counterproductive. Marketplaces require rational consumers who demand ever better products at ever better prices, and producers who are rewarded for supplying both. The health care marketplace, by contrast, is distorted by third-party reimbursement that does not reward rational behavior by either consumers or producers, and in many cases actually penalizes it.

Because the consumer of the medical product is not the purchaser of that product, the consumer has no motive to determine its real value. Such a consumer does not have any incentive to question their innate need for the good; nor any incentive to challenge the seller's motives for providing it; nor any incentive to shop for the best price. In the fee-for-service system that has characterized the U.S. health care system for the past century—and still does for the most part—consumers enter the health care system wielding blank checks, which providers are all too willing to cash.

Because the producer of the medical product determines the need for that product and is paid more for producing more of it, the producer has no motive to reduce cost. Fee-for-service medicine is extremely perverse; it rewards physicians and hospitals financially for overtreatment, heroic treatment, redundant treatment, or any treatment at all, regardless of economic or scientific merit. At its most perverse, this system actually *rewards* minor botches, undetectable by the patient, who then returns to the same physician or hospital to fix, for a fee, what that provider failed to fix in the first place. This is *not* to say that the typical provider delivers care with an eye to maximizing income; it *is* to say that the incentives are in place not to deliver it efficiently.

The fee-for-service system is the logical financing mechanism for the culture of medicine in America. As a society, we have grown up believing that every American—or at least every insured one—has a birthright for immediate and unlimited access to all the medical technology and resources the health care system has at its disposal. Fee-for-service medicine cleaves to a nation's belief in the supremacy of individual rights, self-determination, and unlimited technological progress and availability.

But such beliefs are not cheap. Sooner or later, the bills start coming in.

YOU CALL THIS A SYSTEM?

The U.S. health care system is a mess because perennially unresolved power struggles among hospitals, physicians, and third-party payers—stretching back to the beginning of the 20th century—have rendered it a fragmented, unintegrated, uncoordinated disaster. The one aspect of American medicine more literally incredible than the genius behind its mind-bending technologies is the stupidity of how those technologies are deployed for the average patient.

Medical delivery in the United States is a miracle of disorganization, held together through the sheer collective will of overworked professionals tasked with managing tens of millions of patients by memory, pen scrawl, Post-It note, and telephone call. Indeed, it is overly generous to call this a "system" at all, when it more accurately resembles a chaos of small boats tossed about on a roiling sea of paper. The wonder of health care in the United States is not that so many patients fall through the cracks, fail to comply with medical orders, receive conflicting therapies, and so on. The wonder, given the situation, is how *few* do.

For all our advances in medical science and practice, our providers' abilities to manage the delivery of care over time and geographic space are crude at best, non-existent in the norm, and borderline negligent at their worst. This disaster of inefficiency is a legacy of the history of American medicine, based on a simple but, until recently, wholly unalterable clinical apartheid: physicians practice autonomously from facilities.[14] The United States is almost unique in the world in that physicians are separate economic entities from hospitals, but at the same time continue to treat their patients once admitted into the hospital. This arrangement makes running a hospital extremely complex: those decisions with the greatest impact on the institution's costs and profits—and its quality and reputation—are made by a class of people usually not employed by that institution.

This clinical apartheid is complicated further by the financial one created by third-party payment. The looming, bureaucratic, once monolithic health insurance industry is the third leg—cut to yet a third length—of the wobbly stool that is medical delivery in the United States. It mattered less that an external party was responsible for paying a patient's bills when medical cost inflation was not a significant issue prior to the late-1980s; the insurers just paid them—even if it did take three times longer than any other entity in America to pay its bills.[15] It became a serious problem when insurers began to insinuate themselves into the clinical process, further complicating all transactions and interactions, pitting provider against insurer, patient against provider, and insurer against patient. Only the pioneering HMOs like Kaiser and Group Health of Puget Sound successfully integrated the financing and delivery of medical care; the rest of the industry devolved into an elaborate and costly paper chase that nobody would ever win.

By default, it became chaos as usual across the U.S. health care system. Small wonder that there are enormous, inexplicable variations in the patterns of medical care delivered to patients. Variations by region, physician type, and patient's insurance status infest the entire spectrum of medical care: surgery versus drugs for the same condition; hospital admission rates; hospital lengths of stay; traditional versus leading-edge surgical technique; diagnostic imaging and lab testing frequency; specific drug selection; the list goes on, *ad infinitum*. When viewed in the aggregate, such variations are far more than just costly from a financial and human perspective; they often border on the scandalous.

One of the more egregious examples, noted frequently by researchers if only because of the enormous cost impact, is the arbitrary use of Cesarean section procedures to deliver newborns. The rate of C-sections as a percentage of total deliveries varies from as low as 11 percent to as high as 40 percent for identical populations. The explanation for the variation in many cases? The patient's insurance coverage. As the average hospital charge for a C-section in 1995 was $6,243 versus $2,918 for a normal delivery, good insurance means a woman is far more likely to "require" a C-section.[16] In

Pennsylvania, for example, the largest Blue Shield plan shifted reimbursement for all deliveries to a global fee, regardless of which technique was used. Physicians were paid the same fee for either method of delivery. Within a year, the C-section rate was cut in half.[17]

In health care in the United States, this phenomenon is, unfortunately, not phenomenal. A 1996 study in North Carolina on hysterectomy rates—not a trivial procedure in terms of financial or emotional cost—discovered that for risk-adjusted populations, one group of gynecologists performed the surgery 60 percent more frequently. The difference in the two groups of gynecologists? Their gender.[18]

The gender of a patient's physician should not matter! Clinical decision making should be an objective process, particularly when it has huge economic and psychological implications. And yet study after study reveals enormous variations in the delivery of medical care. What is the sum total of these variations?

MANAGED CARE TO THE RESCUE

The sum total of clinical variations is aggressive intervention by an emboldened third-party payer, positioning itself as the champion of medical necessity and clinical consistency, and driven by its own financial self-interest to bring some predictability to the system. This third-party payer is the managed care organization (MCO)—harsh medicine for health care's bad economics and bad history.

The MCO functions like a near-lethal dose of chemotherapy for a sick health care market. As chemo poisons the body to return the cancer victim to health, so too the U.S. health care system is undergoing the harshest of treatments to rid itself of the cancers that have slowly grown to afflict an otherwise viable, energetic, promising patient. Those cancers include the distorted behaviors and flawed incentives afflicting the medical marketplace, the absence of systems for coordinating patient care over geographic space and time, inexplicable variations in clinical care, and a host of other ills a century in the making.

MCOs have shocked the system into removing excess and costly capacity; shaken providers out of their ignorant bliss about health care costs; created the first-ever expectations about price/performance for employers and other purchasers; developed tools for measuring and monitoring clinical outcomes; and forced hospitals and physicians finally to integrate, coordinate, and rationalize what they do. In the process, managed care has awakened all players in the health care system—physicians, hospital administrators, employee benefits executives, drug and device makers, researchers, and all but the most politically extreme among those involved in health policy—to one simple fact: the health care industry needs to be organized and run like any other industry. If health care is a business, then the tools that have fixed other businesses will fix this one as well.

Managed care as currently practiced is the essence of the health care business in overdrive. The compete-or-die, profit-seeking orientation that managed care brings to medical delivery has emerged as the nation's readily available alternative to a government-led solution to fixing endemic health care system problems. This clear preference for market-based reform is the nation's collective recognition that if government were capable of administering a national health care system—one that worked well, promoted innovation, and met the needs of consumers—there never would have been the need for the private sector to create a Federal Express. Under a government-run health care system—the typical health care purchaser seems to have recognized, if only unconsciously—getting a doctor's appointment, lab test, X-ray, or prescription filled would surely be as quick, easy, and convenient as doing your taxes or getting a new drivers' license. This is a lesson the Clintons had to learn the hard way.

As alien or offensive as this fact sounds to those still clinging to the ideal that health care is a public rather than market good, it is still a fact, one galvanized by an accident of history: private employers drive much of the U.S. health care system and will—for better or worse—for the foreseeable future. Why? Because employment-based insurance is too deeply entrenched in the system, too woven

into union contracts and retirement benefit plans, and too well po-
liced by the dynamics of highly competitive markets for skilled labor. Thus, it was a cultural inevitability that the values and behaviors
of corporate organization would eventually come to dominate the
health system as it struggles to reinvent itself.

Corporate America certainly has a vested interest: total health
care costs for U.S. companies now exceed their net income by 8
percent.[19] Consider the impact of this on the nation's largest employer, and therefore largest private health care purchaser. In 1995
General Motors spent $3.6 billion on medical care, an amount
equivalent to more than $1,200 per car.[20] Not only is this shockingly
high, it is also shockingly disadvantageous: foreign auto companies
spend as little as $100 per car on health care, due to their younger,
healthier workforces and dearth of retirees.[21] For Detroit, this competitive problem will grow only worse as unionized workforces with
guaranteed health benefits continue to age, retire, and consume
medical services. How much worse? To fund the eventual health
care needs of its current and future retirees, Ford needs to set aside
on its balance sheet—for each additional percentage point of medical inflation—an additional *$2 billion.*[22] (This is the miracle of com-
pounding that financial advisers like to talk about, but to a somewhat
different end.)

As a result, the steps taken by corporate America to cope with
systemic health care problems are far more focused and effective
than anything the government—with its tangle of special interests,
conflicting objectives, and lack of any meaningful accountability—
can manage. This wholly explains the movement of numerous government programs to piggyback onto employer-based health systems: these range from the rapid movement of Medicaid and
Medicare populations into managed care plans; to focused experiments like Medicare Insured Groups, under which retirees continue
to use their employer's health care systems instead of Medicare, saving the employers money through greater leveraging of those systems while saving the government money through the efficiencies of
privatization.[23]

The typical large employer's vested interest in managing the long-term health (and thus long-term costs) of its employed population has created an enormous market opportunity for the promise of "managed care," a once exclusively enlightened alternative to unmanaged indemnity insurance. The temporary but ultimately necessary medicines of managed care—beating price concessions out of providers, aggressively controlling utilization, and challenging the clinical decision making of physicians and hospitals—have alleviated the worst symptoms of the health care cost crisis in the closing decades of the century.

But the long-term view of employers—and the infinite-term view of consumers—clashes inevitably with the short-term fixations of managed care as practiced today. This clash spells the certainty of managed care's doom in a market churning with both anxiety and innovations.

NOW...RESCUE US FROM MANAGED CARE

In the course of administering its emergency medicine to the health care marketplace, managed care has exacerbated the confusion and complexity of the system, replacing the chronic disorganization of health care delivery with acute over-organization. The managed care industry has developed and installed a pervasive infrastructure of heavy-handed and cumbersome command-and-control systems that manage cost, not care. Window dressing about quality and other marketing claims notwithstanding, the primary goal of such systems has been singular: reduce direct costs associated with medical decision making, regardless of quality, outcomes, and even long-run economics.

The harsh medicine that is the essence of managed care works, if only because the patient was so desperately ill. But in the end, managed care's methods hardly qualify as stand-alone "products" of sufficient value to justify the continued existence of HMOs, PPOs, and other types of managed care organizations, collectively referred to for the remainder of *Bleeding Edge* as "MCOs." After prices are adjusted to reflect competitive bidding by MCOs—and after the most obvious excessive utilization is pruned from a population's medical experience—what is left for the MCO to do?

In the early to mid-1990s, the MCOs attempted to differentiate themselves as managers of chronic disease like asthma, heart disease, and diabetes.[24] But it quickly became clear to the MCO that the last thing it wanted was a reputation in the community for its "diabetic-friendliness"; the end result would be more diabetics enrolling, and fewer disenrolling. For all its disease management acumen, abnormally high rates of disease incidence still cost a health plan far more than a normal population. This became more problematic by 1995 as the MCOs turned their marketing efforts toward older, less penetrated target populations—populations more likely to have developed chronic disorders. To make matters still worse, at roughly the same time the Internet began to stitch together virtual communities of people suffering from the same disorder. With a few keystrokes a boy with multiple sclerosis (MS) can now sing the praises of how well his MCO helps him get all the care and drugs he needs—and the next days, the family of every MS patient in town is calling to sign up.

With the disease management initiatives backfiring, the MCOs were forced to retreat to their original premise of prevention and wellness.[25] As the manager of a population's collective health status, the MCOs believed they could make money by aggressively vaccinating babies and the elderly, screening for high-risk pregnancy, diagnosing previously undiagnosed hypertensives and depressives, and getting their members on cholesterol-lowering medications. What the MCOs failed to recognize is that these measures usually cost more in the short-run than they return. For example, the standard cholesterol-lowering regimen costs roughly $1,000 per patient per year, but for the average patient the cost benefits do not show up for more than a decade.[26] With an average turnover rate of 20 percent of its population per year, the MCO that invests in preventive medical care is merely saving its competitors medical costs in subsequent years. With both disease management and prevention strategies paradoxically detrimental to the financial performance of the MCO, its only recourse is to redouble its efforts to impose cost-effectiveness guidelines on the physicians who treat their general populations. It can push the rock that much harder.

Unfortunately, the hard place just got harder too.

A 1998 study in the *Annals of Internal Medicine* found that guidelines designed to maximize cost-effectiveness for an entire population do *not* maximize cost-effectiveness for most types of care studied.[27] This signifies a fatal structural defect in the very heart of today's managed care industry: physicians are sworn to their conscience—and their medical malpractice insurers—to do what is best for every individual patient; managed care operators are sworn to their shareholders to do what is cheapest for the entire population. People are not populations, at least not in the United States. This is a problem.

Given this innate and irreconcilable conflict, is it any surprise that MCOs are generally viewed—at least in the media backlash of the mid- to late-1990s[28]—as hostile to individual patients and hostile to individual physicians? *Is it any wonder that managed care has been viewed as anathema to a medical culture compelled by training, disposition, and legal precedent to use t-PA for heart attack patients?*

The MCO's perceived hostility to physicians translates directly into perceived hostility toward patients, hence the backlash. Bad business strategy makes for even worse politics. Among the many political blunders of the Clinton administration in its attempt to overturn California's legalization of marijuana for medical purposes, the biggest was its threat of reprisal to physicians: prescribe marijuana for your patients who need it, and we will take away your DEA control number, effectively shutting you out of practice.[29] Public outrage at Washington's meddling—previously restricted for the most part to California—swept across the nation, and the law still stands. In its zeal to overturn the law, the Clinton administration went after patients suffering from often agonizing diseases, and their doctors for trying to help them. MCOs should heed the example.

The object lesson from this episode? The nation reveres physicians and resents challenges to their autonomy, clinical hegemony, and judgment. Their moral authority—earned through years of training and personal sacrifices that most Americans can comprehend only enough to be awestruck by it—is reinforced by the generally noble portraiture of physicians, warts and all, in generation upon generation of medical television shows. Physicians have an intellectual incumbency that will reign in the end, which stands in sharp relief to the naked ambitions and hollow advertising of MCO marketers.

Try as MCOs might through their mawkish image advertising, Americans equate their personal medical experience with personal encounters with their physicians. Why? Because a patient's or family member's life-and-death hopes rise and fall with their physician's gestures; their best hopes and worst fears hang on their physician's words and asides; and they are quick to rage at their physicians for bad results. Is it any wonder, given this relationship, that physicians have trained themselves to be so circumspect in communicating diagnoses and prognoses?

In glaring contrast to the intensity of emotion involved in the physician/patient relationship, the MCO/"covered member" relationship is a petty nuisance. Why? Because MCOs don't diagnose or treat people; they process them. Hospitals are only slightly better, but are still generally considered large, impersonal machines through which people move when sick, guided not by the hospital's protocols, but by their physician's training and instincts.

Managed care, at least as currently practiced and very much like the economic chemotherapy that it most resembles, has little usefulness beyond removing the system's underlying cancer so that the system can proceed symptom-free and wiser in its habits for the experience. But if managed care has accomplished nothing else, it has succeeded in accelerating the inevitable: it has underscored the fact that the health care business is indeed a business, and as such is not entitled to unlimited subsidy by the rest of the economy; and it has succeeded in pointing out this inevitability to most players in the health care system. Managed care is the profit-seeking architect of the new health care system, its consummate taskmaster, its *de facto* business school professor.

Yet there is one business principle that managed care would rather not articulate, if only because managed care itself will turn out to be its biggest victim: all businesses, like all civilizations, evolve along historic arcs. They begin as cottage industries, a fragmentation of individual producers and purchasers; eventually marketplace and economic forces transform them into rationalized, appropriately scaled industries. Economies of scale, organization, distribution and transaction all emerge, and the collective behaviors of rational producers and consumers create equilibria of price, quantity, and quality. For numerous reasons unique to the nature of health care as a product—all of which will be explored in this book—it took until the 1990s for the U.S. health care industry, prodded by the market-rationalizing forces of managed care, to initiate this transformation. When the transformation is complete, managed care as we currently know it will have self-destructed, leaving in its wake a wholly reorganized and more functional health care industry.

TREATMENT PLAN

Bleeding Edge seizes upon the present, historic moment in health care. It applies various tools of traditional management theory—competitive strategic analysis, operations research, organizational design, and the like—to a $1 trillion business finally subject to the rules, traumas, and triumphs of any other industry.

In the process, this book identifies, formulates, and follows to their full consummation five forces of health care transformation. These forces are deeply rooted in the historic development of—and current challenges facing—today's health care system and the culture. They are working in concert to drive down health care costs today; simplify and streamline the health care system tomorrow; and ultimately liberate providers from managed care when the transformation is complete.

With their interrelationships illustrated in Figure I–1, these five forces are

1. risk assumption, to correct fundamental problems in health care consumption and market economics
2. consumerism, to neutralize distortions in the health system created by the self-interest and faulty paternalism of MCOs and other insurers and galvanize competition among providers
3. consolidation, to scale the health care infrastructure properly, mobilize capital, spread risk across broader populations of patients and providers, and allocate health care resources more efficiently
4. integration, to correct the fragmentation and other structural defects built into the medical delivery system
5. industrialization, to rationalize the haphazard use of services, increase economic predictability, improve quality, and reduce costs

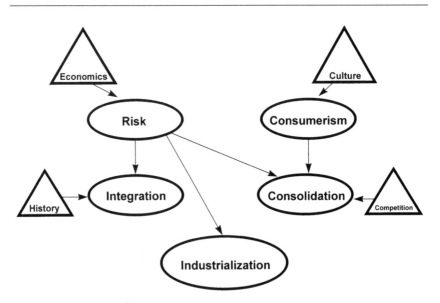

Figure I–1 The Five Forces of Health Care Transformation.

After codifying and projecting the combined effects of the five forces of health care transformation in the new century, this book traces the slow but inevitable ascendancy of a new business entity— the emerging health care organization or EHO. The rudiments of the EHO can be found in the networks of physicians and hospitals currently forming in every major health care market in the United States. The typical market of 10 to 12 hospitals and 200 to 300 small physician group practices is currently sorting into two to four organized "integrated delivery systems" or future EHOs. Most of these entities are striving to consolidate excess capacity, vertically integrate care settings, and raise capital. Over time, these EHOs will eventually develop the critical mass and organizational sophistication sufficient to assume financial risk and industrialize their processes of care to manage that risk profitably.

When fully consummated, the EHOs will have eliminated the MCOs, providing all medical services for fixed fees to covered populations from employers and government. The use of EHOs both to insure and deliver health care removes all the mistrust, antagonism, and ultimately costly, cumbersome nature of the relationship between providers and MCOs. When this transformation is complete, the answer to that most menacing of questions "do you know who controls your health care?" will be—surprise, surprise—your doctor.

Indeed, as you will discover in this book, the rise of the EHO will spare the industry from many of the fashionably gloomy predictions about the destinies of both the medical profession and the hospital community. The analysis at the heart of the chapter on physicians (Part IV, "MD, MBA") concludes that the future U.S. health care system will need at least as many physicians as are practicing today, not fewer, and that the system will also need a higher percentage of specialists to primary care physicians, not the lower percentage that policy makers and others have theorized for years. The analysis included in the chapter on hospitals (Part IV, "The Un-Hospital") illustrates how EHOs will provide today's hospitals with the opportunity to transform themselves from archaic facilities into futuristic care-delivery and coordination sites, central nodes in a system that provide as much outpatient care as inpatient, and that enjoy leadership positions within the EHO due to their legacy capital structures and information systems.

The rise of the EHO will also accelerate the current segmentation of health care markets along the dimensions of consumer preferences. In the typical local market in the new century, each competing EHO—after combining the marketing of health insurance with the marketing of health care providers—will be defined by its unique market and price positioning. Inevitably, there will be an "upmarket" EHO built around the prestigious local academic medical center. This EHO will serve as a constant differentiation check to the price-positioning of the two or three competing EHOs in the same market: the upmarket EHO will promote itself based on an association of its reputation and heritage with higher quality; the other EHOs will position themselves as the lower cost and/or broader market providers.

As we shall see, the differentiation of EHOs within individual markets—while flowing from supply-side logic regarding the evolution of providers—is reinforced by growing differentiation on the demand side, as consumers shoulder an increasing proportion of the financial burden associated with their health care. The main differentiating currency in health care markets, then, will be *choice,* and people will approach health care purchasing like they approach cars: some will have the money and inclination to drive Mercedes; others will be happy (or reluctant) to drive Fords; and still others will be forced by frugality or economic misfortune to take the bus.

The obvious conclusion of this analysis is the inevitable demise of the national managed care company in its current form. When the transformation described in *Bleeding Edge* is complete, MCOs will suffer the same fate of the indemnity insurers of the previous generation. What remains of a national MCO after relinquishing control of care delivery by pushing medical risk down to providers is described as a "Post-MCO." The typical P-MCO will be the middle-market health plan of today, reduced to an organization that vends its marketing, sales, reinsurance, and administrative functions to EHOs organized from the ranks of its former medical contracting providers. By contrast, today's better MCOs will have transformed themselves from insurers of medical risk into vendors of medical management intellectual properties. In addition to selling P-MCO services to EHOs, these companies will market the best of the proprietary tools originally developed to manage the care delivered to covered populations: risk assessment tools, protocols for illness prevention, disease management programs, and outcomes measurement systems.

Such is the end result of the wholesale introduction of business principles into the delivery of health care via the five forces of health care transformation: a short decade into the next century, and the health care system will finally start to look like any other industry. But change of this magnitude is a slow process. Even relatively simple developments within industries take time to establish themselves, work out their kinks and their economics, and gain sufficient consumer awareness and trust to modify ingrained cultures and behaviors. Federal Express emerged as a solution to the unreliability of a government-managed package delivery system in the early 1980s; while quickly conquering the business-to-business market, it took nearly a decade and a half for FedEx drop boxes to make their first appearances alongside mailboxes in residential settings.[30]

Indeed, revolutionizing the movement of packages is a fairly straightforward business. By contrast, consummation of the level and depth of change needed in an industry as large and complex as health care will take time, patience, commitment, and leadership. Transformation of 15 percent of the world's largest economy cannot happen overnight; it is tantamount to turning an oil tanker around in a moving waterway.

REFERENCES

1. P. Starr, *The Social Transformation of American Medicine* (New York: Basic Books/HarperCollins, 1982), 4.
2. E. Topol et al., "An International Randomized Trial Comparing Four Thrombolytic Strategies for Acute Myocardial Infarction," *New England Journal of Medicine* 329, no. 10 (1993): 673.

3. M. Chase, "Genentech Says Its Clot Drug Regains Market Share of 66% after Major Study," *Wall Street Journal*, 3 September, 1993.

4. Derived from calculating t-PA's mortality improvement (1%) times the net difference in the per patient cost of t-PA versus streptokinase ($2,200 – $350 = $1,850).

5. K. Levit et al., "National Health Spending Trends in 1996," *Health Affairs* 17, no. 1 (1996): 38.

6. G. Anders, *Health against Wealth* (New York: Houghton Mifflin, 1996), 22.

7. "National Health Expenditures in Canada, 1975–1984, Summary Report," Policy and Consultation Branch, Health Canada.

8. World Health Organization statistics for 1995.

9. The median acute care nonfederal U.S. hospital had a 49 percent occupancy rate in 1995, according to data published in *The Comparative Performance of U.S. Hospitals: The Sourcebook* (Baltimore: HCIA Inc., 1997), 82.

10. Based on a widely cited analysis—which will be disproved in Part IV ("MD, MBA")—of the following census calculations: one licensed physician per 400 U.S. citizens versus one staff physician for every 800 enrolled members of Kaiser Permanente, the oldest and largest closed-end HMO in the United States.

11. Based on a survey of physician-patient encounters published in *Health Care Strategic Management,* February 1997, p. 14. The calculation is 95 patient encounters per week, divided by five work days.

12. 1996 estimate for total uninsured U.S. residents by the Employee Benefit Research Institute, as reported by E. Weissenstein, "What about the Uninsured?" *Modern Healthcare*, 7 April, 1997, 122.

13. A. Stoline and J. Weiner, *The New Medical Marketplace: A Physician's Guide to the Health Care System in the 1990s* (Baltimore: The Johns Hopkins University Press, 1993), 41. © 1993. The Johns Hopkins University Press.

14. This a major theme pervading P. Starr's landmark, Pulitzer Prize–winning social history of the U.S. health care system, *The Social Transformation of American Medicine* (New York: Basic Books/HarperCollins, 1982).

15. Days in net accounts receivable for the median U.S. hospital was 67.2 days in 1995, according to data in *The Comparative Performance of U.S. Hospitals: The Sourcebook*. The standard for most nonmedical businesses is generally thought to be between 20 and 30 days, which is why most initial collection actions commence at 30 days.

16. Mean charges for the hospital component of normal delivery versus C-section delivery (ICD-9-CM 73.59 versus 74.1), according to data in the *National Inpatient Profile* (Baltimore: HCIA Inc., 1996).

17. From a presentation given by Charles Inlander, president of Consumers Medical Society, Allentown, PA, 1993.

18. N. Bicknell et al., "Gynecologists' Sex, Clinical Beliefs, and Hysterectomy Rates," *American Journal of Public Health*, October 1994.

19. Stoline and Weiner, *The New Medical Marketplace: A Physician's Guide to the Health Care System in the 1990s*, 41.

20. R. Blumenstein, "Auto Makers Attack High Health-Care Bills with a New Approach," *Wall Street Journal*, 9 December, 1996.

21. Blumenstein, *Wall Street Journal*.

22. J. Fischl, "Reversal of Fortune," *Financial World*, 21 January, 1997, 32.

23. J. Kleinke, "Employers Can Do It without Mandates," *Wall Street Journal*, 11 May, 1994.

24. One was hard pressed to attend a health care industry conference between 1994 through 1996 *without* seeing a presentation by an MCO medical executive on the MCO's new disease management program.

25. This change in marketing strategy was reported during interviews with national medical directors from several HMOs who requested anonymity; it was confirmed by almost universal shifts in the content of national advertising campaigns by MCOs.

26. E. Rosenthal, "The HMO Catch: When Healthier Isn't Cheaper," *New York Times*, 16 March, 1997.

27. A. Granata and A. Hillman, "Competing Practice Guidelines: Using Cost-Effectiveness Analysis To Make Optimal Decisions," *Annals of Internal Medicine* 128, no. 1 (1998): 56.

28. M. Brodie et al., "Media Coverage of Managed Care," *Health Affairs*, January/February 1998, 13.

29. M. Pollan, "Just Say Sometimes," *New York Times Magazine*, 20 July, 1997.

30. Personal observation; I first noticed FedEx boxes in my neighborhood in Baltimore in late 1996.

PART II

TREATMENT

Teeming with cash flow and mismanagement, health care is an entrepreneur's paradise.

Sandy Lutz and E. Preston Gee
The For-Profit Healthcare Revolution[1]

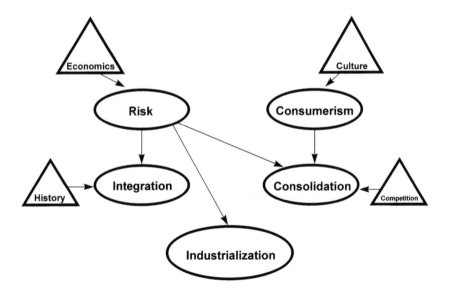

23

If greed generally "works" in the development of a nation's economy, then there is no reason it cannot work in the development of 15 percent of that economy, regardless of its complexity. This is the central principle driving the transformation of the U.S. health care system at the close of the 20th century. Even a cursory look at the industry reveals a massive conversion of the health care community to a for-profit enterprise, in principle and in practice, if not in name.

This is equal parts cultural inevitability and competitive dynamics. Health care is big business in the United States: for-profit hospital systems are considered "growth" firms by Wall Street; most health insurance is marketed by for-profit HMOs or publicly traded insurance companies; and the entire pharmaceutical and technology supplier industries—which bear nearly all of society's responsibility for translating basic biomedical research into usable products—are the darlings of investors the world over. The bloodless pragmatism of these organizations cannot help but inspire rational marketplace and organizational behaviors in the majority of hospitals and MCOs that remain not-for-profit.

The second largest Catholic hospital system, Daughters of Charity, with 49 hospitals in 12 states, routinely closes hospitals unable to compete in local markets. As a result of such closures, the number of hospitals managed by the system has decreased nearly 20 percent over the past years.[2] The Daughters of Charity system and numerous other consolidators of hospitals across the United States have arisen specifically to match the market consolidation and other business strategies of for-profit systems like Columbia/HCA Healthcare Corporation, Tenet Healthcare, Vanguard Health Systems, and others.[3]

The academic medical centers, also of a not-for-profit philosophical bent by tradition and temperament, are similarly prodded toward competitive countermoves—thanks to the market disciplines brought to their communities by for-profit MCOs and competing systems. A good example is the 1996 merger between two esteemed research and teaching institutions, Brigham and Women's Hospital and Massachusetts General Hospital, as a strategy to protect market share. As Jeffrey Otten, the chief executive officer of Brigham and Women's commented in a *New England Journal of Medicine* report on Columbia/HCA, the for-profit companies "exert competitive pressure on us to become more cost-effective. It makes us re-examine how we are providing care. Academic medical centers are very reluctant to close capacity. We haven't been able to do it through planning; perhaps having an external force like Columbia might be the only way to do it."[4] Or, as the medical director for a Columbia/HCA hospital told the *Wall Street Journal* during the government's investigation into the company's business practices, "if you're with Columbia, you're afraid you'll suddenly be investigated. If you're with the local not-for-profit, you're afraid it's so far behind the times it won't make it."[5]

While the government's investigation into allegations of fraud pervading Columbia's billing and accounting practices continues as of this writing, the impact of the company, the other for-profit systems, and for-profit payers continues to reverberate through entire markets. Countermoves by academic medical centers and not-for-profit systems like the Daughters of Charity are typical responses. According to a *Wall Street Journal* report on the ambitious, acquisitive, business-minded growth initiatives of Catholic Healthcare West (CHW), the "nuns can be just as aggressive as their for-profit rivals when fighting to gain market share."[6] The nuns who run CHW certainly have a track record of profitability to defend. Ostensibly a non-profit organization, even after providing charity care worth $174 million, CHW netted $160.5 million on $2.69 billion in revenue in fiscal year 1996.[7] This amounts to a total net margin of 6.0 percent, compared to 5.1 percent for the median not-for-profit hospital in the United States.[8]

Operating margins for not-for-profit hospitals and HMOs are typically reported in the media as such, and are typically not much different from the numbers posted by the for-profits. One of the most vocally "not-for-profit" organizations in the United States is Kaiser Permanente, the gigantic HMO based in California. It rocked the industry by reporting its first ever "loss" of $270 million for 1997—

versus "earnings of $265 million in the previous year," according to a report in *Modern Healthcare*.[9] Not-for-profits report "profits" because the number represents an important barometer of the productive capacity of society's health care resources; they are the numerators in the all-important calculations of "return on equity" and "return on total assets." Such measures are critical because all five forces of transformation described in *Bleeding Edge*—the assumption of medical risk, the development of consumer-driven markets, consolidation and rationalization of capacity, the integration of services, and industrialization—demand the mobilization of substantial capital and deployment of professional management. As capital and professional management both require healthy returns, the "profitization" of health care is a historic inevitability, a key part of the successful healing of health care's underlying disorders through heavy and sustained doses of the medicine of the marketplace.

Given the abuses, inefficiencies, and structural problems that have characterized health care financing and delivery in the United States for decades, it is easy to argue that the system is indeed begging for the accountability that for-profit culture brings to any industry. No government investigations can shake up a company as quickly or as thoroughly as a plunge in its stock price when it has strayed from its primary mission of making money.

CAPITALISTS' PROGRESS

Conversion of the culture of health care has been a work in progress since the advent of managed care in the late 1980s. The heavy for-profit capitalization of the 1990s is simply following this cultural revolution, not causing it. Since the early 1990s, not-for-profit hospitals have been competing ferociously with for-profit hospitals for contracts, and dozens of Blues plans have set up for-profit managed care subsidiaries to compete with MCOs. This sudden conversion and capitalization is a necessary underpinning for the transformation of health care, a catalyst for change that has been imminent for years.

But technically speaking, there has always been for-profit medicine at the hospital level, if only in the regions that lagged behind the rest of the United States in hospital construction. In the South, where hospital construction was stunted by the sustained economic paralysis following the Civil War,[10] and in the West, with fewer of the cultural and social institutions responsible for building not-for-profit hospitals, the importance of for-profit hospital formation was more critical. Given this early presence of for-profit medicine on the West Coast—and the historic coincidence that the MCO industry also germinated there—it is of little surprise that the health care industry looks to its individual markets as a leading indicator of health system change for the rest of the United States.

What has stunned the public (and emerged as a major public policy issue in the late 1990s) is the sudden conversion to for-profit status by hundreds of health care organizations across the United States, including hospitals, MCOs, and other insurers. All are seeking this change of status for the simple goal of raising capital to pursue the development initiatives discussed in this book: the assumption of medical risk, the consolidation of facilities, the development of fully integrated systems, and the creation of industrialized processes for delivering care. The for-profit hospital chains have found willing sellers around the country: most stand-alone hospitals simply cannot finance out of operating cash flow—or out of already strained debt capacity—the purchase and integration of physicians, the solvency funds required to assume risk, and the acquisition of nonhospital medical businesses. As a result of this movement, by 1997 more than 100 nonprofit hospitals had been acquired by the for-profit chains.[11]

The "profitization" of hospitals has created a sort of moral crisis for stalwarts of the pretransformation days foolish enough to believe that the reality of health care delivery somehow should transcend the often muddy fights of the business world. This "crisis" affects not only the small community hospitals that are the first targets of the for-profit chains, but often the largest, most prestigious hospitals in whole communities. As reported by Sandy Lutz and Preston Gee in

The For-Profit Healthcare Revolution, in their insightful history of the for-profit systems:

> The board of Wesley Medical Center, a 760-bed teaching hospital in Wichita, Kansas, agreed to sell the not-for-profit hospital to HCA [later became part of Columbia/HCA] for $265 million in late 1984. The buyout stunned administrators at not-for-profit hospitals, especially those at the VHA [the group purchasing organization for not-for-profit hospitals across the United States]. VHA's member CEOs ran large not-for-profit hospitals and wanted some of the same advantages as investor-owned chains. Clearly, VHA was designed to help hospitals such as Wesley compete with for-profits such as HCA. Now, here was Wesley caving in to the "enemy."[12]

The economics of "caving in to the enemy" are compelling. As discussed in the chapter on consolidation, "by selling to Columbia, tax-exempt hospitals could join a network and get 30 percent better prices on medical supplies. That's better than the buying groups [like VHA] of tax-exempt hospitals, Scott [Columbia's chairman] argued."[13] Lutz and Gee point out that "by taking this business approach to health care, investor-owned chains were able to immediately realize economies of distribution and delivery that had not been tested (or exploited as some might say) by the not-for-profit participants who had a slightly different philosophical bent."[14] This "philosophical bent" is proving highly anachronistic in an industry that is converting to a for-profit enterprise in a few decades and represents one of the lingering problems in health care: lack of management discipline.

Nonetheless, there is tremendous entrenchment across the health care industry, one that will require years of market turbulence to shake out fully. It requires nothing short of a true managerial revolution, as described by Lutz and Gee. "By focusing on the bottom line, tax-paying executives were able to identify and isolate a core objective that was viewed as incidental by many executives in the industry. This contrast in priorities remains an unbridgeable chasm for many of the veteran administrators in the field."[15]

If part of this "unbridgeability" stems from a belief in the cultural divergences between the for-profits and not-for-profits, yet another entrepreneur is rushing to meet the latter's demands for investment capital in a unique way. Joshua Nemzoff, a veteran adviser to not-for-profit hospitals in the process of selling out to for-profits or others, launched MissionHealth in early 1998. The goal of the company is to provide not-for-profits with the working capital they need—and would otherwise be forced to raise through conversion or sale to a for-profit system—to modernize, integrate with physicians, industrialize its operations, and compete for business. MissionHealth buys an equity interest in the hospital for cash; in return, it has a claim on a percentage of the hospital's excess cash flow.[16] Sounds a lot like what a shareholder gives and gets with a for-profit company, no? Once again, a frothy market blurs the distinction between the behaviors and culture of the for-profits and not-for-profits: different mechanism and different label, but the same end.

There is a similar rush toward capitalization in order to bolster competitiveness in the payer community. Since 1982, market share for investor-owned versus not-for-profit MCOs has increased from 20 to nearly 60 percent.[17] Since 1995, five Blue Cross and Blue Shield plans—historically the embodiment of not-for-profit insurance—have converted to for-profit status and issued shares to the public, or are in the process as of this writing.[18] The loss of the community service that the Blues plans have provided as "insurers of last resort" will, at least in theory, be offset by the recipients of much of the proceeds of the stock offerings—the public foundation set up and capitalized by their conversion. Capital allows the Blues plans and other payers to accelerate their own consolidation as an industry; it also funds the development of the complex information systems and marketing programs necessary to compete in the new health care marketplace.

The profligate capitalization of health care organizations will turn out to be a self-fulfilling prophecy: everyone needs capital, if only to compete with all the other well-capitalized players. Lutz and Gee put it most bluntly: "as hospitals are passed back and forth like children of divorced parents, one might wonder, Doesn't it matter who owns these institutions? Perhaps not. The leaders of investor-owned hospital companies aren't managing hospitals as much as they're managing money."[19] Indeed, in light of their generally decentralized operating structures, for-profit systems like Tenet, Columbia, and Vanguard—and the not-for-profit systems like Daughters of Charity and CHW—may prove, in the end, to be nothing more than a combination investment banker and group purchasing organization.

Daughters of Charity has proven particularly adept on the money management side. It sits on a pile of cash and investments worth $2 billion; and it keeps interest rates on its bonds low by consistently earning investment-grade bond ratings from an investment community that it works with slick "road-show" type presentations to bankers and investors—the type commonly used by publicly traded corporations. For its acumen the system has also earned a nickname among Wall Street financiers—"Daughters of Currency."[20]

ENTREPRENEUR'S PARADISE

As the many examples in this book will illustrate, all significant innovation in health care financing and delivery stems not from government programs, but from entrepreneurial inspiration. This pattern has repeated itself dozens of times over the past decade and a half. Within the current health care system, the entrepreneur identifies a major and expensive flaw of medical delivery, creates a fix for that flaw, finds the money to finance the development and launch of that fix, and rewards the financing with heady profits.

The entire home health care industry—the most clinically important driver of the reduction in expensive hospital stays—was the vision of a former hospital clerk with a business degree. In 1979, James Sweeney pitched his idea of providing home infusion, IV nutrition, oxygen therapy, and other key medical services to people in the comfort of their own homes, rather than in a high-priced hospital room.[21] The idea was such a threat to Sweeney's employer, McGaw Laboratories—which at the time enjoyed the cozy and profitable business of supplying those hospital rooms—that he was fired. He decided to establish the business himself, growing it into a company he sold eight years later for $586 million to health care conglomerate Caremark. Seven years later, he bought the business back from Caremark when it was embroiled in a variety of problems, mostly of its own making. Sweeney operated it for a year and a half as Coram, and sold it again to Integrated Health Services in 1996.

HealthSouth is another of health care's many Horatio Alger stories. Founded by Richard Scrushy in the mid-1980s to ride the wave of surgery as it shifted from inpatient to outpatient settings, HealthSouth grew into a $2.5 billion-per-year business in 12 years. It is now the largest provider of outpatient surgery and rehab services in the country.[22] Just like home health and subacute care, HealthSouth's outpatient facilities—unburdened by the large fixed costs of hospitals—can provide inpatient-type medical services far more cheaply. The emergence of HealthSouth is typical of what Anita Sharpe of the *Wall Street Journal* calls the health care "honey pot that technology has been since the early 1980s."[23] Sharpe writes that health care "adventurers are building big companies from little ones, and fortunes are being won—and sometimes lost—by those bold enough to bet on innovation."[24]

Fueled by Wall Street money and its growth accelerated by acquisition, HealthSouth is timed to exploit most of the forces of health care transformation: cost containment, consolidation, industrialization, and masterful exploitation of the increasingly important role of consumer awareness in the marketing of health care options. HealthSouth aggressively develops awareness of its "brand," and markets all the requisite elements of standardization and quality control that are central to the concept of brand management. Of course, feverish acquisitions, aggressive marketing, and product standardization all require capital; Wall Street has readily provided this to HealthSouth, beginning with an initial public offering (IPO) of stock in its second year of business and a market capitalization by the end of 1996 of $6.6 *billion* after 12 years in business.[25]

But at rock bottom, the source of the success of these companies is their ability to lower costs. The cost-driven focus of managed care has unleashed this as a rallying cry for capital formation for new businesses, and as the core strategy for marketing everything from clinical reengineering services to new ways of packaging supplies. This is the spillover effect of the cost-driven competition that now pervades the entire system. While highly disorienting for many in health care—particularly physicians—such competition is a critical component of the general transformation of health care into a full-fledged industry. Price competition drives cost minimization, product standardization, and ultimately innovation. The pressures of competition result in the aggressive pursuit of risk-assumption contracts, which in turn force an elimination of excess capacity, compel the integration of care, and accelerate the processes of health care industrialization.

Competition is also good because it brings with it information, the currency of real health care reform, and one that purchasers and consumers of health care have always lacked. The introduction of data and analytical tools on competing providers' business and clinical decision making helps improve the entire industry by continually raising performance standards. It also serves as a defensive strategy against empirically unfounded judgments by an MCO regarding an individual provider's utilization patterns and clinical performance. This process is fully consistent with Michael Porter's observation in *Competitive Advantage* that "competitors can enhance a firm's ability to differentiate itself by serving as a standard of comparison. Without a competitor, buyers may have more difficulty in perceiving the value created by a firm, and may, therefore, be more price- or service-sensitive."[26]

Another of Porter's observations regarding the benefits of competition is particularly relevant to health care, as such competition promotes consumer education and heightens a market's awareness of choices, values, and the overall contributions of health care providers. "Competitors can lower a firm's cost of market development, particularly if competitors spend disproportionately on it relative to their sales and if their market development efforts are in areas that represent industry-wide problems."[27] The suddenly aggressive competitiveness of the for-profit hospital chains provides precisely this type of cultivation of health care markets across the United States. The most profound effect of all is competition's spillover effects on organizational behavior across the health care industry. When confronted with competition by the for-profit systems, the not-for-profit hospital systems respond in kind, seeking to develop the same efficiencies, marketing themselves as aggressively, and the like.

A DASH OF IRONY FOR THE NAYSAYERS

Many in health care find its "profitization" extremely offensive. They believe that medicine is sacred; that it is morally wrong to profit from the medical misfortunes of others; and that hospitals and physicians should be cloistered from the harsh discipline of the market. Such sentiment ignores the fact that hospitals are organizations like those we all work in and are thus subject to the same rules, behaviors, and problems. It also ignores the fact that—and notwithstanding their possession of the most critical and noble of all human skills—for all their training and dedication, physicians are human and wage-earners like the rest of us; and it ignores the fact that commercial scientific research has a ghastly appetite for funding. The health care industry, for all its unique complexities and problems, is an industry no different than any other. Judging by their politics in general, it is clear that those most offended by the "profitization" of health care are no doubt just as offended by profit-seeking behavior for any other industry that serves human needs, from food production to home construction to gambling.

One thing is certain: had the U.S. health care system been built exclusively by for-profit forces over the past century, there is little doubt the industry would be in its current shape. Perverse government policies and marketplace intrusions, driven by professional and institutional lobbying, created overcapacity;[28] unique professional monopolies and collusive unity created the artificial separation of physicians and hospitals;[29] and a highly dysfunctional market structure created a miasma of inconsistent practices and out-of-control costs. None of these problems would have occurred—to such an extent and for such a sustained period of time—had the industry been permitted to evolve like any other. But, for better or worse, the government was and still is the single largest purchaser of health care services, a near monopsony buyer, thus creating a distorted market structure that is only now righting itself.

As a purchaser, the government does not feel any of the margin performance pressures imposed by real shareholders. (Taxpayers as shareholders have the most contorted of all shareholder "voting rights" and thus more closely resemble hostages than shareholders.) As a consequence, government has for decades been a remarkably inefficient purchaser of health care services—a sharp contrast to the purchasing behavior of for-profit MCOs. Driven by the vigilance of shareholders and other free-market forces, MCOs have pioneered methods of contracting, risk management, and reimbursement that the government is only now finally acknowledging that it has needed all along. It is no accident that as health care transforms itself through private market forces at the close of the century, the only viable proposal for reforming Medicare and Medicaid is a wholesale migration of both programs into private health care systems.

That's how we got here. What happens next is another story.

The long-term prognosis for aggressive "profitization" of health care services, once the transformation of the U.S. health care system is complete, is more complicated. Why? Because the entire "profitization" movement in health care will prove, in the end, as transitory as "managed care" itself—necessary to help fix the health care system's worst problems, but not necessary to sustain it.

In the new century's health care system, nothing will prove more paradoxical than the ultimately self-defeating nature of the system's profitability. Indeed, there is little in the delivery of medicine at the local level that will drive down health care profits faster than the full emergence of for-profit medicine. In the typical health care market of today, there are too many competing entities; it is too easy to develop substitute financing goods; there is too much capacity; consumers have too much mobility; and there is too much information about costs, profits, and quality for highly profitable arrangements to persist for long.

This is not to say that the behaviors learned under the task-mastering culture—the financial accountability, quantification of job performance, etc.—of the for-profits will go away. On the contrary, it will be precisely this taskmastering that will keep costs from ever getting out of control again. Profit-seeking behavior and competition are changing economic behaviors, eliminating efficiencies, and correcting flawed operating structures. Once these corrections are made, the only difference between today's and tomorrow's enterprises will be the size—and use—of their margins.

The high level of MCO profits up until 1997—and their lockstep crash that year—are all part of this process, and underscore the generally transitional nature of the MCO phenomenon itself. National MCOs represent the creation of a new industry, formed specifically to rationalize one of the oldest nonindustries; the risk/reward profile generated by this moment in economic history attracted significant capital and worked to achieve the goals of the new industry. But this process merely accelerates its own end.

To the naysayers who detest profitability in health care generally, you can have the first dance at the funeral for the for-profit MCOs. And consider yourself lucky—there will be countless physicians and hospital administrators standing in line for the next one.

*   *   *

The remainder of this section describes the major modalities of treatment for the health care system's ills that are making this position not only plausible, but one that will predominate in the new century's health care system. These five types of treatment—five forces of system transformation—are

1. risk-assumption, to correct fundamental problems in health care consumption and market economics;

2. consumerism, to neutralize distortions in the health system created by the self-interest and faulty paternalism of MCOs and other insurers, galvanize competition among providers, and drive product and process innovation;
3. consolidation, to scale the health care infrastructure properly, mobilize capital, spread risk across broader populations of patients and providers, and allocate health care resources more efficiently;
4. vertical integration, to correct fragmentation and other structural defects built into the medical delivery system; and
5. industrialization, to rationalize the haphazard use of services, increase economic predictability, improve quality, and reduce health care costs.

Four of these five forces are critical to the developmental state of *any* industry.

Consumerism is the wellspring of all major innovations in the economy, from the advent of the shopping mall in the 1970s and its eclipse by the superstore in the 1990s, to lightning-strike product markets like VCRs and cell phones, to demographic phenomena like the minivan.

Consolidation is a function of cost-economics, the same force that has decided the world can support only three U.S. automakers and a handful of fully international airlines; as a result, both of these industries consolidated to this degree decades ago.

Vertical integration describes the success of a company like Barnes & Noble as both publisher and retailer, the mushrooming of shopping via mail-order catalog and factory outlet store, and the proliferation of private label brands in every major supermarket chain in the United States.

And the impact of industrialization on pure service businesses explains the origins and competitiveness of industries ranging from fast food, to package delivery services, to automotive repair.

Only one of the five forces—risk-assumption—is truly unique to health care. Why? Because the flawed market dynamics and consumer behaviors permanently associated with the consumption of medical services are forcing the industry to circumvent the demand side of the health care equation. Risk-assumption seeks instead to change *producer* behavior, working the supply side of the equation through the reformulation of the entire medical product into the buying and selling of the medical/financial risk for patient care. Risk-assumption thus stands as a prerequisite to any meaningful reform of the entire health care system.

Each of these five forces is highly interdependent, and driven by the dynamics of a suddenly rational and emerging health care marketplace. Each is consistent with principles of classic strategic industry analysis. And each provides a critical, if belated, curative to the many afflictions of the traditional health care system. For success in the new century's system, every health care organization needs to embrace each force fully—or be rendered fully disabled.

REFERENCES

1. Epigraph from S. Lutz and E. Gee, *The For-Profit Healthcare Revolution* (Chicago: Irwin Professional Publishing, 1995), 70.
2. J. Kleinke, "Deconstructing the Columbia/HCA Investigation," *Health Affairs*, March/April 1998, 12.
3. R. Rundle, "Catholic Hospitals, in Big Merger Drive, Battle Industry Giants," *Wall Street Journal*, 12 March, 1997.
4. Remarks of J. Otten, Chief Executive Officer, Brigham and Women's Hospital, to R. Kuttner, "Columbia/HCA and the Resurgence of the For-Profit Hospital Business," part 2 of 2, 8 August, 1996, 450. *New England Journal of Medicine.*
5. Comments by M. Alvarez, MD, Medical Director of Columbia Dauterive Hospital, in "Hospitals and Doctors Fight for the Same Dollars in Louisiana Town," M. Langley, *Wall Street Journal*, 11 November, 1997.
6. Rundle, *Wall Street Journal.*
7. Rundle, *Wall Street Journal.*
8. Data on hospital profitability for the median, acute care, nonfederal U.S. hospital in 1995, according to *The Comparative Performance of U.S. Hospitals: The Sourcebook* (Baltimore: HCIA Inc., 1997).

9. L. Kertesz, "Enrollment Albatross," *Modern Healthcare*, 23 February, 1998, 12.

10. P. Starr, *The Social Transformation of American Medicine* (New York: Basic Books/HarperCollins, 1982), 170.

11. "As Big Hospital Chains Take Over Non-Profits, a Backlash Is Growing," *Healthcare Trends Report*, December 1996, 6.

12. Lutz and Gee, *The For-Profit Healthcare Revolution*, 15

13. Lutz and Gee, *The For-Profit Healthcare Revolution*, 95.

14. Lutz and Gee, *The For-Profit Healthcare Revolution*, 56.

15. Lutz and Gee, *The For-Profit Healthcare Revolution*, 56.

16. D. Bellandi, "Dealmaker Changes Tune," *Modern Healthcare*, 2 February, 1998, 22.

17. "Will For-Profit Trend Hold Up as MCO Margins Decline?" *Medicine & Health Perspectives*, 25 November, 1996.

18. L. Kertesz, "This Is Not Your Father's Blues Plan," *Modern Healthcare*, 14 October, 1996, 64.

19. Lutz and Gee, *The For-Profit Healthcare Revolution*, 135–136.

20. M. Langley, "Nuns' Zeal for Profits Shapes Hospital Chain, Wins Wall Street Fans," *Wall Street Journal*, 7 January, 1998.

21. T. Burton, "Combine Simple Ideas and Some Failures; Result: Sweet Revenge," *Wall Street Journal*, 3 February, 1995.

22. A. Sharpe, "Medical Entrepreneur Aims To Turn Clinics into National Brand," *Wall Street Journal*, 14 December, 1996.

23. Sharpe, *Wall Street Journal*.

24. Sharpe, *Wall Street Journal*.

25. Sharpe, *Wall Street Journal*.

26. Adapted and reprinted with the permission of The Free Press, a Division of Simon & Schuster from *COMPETITIVE ADVANTAGE: Creating and Sustaining Superior Performance* by Michael E. Porter. Copyright © 1985 by Michael E. Porter. p. 203.

27. Adapted and reprinted with the permission of The Free Press, a Division of Simon & Schuster from *COMPETITIVE ADVANTAGE: Creating and Sustaining Superior Performance* by Michael E. Porter. Copyright © 1985 by Michael E. Porter. p. 209.

28. J. Kleinke, "Deconstructing the Columbia/HCA Investigation," *Health Affairs*, March/April 1998, 11.

29. This is a main conclusion of the historic analysis central to Paul Starr's *Social Transformation of American Medicine*.

1

RISK-ASSUMPTION

What do I care? I get paid whether I operate or not!

Capt. Benjamin Franklin Pierce, MD
United States Army, M*A*S*H 4077th

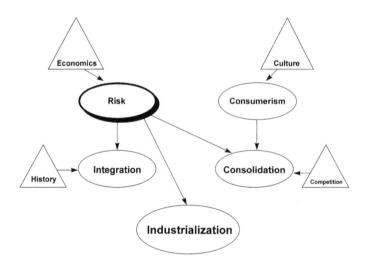

The health care system has not worked because its own economic incentives have always worked against it. The economic behaviors motivating the way providers and patients carry out health care transactions have been backwards since the origins of the industry. Under the fee-for-service system that pays physicians and hospitals for each medical service delivered, the sicker a patient is (or, more accurately put, the sicker a patient is diagnosed to be) the more money the provider makes. The typical patient is incapable of challenging the physician; the typical patient is also economically unmotivated to—because someone else is paying most or all of the bill and, more importantly, because one's physical health and well-being are priceless, at least in their absence. Under the fee-for-service system, providers are, in effect, financially penalized for keeping patients healthy. Prevention of illness in their patients costs physicians money in the long run. Practicing better medicine ultimately means less chance that the patients will return; under fee-for-service medicine, good doctoring does not pay.

The problem has grown only worse under managed care. The first strategy of managed care was to pool purchasing power under one plan, using it to leverage doctors and hospitals to accept reduced prices. This would have worked fine at reducing health care costs, if price were the only moving part in the machine. But there is the nagging problem of utilization: cut the price you pay for something and the producer simply produces more units, so as to generate the same total paycheck at the end of the week. The health care version of this behavioral truism is embodied in a theory developed by health economists that physicians have a "target income" and simply modify their clinical behavior to reach it.[1] The idea of the "target income" and its impact on clinical behavior has been so thoroughly accepted as doctrine that the federal government actually incorporates it into its health care budgeting process. In calculating spending estimates, the Health Care Financing Administration assumes that for every 1 percent reduction in physician fees for a given service, the total volume of the service will increase by 0.5 percent.

The takeaway? If you want to control health care costs, you have to control both price *and* utilization.

UTILIZATION MANAGEMENT: DR. THROTTLE AND MR. BRAKE

The magnitude of the utilization problem under fee-for-service reimbursement goes well beyond the perverse incentives that exert upward pressure on physician costs. Because physicians hospitalize patients, recommend surgery, prescribe drugs, and order diagnostic

tests, their decisions directly affect from 70 to 90 percent of *all* out-
lays for health care in the United States.[2] This discretionary power,
and the hundreds of billions of dollars it drives, has prompted the
intensive scrutiny and micromanagement of managed care, manifest
in a costly, labyrinthine layer of managed care activity known collectively as "utilization management."

Utilization managers are clinical auditors: they hound clinicians
for justifications. Why this drug for her? Do you really need to do
that surgery on him? Why this lab test again? Can't you discharge
her from the hospital yet? They check, question, doubt, verify, con-
firm, and badger. Even if they are not successful at modifying a
physician's behavior today, as with any auditors, the menace of their
very presence is designed to induce self-modification tomorrow.
Utilization management is an attempt to slam the brakes on the fee-
for-service engine, and keep them on as long as physicians still have
every incentive—economic, legal, and cultural—to throttle the engine. The premise underlying utilization management is extremely
cynical: it presumes physicians will overtreat, overhospitalize, over-
test, and overmedicate, and do so to such a degree that the expense of
utilization management pays for itself many times over in reduced
"waste."

Utilization management is a ham-fisted "fix" doomed to failure.
The real waste is not overtreatment: it is managed care's overreaction to overtreatment; its self-serving failure to correct *under*-
treatment, which results in greater costs in the long run; and all the
additional costs heaped on the system by providers attempting to
cope with utilization management itself. Physicians and hospitals
have developed elaborate strategies for coping with managed care's
many, varied, and complex utilization management techniques.
These include the spawning of a two-headed software industry: one
half assists providers in maximizing fee-for-service reimbursement
through "optimization" of the medical coding on claims; the other
half assists payers in minimizing reimbursement through identifying
such manipulation. All this despite mounting anecdotal evidence—
namely, the proliferation of media accounts, lawsuits, and state and

federal legislation—that the public has grown weary of external care denials or restrictions under utilization management; that second-guessing one's physician is not only morally wrong, but medically dangerous; that utilization management exists only to help a self-insured employer or at-risk managed care organization (MCO) or other insurer breach its contractual promise of guaranteed health benefits.

Nonetheless, utilization management techniques continue to exist, if only because of a consensus fear that removing them after a decade would be to court economic disaster. As with the anxiety that surrounded the lifting of wage and price controls in the early 1970s, to take the utilization management lid off a still predominantly fee-for-service system would result in an explosion of artificially restrained economic behavior; surely all the cost reductions of the past five years will catch up with us, if not with interest! While that view may seem a bit extreme, it points to the obvious: in the end, the elaborate and expensive command-and-control systems that comprise utilization management do nothing to change the fundamental behavioral problems associated with fee-for-service medicine; they merely weed out the worst excesses of those behaviors, and maintain vigilance against any weeds that may grow back.

But beyond rooting out extreme behavior, utilization management is an ultimately futile attempt to apply brakes to the law of gravity. The more enlightened MCOs have come to acknowledge this, found mechanisms to work their way around it, and in many cases use these mechanisms as a source of cost and therefore, competitive advantage. Such mechanisms acknowledge the reality of physician target income—and its associated behavioral modifications—and strive to work *with* rather than *against* it. The key design behind the most inspired of these mechanisms seeks to align the financial self-interest of the provider with the financial self-interest of the MCO.

The essence of this design is the sharing of financial risk, the rudiments of which are now in wide practice across the U.S. health care system. The crudest form is simple contractual withholding: a portion of a provider's total fee-for-service reimbursement is withheld until the end of a contract period; if the provider delivers services within budgeted targets, the extra reimbursement is paid out. The next crudest forms involve the payment of special bonuses for improving total productivity, and reducing utilization of nonphysician resources, such as inpatient care, and other costs. A more progressive form of risk-sharing involves special "global set-asides," a withholding of a portion of the total budgeted provider payments for keeping down *total* utilization and *total* costs within a contract period.

The "global set-aside" contractual structure signifies an important departure from fee-for-service: it breaks the grip of all the faulty incentives built into the traditional system. Under this arrangement, providers are paid more to provide less, signifying a critical reversal of the dysfunctional economics of fee-for-service delivery. This arrangement, however, represents a less-than-perfect system. It can easily backfire on the self-insured employer, MCO, or other purchaser who bears long-term financial risk for the patient's total health, while rewarding physicians in the short term for doing as little as possible to promote that health.

THE WONDER DRUG OF CAPITATION

The only fix for the residual mismatch of incentives under global set-asides is called "capitation." Capitation, based on the Latin word "caput" for "head," pays physicians and hospitals a fixed dollar amount per person (per head) for every person in a given population. The banking of these up-front payments by providers is used to cover their costs of providing all the health care services that every person in that population may require over a specified period of time. Payments to providers on a capitated basis represent the wholesale transfer of insurance risk from the traditional purchaser of care to the traditional provider of care.

The source of capitation's greatest strengths—and its greatest perils—is the immutable fact that this type of reimbursement carries with it all the economics, risks, and rewards of insurance. This simple fact is the axis upon which the entire restructuring of the health care system will turn as it moves into the new century: it explains why providers need to consolidate (to pool risk and reduce financial exposure); integrate (to offer the lowest cost settings); and industrialize (to reduce costs and improve predictability).

A capitation payment to a group of providers is an insurance premium and it is meant to cover the entire insured population. A small minority of patients in the capitated population will require far more care than the fixed payment amount covers, and providers are obliged to deliver that care without additional payment. But that care is subsidized by the capitated payments banked by the providers for all the other patients in the population who require little or no care. Capitation is the logical endpoint of a system that will fix its underlying economic problem only when it has shifted all of its health insurance risk fully onto providers.

Under capitation, a hospital's and physician's entire income is based on their success in keeping patients healthy, rather than on maximizing the number of medical services delivered to those patients. As a consequence, capitation turns a number of key aspects of health care delivery inside out:

- the least busy physicians and emptiest hospitals are the most profitable ones;
- excessive or unnecessary interventions cost the physicians and the hospitals money, not the patient or the payer;
- expensive medical technologies are liabilities to be used judiciously to minimize costs, not assets to be exploited to maximize fee-for-service reimbursements; and
- physicians and hospitals readily provide their own utilization management.

How drastically does capitation change the singing of old tunes? Under fee-for-service reimbursement, the daily obsession of a hospital administrator is the daily census, or the number of patients in the hospital at a given point in time. A big number is a good number. The store is full, and we can send out lots of bills at the end of the month. By contrast, under capitation this obsession does not change;

rather, the favorable value inverts. The store is empty, so we are not running down any "inventory" we would have to stock up at the end of the month.

Though capitation was not widely put into practice until the early 1990s, its clearly superior economics have a snowball effect on any given market, and thus on the health care system in general. Once introduced into a market, few groups of physicians or hospitals can compete on something as old-fashioned as price with those willing to assume all medical/financial risk. Why? Because under capitation, all the resource consumption patterns (i.e., the 70 to 90 percent of total health care costs that physicians control) change radically. Physicians under full capitation manage patients better, hospitalize them less often, and ultimately allocate total medical resources more efficiently. A landmark *New England Journal of Medicine* study of capitation in California found that between 1990 and 1994, the number of MCO enrollees covered under capitation increased 91 percent. In 1993, near the end of this period, the authors calculated that the number of inpatient days per 1,000 non-Medicare enrollees among the capitated groups ranged from 120 to 149 days, versus 232 for all of California and 297 for the total United States.[3]

With total hospitalization days running at half the rate, capitation sets up a medical cost downdraft that rushes through entire markets. In order to compete in such markets, all providers are compelled to convert to capitation, often in one or two insurance purchasing cycles. As a result, more than half of organized physician networks around the United States now compensate their physicians through some form of capitation.[4] And those are the *organized* networks. As for the entire universe of physicians, 81 percent expect to accept capitated patients by the year 2000.[5] Those who already do accept them anticipate that half their practice revenues will be derived from capitation.[6]

The Greedy Docs Who Keep Their Patients Healthy

The use of capitation removes all the clumsiness, inefficiency, and antagonism inherent in the three-ring circus typical of providers, patients, and "utilization managers" in traditional managed care settings. Pushing all the financial risk and associated medical responsibility for an insured population past the MCOs and squarely onto hospitals and physicians greatly simplifies the process of "managing care," rendering the phrase a long overdue redundancy. Most importantly, capitation aligns the incentives of providers with those of patients. Under capitation, physicians and hospitals

- have a heavily vested interest in maintaining the health, rather than treating the illnesses, of their capitated patients;
- are forced to balance profit-seeking behavior and the clinical needs of patients; and
- are finally required to act like all other free-market producers of goods, motivated to focus not only on maximizing revenues, which they have done with abandon in the past, but also on the cost of goods sold.

Critics of capitation argue that the system introduces a new economic tension into the relationship between providers and patients. They claim that capitation forces physicians and hospitals to choose between their own financial enrichment and the health of their patients, introducing an insurmountable conflict of interest into the health care system. Under capitation, they argue, the foxes are guarding the henhouse.

This is a knee-jerk reaction, borne of a naiveté jolted from its ignorance over the reality of fee-for-service medicine. How exactly is capitation's conflict of interest any different from its inversion? How is the physician who, under fee-for-service, is paid handsomely for performing a surgery, *not* subject to the same conflict of interest when making the decision to operate or not operate? The reality is there is no difference whatsoever. It is simply a reworking of an unchanging equation; with the plus and minus dollar signs on either side reversed, the other variable —namely utilization—moves in the opposite direction, and total health care costs are reduced.

Those most scandalized by the bloodless pragmatism underlying a support for the economics of capitation are not going to be convinced by either theory or empiricism. They are professional naysayers who suspect profit motives of any sort when applied to medicine. Such cynics would be just as scandalized had an accident in the development of medicine reversed the process. Suppose that during the initial industrialization of the United States, the very earliest modern physicians were reimbursed directly by employers on a capitated basis. (This actually very nearly happened.) As a result, at the turn of the century, capitation emerges as the model for health care financing across the country. And then suppose that, for whatever reason—say a shortage rather than oversupply of physicians, combined with an aging of the population—physicians were able to bid capitated rates up high enough to constitute a cost crisis in the 1980s. What happens next? As a "reform," a few physicians break from the pack and offer not to take the full capitated fees for covered populations, but to provide services on a newfangled "fee-for-service" basis and only when those services prove medically necessary. Critics of the new reimbursement mechanism would quickly recognize that physicians were setting themselves up to put their incomes ahead of their patients: they would treat patients and perform surgeries simply because they could and would be paid to do so. Such a conflict of interest! Such a scandal!

Capitation is scandalous because it is new, and because it questions our faith in the purity of medical science and the motives of our personal physicians. Capitation forces people to confront the reality that physicians are self-interested economic agents, just like the rest of us, and that perhaps a lifetime of our own medical care may have been delivered to us only because we had the ability to pay and not because of the dedication of "our" physicians to us personally. But the fears embodied in such criticism—primarily those of patient underdiagnosis, undertreatment, and neglect—are groundless. The medical malpractice community has, since the 1950s, provided the nation's health care consumers with vigilant service in the fight against what it alone managed to identify as the teeming and widespread incompetence of physicians. These lawyers will no doubt prove even more effective in defending patients against capitated physicians who fail to provide needed care, given the legal profession's general familiarity with self-serving economic motives. As the specter of professional liability and, failing that, professional conscience police against the withholding of needed patient care under capitation, even better safeguards exist with the long-term financial interest inherent in the capitation system itself. Herein lies the purest elegance of capitation as an economic tool. A capitated hospital that prematurely discharges a patient to improve its own profit on that patient will lose this profit many times over when the patient returns with complications associated with the premature discharge. If the patient does *not* re-admit, then the discharge, however inconvenient or unpleasant, was obviously not medically premature. Similarly, capitated physicians who line their pockets by denying needed treatment to sick people under their capitated care will be contractually obligated to treat those people when they become *very* sick. Under capitation, the foxes may be guarding the henhouse but they are also responsible for egg production.

The public policy debate notwithstanding, capitation is the system that the market—no longer tolerant of runaway health costs—clearly wants. Not only does this explain why managed care uses capitation aggressively to isolate and predict its medical costs; it describes the very origins of managed care as an organization. The original concept of the MCO is based on the principle of capitation: it theorizes that an organization designed specifically to maintain people's health will be able to resolve all the medical needs of a population for a fixed fee per member; it also theorizes that the organizations that do so effectively will earn a profit for their efforts.[7]

Physician Resistance, Redux

While the market clearly prefers capitation, there is a major obstacle to full conversion to this method of physician compensation: the physicians themselves. Provider resistance to the economic accountability inherent in assuming medical/financial risk is not new, merely recast as resistance to the tools of managed care. Precisely this same resistance was brought to bear decades ago, as the modern health care system was taking shape in the 1920s through 1940s. At that time, physicians were in much better position to shape it to their own desires.

The original version of capitation was called "contract practice." It involved fully prepaid health care for groups of covered employees, with its earliest origins along the railroads and in mining camps where single employers needed to employ physicians to care for their workers. With predefined labor populations and their accompanying physicians functioning as an isolated, autonomous group, fee-for-service medicine was completely impractical; as a result, a nascent form of capitation won out by default. But any attempt to re-create this arrangement in less captive communities in the first few decades of the 20th century was resisted fiercely by physicians, who viewed the willingness to work for a prepaid amount of money as traitorous. Physician resistance then, like the small but vocal pockets of physician resistance to capitation under managed care now, was fierce.[8] Reprisals by physicians against those who broke ranks were so well organized under the American Medical Association that it was eventually indicted for violating the Sherman Antitrust Act in its attempts to block the formation and operation of an early prepaid group practice, the Group Health Association of Washington, D.C.[9]

Despite these efforts, the origins of capitation occurred in an isolated number of well-defined geographic and economic hotspots. These early experiments were spawned not by providers but—like one of the key drivers of health care transformation today—by large employers functioning as purchasing blocs. In 1929, such a plan was developed for the Los Angeles Department of Water and Power. The plan was unusual from even earlier experiments with contract practice as it was the first to combine hospital as well as physician care. As Paul Starr describes it in his *Social Transformation of American Medicine*, "soon other employee groups, mostly from governmental agencies, joined the program, and by 1935 the Ross-Loos Clinic had enrolled more than 12,000 workers and 25,000 dependents. Each subscriber paid $2 per month, plus some additional fees. As of 1934, subscribers paid an average of $2.69 a month."[10] The economics were as much a departure from the fee-for-service system of the 1930s as capitation is today for the same reasons. According to Starr, total costs were "less than half the cost incurred by similar urban families according to a California State survey that year."[11]

Early experiments with even more formalized structures mirrored this performance for large employers. In 1933, Sidney Garfield, a California physician, created the first large capitated group practice, which provided comprehensive care for $1.55 per worker per month, for all workers building an aqueduct.[12] These experiments gave way to plans that offered coverage beyond the confines of single employers, including the nation's two pioneering MCOs, Group Health Cooperative of Puget Sound and Kaiser Health Plan, still two of the largest and most prestigious MCOs in operation today. Group Health grew rapidly and aggressively, financed by the sale of bonds to those it covered.[13] Such employer-dedicated prepaid plans had almost closed when, in late 1945, their leaders decided to resuscitate them by opening the plans to the public. Most notable among them was Henry Kaiser's dream. The largest employer in the Oakland area, he had created the Kaiser Health Plan to provide care to the thousands of workers who built his ships for the war effort. As Starr describes it, "with an almost missionary zeal, Henry Kaiser believed he could reorganize medical care on a self-sufficient basis, independent of government, to provide millions of Americans with prepaid and comprehensive services at prices they could afford."[14] It is interesting to note that nearly all of these experiments occurred on the West Coast, as the innovations of West Coast health care markets continue to serve as leading indicators for where the rest of health care in the United States is headed.

Despite the success of Group Health and Kaiser—or perhaps because of it—the medical profession was able to block the emergence of subsequent cooperative and prepaid group practice plans.[15] Why did physicians resist the assumption of risk as a compensation mechanism, and why did they so vigorously police their colleagues against doing so? The easy explanation is to blame the profession for outright collusion. Who wants financial accountability for their job performance if they can avoid it? To take prepayment in the 1940s— or capitation today—is to assume risk for the outcomes of one's clinical practices. Why assume risk when you have the market power to avoid it altogether?

A more realistic explanation for physicians' uneasiness over the assumption of medical/financial risk—then and now—is a certain economic anxiety, driven by an intimate familiarity with disease and its often catastrophic economics. Who better than a physician knows how easily out of control a disease can rage, how ugly and immutable its course, and how horrendous (and often pointless) the expense of trying to reverse or even slow it?

The assumption of risk by an MCO, group of providers, or any other entity is an acceptance of the uncertainty associated with the incidence of disease and the costs of treating it. The physician community's fierce opposition to "contract practice" in the early part of the century—and to every major type of health insurance emerging in the coming decades—was an abandonment to patients of the risks and vagaries of disease incidence and its associated cost. By rejecting prepaid practice and purging it from the ranks of their peers, the nation's physicians successfully pushed financial accountability back onto the least capable bearers of medical risk—the patients themselves. In so doing, they opened up history for the germination and rapid flourishing of third-party health insurance in the 1940s through 1980s. This in turn created an economic crisis resolvable only through the return of financial accountability to the doctors themselves, in the form of capitation.

RISK AS CURRENCY: PROVIDERS' TRUMP CARD

The history of the U.S. health care system is a story of economic determinism, but one in slow motion. The market dysfunction and mushrooming costs associated with medical services delivered on a fee-for-service basis should spell a quick end for such a system, right? Indeed, with a surplus of hospital beds, technology, and (supposedly) physicians, those providers who would break ranks and assume financial risk, rather than be paid on an *a la carte* basis by insurers, would quickly prosper and change the rules for everyone else. In retrospect, the process seems to be equal parts historic and economic inevitability, and so is proving to be at the close of the century.

So why did it take so many decades and so many hundreds of billion dollars of excess cost to come to fruition? Because collective physician power and their earliest negative experiences with contract practice set physicians against *all* third-party payment systems. Early exposure to prepaid medicine was, according to Starr, "sufficient to persuade [physicians] that any financial intermediary would like nothing better than to pay them as little as possible. So their own past strongly biased them against any extension of organized financing."[16] How paradoxical, then, that capitation—the modern embodiment of the economics of contract practice—is allowing providers to circumvent the greatest behemoths of "organized financing" of all: the national MCOs and health insurers.

In today's most progressive markets, "global capitation"—a fixed dollar amount for all necessary care—is the premium rate that physicians and hospitals, when consolidated and integrated sufficiently to assume risk, now charge consumers for health care coverage. They market their services for "global caps" either directly in the retail insurance market, via self-insured employers, or through the administrative shells of the traditional insurers and MCOs.

How wonderfully ironic! Capitation presents an enormous opportunity for physicians and hospitals to bootstrap themselves out of the subservience to fiscal intermediaries they sought generations ago to avoid—a subservience that can grow only more onerous under a perpetuation of fee-for-service practice, with utilization management systems as the only check against runaway costs. In this sense, capitation is the vehicle of provider *liberation* (rather than subservience) from the inevitable "organized financing" that arose in the wake of their abdication of risk-assumption through contract practice. Yesterday's curse is today's cure.

The assumption of medical/financial risk by providers sets the stage for a health care industry transformation more profound and poignant than all the incremental layers of managed care put together. As groups of hospitals and physicians assume risk from an MCO, reversing all of health care's faulty economic incentives and correcting a flaw in medical delivery that took over a century to create, the role of the MCO becomes increasingly marginalized. This sets the stage for the *real* managed care revolution—forward integration by providers, who through risk-assumption are ideally positioned to subsume the role of the health insurer.

The willingness to bear risk translates into a readiness to engage directly in the key health care transaction: the prepayment of medical services from consumer and/or employer to provider. Such a forward integration, already occurring in the most competitive health care markets around the United States, represents medicine's version of direct manufacturer retailing. The administrative streamlining, clinical efficiencies, and economic impact inherent in this forward integration—this elimination of health care's middlemen—are self-evident. When fully played out across the system, a simple and powerful conclusion emerges: *in the new century's health care system, the only transactions left will be the transfer and assumption of medical/financial risk.*

Historic ironies and strategic trumping by providers notwithstanding, the economic logic that dooms the traditional insurers and MCOs needs the same grease that these well-entrenched intermediaries have always used (and guarded jealously) to operate their businesses: information. The assumption of risk requires knowing the likely incidence of every disease and injury in a given population, and all the costs associated with each. This places a renewed emphasis on the actuarial side of medicine, which has long been the exclusive province of the insurers; under risk-assumption, it is suddenly the lifeblood of the entire provider industry.

The strategic importance of information is not trivial. Because of their long history of underwriting risk and paying claims, payers typically have better information than providers either seeking to negotiate capitation contracts with them or, more critically, seeking to compete against them directly for an employer's business. Payers thus have more leverage in negotiation *and* in competition. This special leverage is a major force behind the consolidation of providers—especially those who seek to bear risk aggressively—into ever larger groups. Such consolidated groups can mobilize the capital and intellectual resources required to neutralize this advantage.

In addition to compelling the rapid consolidation of physician groups and hospitals for bargaining purposes, the assumption of medical risk also necessitates that providers take other bold steps. As bearers of financial risk for patients' entire medical care, consolidating provider groups need to

- position themselves for aggressive marketing to targeted segments of health insurance consumers, the ultimate customers for at-risk systems of care;
- coordinate the care delivered to those consumers, toppling the legacy divisions that have been built up over time among medical care settings; and
- standardize the delivery of that care to reduce bad clinical and economic outcomes, predict and control total costs, and maximize profit.

These strategic imperatives—in conjunction with risk-assumption and consolidation—constitute the other forces of health care transformation discussed in this section.

REFERENCES

1. A.M. Stoline and J.P. Weiner, *The New Medical Marketplace: A Physician's Guide to the Health Care System in the 1990s* (Baltimore: The Johns Hopkins University Press, 1993), 100.

2. Stoline and Weiner, *The New Medical Marketplace: A Physician's Guide to the Health Care System in the 1990s*, 90.

3. J. Robinson and L. Casalino, "The Growth of Medical Groups Paid through Capitation in California," *New England Journal of Medicine*, 21 December, 1995, 1684.

4. H. Brown and R. Shinto, "Making Physicians Networks Work," *Health Care Strategic Management,* April 1996, 22.

5. Survey conducted by Evergreen Re and reported in *Modern Healthcare,* 5 January, 1998, 50.

6. Survey, *Modern Healthcare,* 50.

7. P. Starr, *The Social Transformation of American Medicine* (New York: Basic Books/HarperCollins, 1982), 395.

8. Starr, *The Social Transformation of American Medicine,* 305.

9. Starr, *The Social Transformation of American Medicine,* 305.

10. Starr, *The Social Transformation of American Medicine,* 301.

11. Starr, *The Social Transformation of American Medicine,* 301.

12. Stoline and Weiner, *The New Medical Marketplace: A Physician's Guide to the Health Care System in the 1990s,* 25.

13. Starr, *The Social Transformation of American Medicine,* 321.

14. Starr, *The Social Transformation of American Medicine,* 322.

15. Starr, *The Social Transformation of American Medicine,* 305.

16. Starr, *The Social Transformation of American Medicine,* 256.

2

CONSUMERISM

Let them eat cake.

Marie Antoinette
Queen of France before the Revolution

In 1997, shares of publicly traded MCOs went into a serious free fall. A succession of negative earnings reports, beginning in early summer and ending in November of that year, knocked $13.2 billion—a whopping 25 percent—off the combined market value of the five largest for-profit HMOs.[1] The news behind each report was numbingly repetitive: market saturation was holding premiums flat against inflation, while medical costs continued to grow.

Why? Because by 1997 most managed care organizations had relinquished a key tool in their ability to manage those costs: they had relinquished significant control over patient access to physicians.

The cultural hard place—our freedom to choose, sense of self-determination, desire for service-on-demand, and other core American values—had proven stronger than the managed care rock. We want *our* doctor, *now*!

Our commitment as a society to freedom of choice is manifest in ways both sublime and ridiculous. It has been used effectively to bolster the defense in the reproductive rights debate; and it is the inspiration for 300 types of shampoo and conditioner lining entire aisles of our supermarkets. Our desire for variety drives everything from continuous product innovation, to brand proliferation, to the emergence of the superstore as mass retailing's logical end point. Combine this cultural fact with the intense sense of privacy (some would say shame) that Americans have about their bodies, a sense steeped in our Puritan roots—compare the number of nude beaches around the world with the outcry one typically inspires in a U.S. community—and you quickly understand why the freedom to choose one's own doctor and hospital is so sacrosanct in America.

The freedom to choose physicians is also consistent with the sheer heterogeneity of the U.S. consumer market. Many women feel that only gynecologists—and female ones—are capable of managing their general health needs, and so chafe against the primary care gatekeeping model of the traditional MCO. Many other people are extremely sensitive about physicians of the same race or nationality; others choose their physician by gender; still others are extremely choosy about their pediatricians, psychiatrists, and obstetricians. These variables complicate an MCO's ability to establish and manage a tight provider network: to accommodate as many diverse members as possible, an MCO is forced to build a network to sufficient size and diversity, while still touting its supposed selectivity as a way to leverage physician groups on price.

But the best network in the world does little to avoid the central reality: the traditional MCO is anathema to the freedom to choose one's physicians, whatever the reasoning behind those choices. It asks consumers to trade their freedom to choose any provider—and their freedom to move about the treatment system—for lower costs.

How little appeal this has for the typical U.S. consumer is embodied in the preponderance of MCOs forced to use—through the Orwellian inversion of reality typical of advertising ("shop and save")—the words "freedom" and "choice" in their plan names. The MCOs have co-opted these phrases because they are delivering precisely the opposite of what they are selling: the existence of a provider "network" means your world of choices has shrunken to the size of the MCO's contracting world.

Until recently, that is. Growing demands by consumers to regain provider choice—once they signed up for the plan and learned the hard lessons about reading fine print—has compelled the MCOs to open their formerly restrictive plans to retain market viability. Almost all enrollment growth for HMOs between 1992 and 1997 occurred within "point-of-service" or POS plans, which allow members to see physicians outside the network, for additional copayments. In 1992, only 5 percent of all insured employees in the United States were covered by POS plans; by 1996 that number had ballooned to 19 percent—almost the same share as the traditional, restrictive types of plans.[2] The share has changed so quickly because POS plans represent the only MCO model to experience significant enrollment growth since 1994.[3] Enrollment growth at Oxford Health Plans—Wall Street's highest flier and biggest crasher in 1997—has embodied this trend in overdrive: by the time the plan's worst news about its loss of control of its financial systems and medical costs hit the street, 86 percent of its membership was enrolled in its POS plan.[4]

While allowing out-of-network coverage under POS plans is a defensive strategy designed to preserve and grow market share, MCOs have been similarly forced to loosen restrictions on mobility *within* their networks. A telling example is the publicizing by United Healthcare that it provides members with direct access to specialists without primary care physician (PCP) authorization in United plans in 18 states—this within a few weeks of Oxford's announcement that specialists rather than PCPs would be managing its chronically ill members. "Such plans are the fastest-growing part of United

Healthcare's non-Medicare business," James Carlson, executive vice-president for the MCO's health care operations told the *Wall Street Journal*.[5]

Direct specialist access is, like the choice of individual physicians, highly cherished by the American health care consumer. This preference is destined to increase as the average consumer grows older and sicker, and as they become more educated about their own health care thanks in some part, paradoxically, to the wellness and prevention efforts of the MCOs themselves.

THE PREFERRED PROVIDER IS YOUR PROVIDER

The proliferation of POS plans and loosening of access to specialists are managed care's capitulation to the reality of the U.S. consumer health care market. As a class, MCOs have failed to *demonstrate* (not the same thing as advertise) to consumers what value they add sufficient to offset their loss of the freedom to choose. The market-driven punishment for this failure is reinstatement of that freedom. With indemnity or fully unrestricted plans still a widely available, if more expensive, alternative, the POS plan does indeed represent a defensive product strategy. The resulting plan design erodes an MCO's key operating strength: its ability to trade patients for price concessions and utilization control.

Perhaps in recognition of this, health care providers have purposefully complicated the situation for the MCOs. While MCOs still tend to focus on the self-insured employer as their customer,[6] provider organizations have rushed to market themselves directly to consumers, either alone or as integrated systems. These marketing efforts are designed for their "pull-through" effect on consumers: *if enough people in a plan demand a high-priced, well-marketed provider—perceived through successful brand management to have superior quality, service, or other features—then the MCO will be forced to include that provider in its network, or risk losing those consumers.* (This consumer "pull-through" strategy mirrors a key trend in the marketing strategies of pharmaceutical companies: in 1997, drug manufacturers spent $800 million on direct-to-consumer advertising, a 1,000 percent increase over spending in 1992.[7] The thinking behind the consumer marketing of prescription drugs? If patients know of and ask for drugs by name, then physicians—the traditional targets of pharmaceutical marketing—will be forced, when minimally appropriate, to prescribe them.)

The consumer pull-through strategy works for providers because it taps into the deeply held consumer belief that physicians—not health plans—are the real providers of care. In a comprehensive and detailed study published in *Health Affairs* on the relationship between sources of consumer information and health care choices, respondents rated physicians as the most important source of reliable information when picking a health plan. The "trust a lot" response topped out at 62 percent of respondents for physicians—greater than the 58 percent rate for friends and family members, and far greater than the 15 percent rate for insurance companies or the 11 percent for "large managed care organizations."[8] This was confirmed by the first national study of managed versus nonmanaged care consumers in 39 different health plans, conducted by the consumer research firm, J.D. Powers & Associates. It found that members' trust in physicians exceeded trust in their health plans by more than 20 percent.[9]

What is the source of this bias?

For an answer, the MCOs need look no further than their own television advertising. With its mawkish imagery of invariably healthy families frolicking through small town America—and their obligatory, banal, unsubstantiated voice-over narratives about the plan's "quality"—the ads center on the special dedication and commitment of "their" physicians. Most of "their" physicians, of course, are in reality independent practitioners who can be (and would almost certainly rather be) accessed by those families through any insurance channel other than the MCO. Indeed, the typical MCO advertising is pure image promotion, all sugar and no protein, the same "identity" labeling used for soft drinks and fragrances.

The hollowness of such ads echoes the hollowness of the MCOs' ultimate contribution to the health care system. The poignancy of this fact is nowhere more evident than in juxtapositions created by some of the MCOs' favorite media buys: police and medical dramas. One would be hard-pressed to conjure up a more illustrative contrast of the relative contributions of MCOs and physicians than a series of ads run by Aetna/US Healthcare during the television show *ER* in 1996: interrupting an episode in which the show's doctors helicopter to a gruesome traffic accident scene and successfully stabilize a mother and infant suffering bloody injuries—is a glossy, feel-good pitch for the $18.5 billion-per-year archenemy of physicians, one that tells viewers absolutely nothing about what Aetna/US Healthcare actually does, aside from sell you health insurance and buy expensive TV time with the premiums.[10-11] (It would probably not make much sense for an MCO to advertise its real contribution to health care—to tell consumers that it has helicoptered to the gruesome traffic accident that was the U.S. health care system and delivered the harsh medicine of managed care.)

The *Health Affairs* study of consumer information found that the quality of physicians in a plan is the most important consideration in plan selection, with 95 percent of respondents ranking it as their most critical criterion.[12] By contrast, cost was rated less important by the majority of respondents than numerous other features.[13] This finding reflects a key opening for groups of providers—best marketed as fully integrated systems of hospitals and physicians—to neutralize the power of MCOs. It also explains why the average hospital spent $195,100 on advertising in 1996, compared to $21,300 in the pre–managed care days of 1984.[14]

Though this phenomenon has not been studied, it makes for an interesting hypothesis: when given a choice of plans—and most people with employer-based insurance do have a choice of plans—consumers will pick their providers first, and then retrofit their health plan to that choice. They will find "their doc in the book" (the plan's directory of network providers) and then choose that plan with the cleanest administrative relationship with that physician. Of course, the cleanest administrative relationship of all involves no claims transactions—a situation possible only under capitation.

This type of consumer behavior explains why many MCOs have been forced to broaden their networks to the point of meaninglessness; it explains the huge popularity of the POS plan; and it represents a major dissolution of managed care as traditionally imposed upon a market of providers.

THE UN-PLAN PLAN

Providers know this about consumers instinctively, if only because they have been forced to staff roomfuls of people to fight MCOs every day on behalf of patients who want to be treated by them. After a decade of managed care's medicine, these providers have come to recognize that their ultimate target market is *not* the contracting MCO, but rather those with the health coverage (or the cash) whom the MCOs are fighting with each other to insure.

All of this spells the inevitable end of the MCO as paternalistic insurer and provider adversary. Resentment over the MCO's interposition between patients and providers has inspired providers to retaliate; their development of integrated networks to effect consumer pull-through is only the first prong in a counterattack; the final prong is the formalization of these networks into full risk-assuming entities, identified throughout this book as "EHOs," or emerging health care organizations. With less infrastructure than the traditional MCOs, these new organizations—the rudiments of which are fully functional in a handful of markets around the United States—are designed specifically to circumvent the traditional MCOs. As will be explored more fully in later chapters, this represents a classic "forward integration" business strategy, under which the producer of the good (the health care service) also becomes its marketer and distributor (the health insurance entity). A perfect example of this strategy are the retail stores operated by Levi Strauss.

The EHO that markets itself directly to covered employees and retail consumers, on a risk-assumption basis, is collapsing the highly inefficient barrier between medical financing and delivery that has existed since the advent of commercial health insurance. This strategy becomes increasingly viable as the health care market becomes increasingly consumer driven: it brings simplicity to the administration of the health benefit, and it provides an unprecedented clarity for consumers as to which providers they are choosing when they choose a health plan. (Because these entities are subject to the same problems discussed above with regard to building physician panels of sufficient size and diversity to accommodate choice, the force of health care consolidation is accelerated by the force of consumerism.)

The integration of health care financing and delivery through the EHO solves the thorniest of problems associated with traditional managed care. The major MCOs all devise and propound their own "care guidelines." Taken together, these clinical rules force physicians to practice one way for one patient, a different way for another patient, and still a third way for another. While this divergence in enforced practices obviously perverts the clinical decision-making process, physicians' collective rage at this perversion has generally received little attention, except from the occasional vigilant reporter or opportunistic politician. But try as they might with intrusive, cumbersome laws meant to strong-arm individual clinical practices, legislators simply cannot make the MCOs abandon the practice in general; consumers can, however, by abandoning the MCOs.

As consumers are only now beginning to discover how violently managed care operators have interjected themselves into the physician-patient relationship, they will vote with their premiums. And where better to take those premium dollars than directly to "your" physician?

THE PATIENT WILL SEE YOU NOW

The sudden surge in health care consumer marketing is not the caprice of a few thousand executives who all attended the same industry conference. It signals the changing demographics of America, as the typical consumer grows older, more affluent, and more educated. Over the past decade, the baby boom generation has, in effect, been subsidizing the managed care system, paying more in premiums than it has taken out in claims.[15] But as this generation ages sufficiently and becomes a net consumer of health care dollars, it will—as it has in numerous product markets (e.g., financial services)—demand more for itself than previous generations ever did.

The coming empowerment of health care consumers, spearheaded by this generation, is ushered in by increased coverage of medical news in the popular media and the proliferation of clinical information and disease-specific support groups on the Internet. And it reaches its full consummation in the purest alternative to traditional and managed care coverage: the Medical Savings Account (MSA).

With pretax money, an MSA lets a consumer set aside nearly the same amount of money that he or she would be spending on health care premiums, and use these funds to purchase and manage their own routine care. The account is coupled with catastrophic insurance with a very high deductible, which takes effect in the instance of a major medical event. Barring such an event, anything left over in the account at the end of the year is the consumer's to keep, after paying taxes on it, or to roll over for the next year. The goal of the MSA is to correct the dysfunctional economics of health care by turning patients into discriminating consumers.

MSAs cede to patients all control over their routine medical spending; as a result, they provide the clearest break of all from the consumer *dis*empowerment inherent in the traditional MCO, which presupposes that consumers are unable or unwilling to manage their own care. Such a clean break with the present, paradoxically, represents a return to health care consumerism's past: when health insurance was first introduced in the 1940s and 1950s, it carried with it what was in those days an extremely high deductible—usually $200—precisely the same deductible standard in today's indemnity insurance plans. Tom Emerick, who directs health care purchasing for Wal-Mart, carries in his briefcase a copy of a hospital bill for a normal newborn delivery from 1951. In the middle of debates over how to fix the health care system, he likes to pull out this bill to make a point about the loss of consumer responsibility for their health care costs. *The bill for the six-day hospital stay is $85.* Combine this with physicians' fees, and having a baby in 1951 still did not cost enough to exhaust the typical health plan's deductible.

As the amount of deductibles has remained frozen in time over decades of inflation, consumers' perceptions of the function of health insurance has mutated accordingly. What was once meant truly as insurance for medical catastrophes has come to represent prepayment for all commonplace medical events and needs. This is like expecting your auto insurance carrier to cover the cost of tune-ups, oil changes, and brake work. (If it did, you wouldn't shop all that hard for a better price on those new tires.) MSAs thus hearken back to the days when people purchased all their own standard health care services, and separately purchased insurance as protection against the unimaginable. It placed them in charge of their own health care and made them responsible for the financial conse-quences—up to a point—of neglecting it. Unlike today, however, patients in 1951 were not in any position to challenge the sovereign authority of physicians. Medical malpractice was unheard of then, and physicians were legally and culturally unassailable. With these important safeguards now in place, isn't it time to give this old way of doing things a new spin?

Many think not. Because MSAs were included as an alternative to traditional Medicare coverage for beneficiaries, an entire Medicare reform bill almost failed to pass Congress in 1997; fierce resistance to MSAs—the Democrats claimed they would favor the wealthiest, healthiest seniors—originated with lobbyists from the traditional in-surers and MCOs. Why? Because they recognized that patient con-trol over the bulk of their own health care financing accelerates the insurers' and MCOs' marginalization. The MSA flies in the face of the outmoded—and culturally unworkable—paternalism upon which so much of the current health care system is predicated.

The consumer culture's willingness to challenge physicians is not the only difference between health care in the 1950s and now. Suc-cessfully managing one's own care under an MSA requires access to reliable, in-depth medical information—and the ability to comprehend and relate that information to the medical matter at hand. Such information has traditionally never been readily available to patients, giving physicians and hospitals an unfair advantage in their dealings with them. This phenomenon is referred to throughout health care business literature as "asymmetries of information"; such asymmetries are commonly held out as one of the major impediments to the health care system functioning like any other normal marketplace.[16-18]

These asymmetries traditionally discolor patients' encounters with their physicians *and* with their insurers. In both cases, they preclude truly informed decision making, and thus provide an enormous rationale for the wealth of medical information suddenly available to consumers on the Internet. There are more than five million pages of medically related text on-line, delivered by more than 7,000 indexed Web sites.[19] "Medline," the clearinghouse for clinical literature used by physicians and researchers for more than a generation, was finally made accessible to public Internet users in June of 1997; within six weeks it was receiving one million "hits" per day. By gaining direct access to the same literature that clinicians have always used, patients no longer suffer from the same degree of information asymmetries that have always put them at a disadvantage. They are empowered by this access, finally able to shop around for better prices and better doctors; give better voice to their symptoms; question and challenge their physicians' diagnoses and treatment choices; and appreciate more fully the directives of their caregivers.[20-21]

So much for the role of the MCO as *de facto* "information broker" between unorganized patients and disorganized providers. One of managed care's more important—if less well articulated—functions has been to neutralize the distorting effects of information asymmetries by challenging providers' decisions, supposedly on the behalf of patients unequipped to make such challenges. In the legacy world of fee-for-service reimbursement—with its dysfunctional market economics and potential for provider conflict of interest—the patient wanders a landscape of undifferentiated providers. The MCO's job is to differentiate those providers for patients, tracking and monitoring provider quality, finding the best combination of cost and clinical effectiveness, and channeling them to the best performers.

As with the conversion of numerous other proprietary activities into public domain intelligence, the Internet and its unimaginable masses of information eliminate the consumer's need for the MCO's information brokering. Such an elimination embodies a broader phenomenon associated with the Internet known as "disintermediation." Disintermediation has a particularly populist appeal, especially when unleashed in industries that have successfully relied on asymmetries of information to confuse consumers. A good example is General Motors' use of the Internet for its "BuyPower" program. The service gives customers detailed information on GM's products, latest prices, and inventories by dealer.[22]

So much for the games car dealers play with car buyers. And so much for the games MCOs play with patients. The end result looks so similar, if only because the same technology is curing the same problem.

JUST HEAL IT

There is probably no greater embodiment of the trend toward consumerism in health care than the creation and promotion of health care "brand awareness." The cultivation and promotion of health care organizations as true "brands" like McDonald's, Disney, or Nike, is inevitable as

- employees pick up an ever larger portion of health benefits costs;
- demographics drive increasingly consumerist behavior in health care; and
- MCOs, at-risk EHOs, and other types of plans align themselves along a continuum of price and perceived quality in response to the first two factors.

Emerging from a monolithic delivery system is a much more discretionary system, one identical to any other consumer marketplace segmented along its own continuum of price and perceived quality.

As functional medical marketplaces emerge around the United States through the forces described in this book, and as consumers shoulder more of the financial burden for their own health care, they will purchase health care—through their benefit selection, directly through the retail market, or through liberalization of the Medicare program—precisely like they purchase cars. And as night follows day, so too does the emergence of the discriminating consumer give rise to the aggressive marketer.

The "branding" movement in health care is clearly an inevitability. Interestingly, it began in the mid-1990s with the MCOs. With little of substance to promote about their products, they were forced to default to pure identity advertising. The almost uniform thrust of these generally inane, saccharine efforts involve lots of shiny happy people, none of whom look like they require any medical care; these of course are the MCO's favorite customers. But when there is substance behind the brand—at least in the form of a heritage of consumer satisfaction—these efforts are well worth pursuing. In a random survey, the Blue Cross & Blue Shield Association found that consumers attributed superior security and quality to any insurance product with the "Blues" name attached to it. It also found that 62 percent of consumers responded more positively to plans with "Blues" as part of their names than to identical plans without it.[23]

As discussed above, providers have been particularly aggressive at promoting their brands. The most expensive and controversial branding campaign was undertaken by Columbia/HCA; this campaign was a major part of the business strategy of the company since deposed founder, Richard Scott. In 1995 and 1996, the hospital system embarked on a highly visible national multimedia advertising campaign, in the first ever attempt by a health care provider to launch a truly national "brand." The company renamed its hundreds of facilities around the country to reflect the name and look of the corporate parent. It also embarked on a well-produced and often amusing national broadcast campaign to the tune of $200 million over two years.[24] The campaign emphasized both the comprehensiveness and ubiquitousness of Columbia.

In a letter to shareholders from Scott, the campaign was launched to "raise awareness about Columbia and the quality services we provide. While patients and consumers recognize the quality at our facilities, few realized that each facility belongs to a broader integrated health care delivery system that serves our communities across the nation."[25] This unique combination of education and promotion was intended to make Columbia a household name, synonymous in consumers' minds with three key elements of the new health care system: consolidation, integration, and standardization. In this regard, Columbia was positioning itself precisely the same way McDonald's did for two decades: as McDonald's was synonymous in the American mind through the mid-1970s with the newfangled way of preparing and serving food, Columbia was attempting to make itself synonymous with the newfangled way of delivering health care services.

Unfortunately for Columbia, it worked *too* well. When the company's fortunes turned—following wide-ranging investigations into its billing and accounting practices by the federal government, numerous state agencies, and the news media—everyone suddenly knew *exactly* who Columbia was. The strategy actually hurt the company, as patients and physicians abandoned this new "household name" suddenly making headlines across the country. This explains why Thomas Frist, Jr., MD, who took over after Scott's ouster, quickly moved to dismantle the campaign.

It also explains why Tenet Healthcare, itself the survivor of a major federal investigation and settlement (of National Medical Enterprises, one of two companies that came together to form Tenet), chose specifically to brand its hospitals much more selectively. Tenet's corporate name is generally secondary to the legacy name of the local facility. This reflects the company's belief that branding is still market specific—and that the long-held axiom, "all health care is delivered locally," will survive the current, historic transformation of the health care system. According to a report in *Modern Healthcare*, the different approaches to the two systems' original branding strategies "reflects Columbia's determination to take advantage of its size and Tenet's intent to cultivate flexibility in each of its markets."[26] Different strategies, different tactics, same end: cultivate and communicate a brand's value in a local market.

Because Columbia's problems have nothing to do with its branding campaign, its efforts have been echoed almost to the note by numerous companies since. Manor Care, the fourth largest chain of long-term care providers, changed the names of all its facilities to reflect the corporate name, embarking on a $1.5 million advertising campaign.[27] And Catholic Healthcare West, the consolidator of Catholic hospitals across the West, is extremely conscious of the importance of managing its "brand." In CHW's case, this entails specifically downplaying its Catholic affiliation, so as not to alienate the large market segment uncomfortable with a health care provider that does not provide truly comprehensive health care services. According to the *Wall Street Journal*, the nuns who run CHW are "mulling a proposal to drop the word 'Catholic' from signs and advertisements, using instead the CHW initials in a move to build a brand name."[28]

And finally there is HealthSouth, the brashest brand manager of all. Its promotions include sports stars, celebrity endorsements, and extensive logo branding on giveaways. The *Wall Street Journal* reports that its founder, Richard Scrushy, "aims to carve a brand-name consumer product...and create a kind of Holiday Inns or McDonalds' of health care, with readily accessible, standardized care across the country."[29] These efforts—aimed wholly at the emerging consumerism of the health care system—may strike many as beneath the dignity of health care providers and not worth the effort and expense.

If so, they should check their closets and count how many of their sporting goods and fashion items bear the Nike logo.

REFERENCES

1. J. Kleinke, "Managed-Care Meltdown," *Barron's*, 22 December, 1997, 51.
2. Kleinke, *Barron's*, 51.

3. Median enrollment growth figures included in the *1997 Guide to the Managed Care Industry* (Baltimore: HCIA Inc., 1996).

4. Kleinke, *Barron's*, 51.

5. N. Jeffrey, "Doctors Battle Over Who Treats Chronically Ill," *Wall Street Journal*, 11 December, 1996.

6. One of the findings in "Consumerism in Health Care: New Voices," a study conducted and published by KPMG, January 1998.

7. J. Kleinke, "Power to the Patient," *Modern Healthcare*, 23 February, 1998, 66.

8. S. Isaacs, "Consumers' Information Needs: Results of a National Survey, *Health Affairs* 15, no. 4, (1996): 39.

9. J.D. Powers & Associates study, as reported by E. Weissenstein in "HMO Picture Unclear," *Modern Healthcare*, 20 October, 1997, 24.

10. Revenue figure taken from *Wall Street Journal* Interactive article on Aetna/ US Healthcare purchase of NYLCare, 16 March, 1998.

11. Television advertisement for Aetna/US Healthcare, aired during episode of *ER* on NBC.

12. Isaacs, *Health Affairs*, 35.

13. Isaacs, *Health Affairs*, 37.

14. Results of the 1996 National Hospital Marketers' Survey, Opinion Research Corporation International (vol. IV, no. 1), 1.

15. A. Gosfield, "Who Is Holding Whom Accountable for Quality?" *Health Affairs* 16, no. 3 (1997): 39.

16. P. Starr, "Smart Technology, Stunted Policy," *Health Affairs* 16, no. 3 (1997): 91–105.

17. D. Blumenthal, interview published on Internet Web site for "Satellite Committee for People with Disabilities," 23 November, 1997.

18. Kleinke, *Modern Healthcare*, 66.

19. B. Chan, "The Digital Revolution of Medical Education," *JAMA*, 3 December 1997.

20. Blumenthal interview.

21. D. Blumenthal, "The Future of Quality Measurement and Management in a Transforming Health Care System," *JAMA* 278, no. 19 (1997): 1622–1624.

22. Described in "Consumerism in Health Care: New Voices," a study conducted and published by KPMG, January 1998.

23. Survey by the Blue Cross & Blue Shield Association, as reported by D. Bellandi in "Paint It Blue," *Modern Healthcare,* 2 March, 1998, 74.

24. B. Japsen, "Columbia's Big Ad Bucks," *Modern Healthcare*, 10 March, 1997, 2.

25. Letter to Shareholders from Richard L. Scott, President and CEO, Columbia/ HCA Healthcare Corporation, 1 September, 1996.

26. B. Japsen, "Low-Key Branding," *Modern Healthcare*, 7 July, 1997, 40.

27. C. Snow, "Manor Care Strives for National Name," *Modern Healthcare*, 9 September, 1996, 24.

28. R. Rundle, "Catholic Hospitals, in Big Merger Drive, Battle Industry Giants," *Wall Street Journal*, 12 March, 1997.

29. A. Sharpe, "Medical Entrepreneur Aims To Turn Clinics into National Brand," *Wall Street Journal*, 14 December, 1996.

3

CONSOLIDATION

*The pavilion's benefactor and other donors who received
crystal bowls at black-tie "Affairs of the Heart," would be
as unknown to a future CEO as a boy riding his skateboard
past the doctors' parking lot.*

Marc Flitter, MD
*Judith's Pavilion: The Haunting Memories
of a Neurosurgeon*[1]

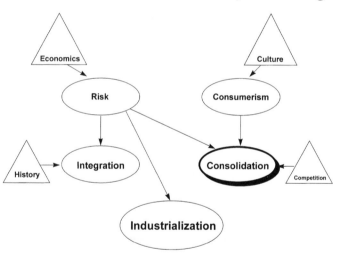

One of the few theories of corporate strategy that has outlasted
an entire business cycle is Michael Porter's work on the five competitive forces of industry structure. Introduced in 1980 in his still
hugely influential work, *Competitive Strategy*, Porter's model is a
crisp and incisive description of how strategic moves among competitors, purchasers, suppliers, producers of substitute goods, and
new entrants engage in a dance of continuous actions and reactions.

As the spectrum of human dance ranges from slow and pensive, to fluid and graceful, to jarring and unpredictable, so too the character of the dance among competing firms constitutes the development of an industry.

It is a testament to the flexibility, durability, and enduring genius of his model that, despite the often bewildering complexity of the U.S. health care system, Porter's forces of competition are nowhere more applicable than to the health care industry. That they apply so readily, with almost no modification, is also the strongest single testament to the central thesis of this book: health care is indeed transforming itself into a business no less exempt from the laws of competition than the auto, airline, or retailing industries.

FROM CHAOS TO CONSOLIDATION

The principles behind Porter's forces of industry competition are responsible for much of the consolidation wave that has engulfed the health care system in the 1990s. This idea is confirmed in the inverse: consolidation proceeds with such speed and comprehensiveness if only because the health care system was nearly devoid of competition for so long. Between 1990 and 1997, 62.7 million covered lives—one out of every four Americans—have been traded as part of transactions among insurers and MCOs.[2] In the same period, nearly 60 percent of the health care delivery system has changed ownership control.[3] And the 5 largest drug companies in 1997 had more revenue than the 25 largest a decade earlier.[4] What was a highly fragmented, disorganized system—with such disorganization inadvertently subsidized and even rewarded by the perverse incentives of fee-for-service reimbursement—is sorting itself into a matrix of horizontally and vertically integrating firms; and competition for suddenly stagnant aggregate revenue is the catalyst.

Before adapting Porter's principles of competitive dynamics to analyze this process, one of the industry's more problematic structural features should be incorporated into his model. There is an uneasy coexistence—part competition, part cooperation—among physicians, hospitals, and ambulatory service facilities. These three types of providers do to some degree compete with each other—either directly or through the provision of "substitute goods" (the same surgery can often be performed in a hospital, outpatient clinic, or physician's office). This is a legacy of the fragmentation of the health care system itself and will be addressed throughout this book.

From an industry-wide perspective, however, "provider" describes any producer of medical services positioned between the hard bargaining of the health care payer or purchaser (the insurer, managed care operator, or self-insured employer) and the hard selling of the health care supplier (the drug company, equipment manufacturer, malpractice insurer, etc.). In this context, hospitals, physicians, and other providers are in precisely the same competitive predicament, and thus are aggregated in the model; this is also the core rationale for their rapid movement into vertical alliances and the subject of the next chapter ("Integration"). Meanwhile, we begin with all providers at the center of the schematic in Figure II–1, which shows Porter's five forces of competition applied to the health care industry.

Again, this schematic presupposes the achievement of a workable coexistence among various types of providers—except when one type of provider represents a "threat of substitute goods." Such "threats" are common in health care delivery; they have served as the source of the health care system's most economically powerful innovations over the past decade, including the seemingly overnight appearance of freestanding ambulatory surgery centers, subacute and rehab facilities, and home health care agencies. Each of these substitute goods supplants the high costs and unnecessarily restrictive use of inpatient resources for resolving patient illness or injury. Because of the compulsion of health care providers to integrate services into a "continuum of care," the competing firms in the center of this schematic have rapidly incorporated these substitute goods into their own product portfolios, either through acquisition, alliance, or imitation.

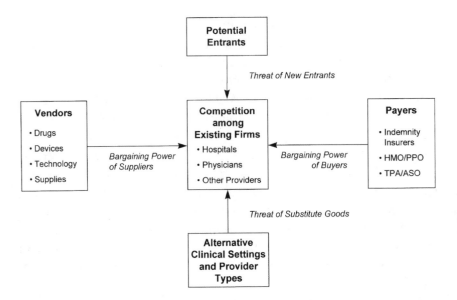

Figure II–1 Porter's Forces Driving Industry Competition, as Applied to the Health Care Industry. *Source:* Adapted and reprinted with the permission of The Free Press, a Division of Simon & Schuster from COMPETITIVE STRATEGY: Techniques for Analyzing Industries and Competitors by Michael E. Porter. Copyright © 1980 by The Free Press.

The ability of provider organizations to assemble and assimilate a vertical system of care summons another key strategic challenge in health care: who is the real "provider" at the heart of this industry analysis? As will be explored throughout the remainder of this book, there are numerous contenders:

- the provider is hospital-based, and employs or contracts with physicians;
- the provider is physician-group–based, and contracts with hospitals;
- the provider is a holding company for the continuum of outpatient services, and contracts with both hospitals and physicians;
- the provider is the payer, and "backward-integrates" through the purchase of hospitals, physicians, and others.

As of this writing, the right answer is "all of the above." All four models are currently competing to assume control of the mantle of "provider-competitor" at the center of this schematic.

For our purposes, it does not matter how this plays out. In fact, it may play out that all four models endure and emerge as competitive alternatives; their very different structures, cultures, and cost economics may prove in the end to be the wellspring of their competitive differentiation. Regardless of form, one critical point endures: competition is a new, significant, and permanent fact among provider organizations, now that the nation's purchasers (employers, government, and consumers) have been stretched to their limits of tolerance for outsized health care spending. As we relate the dynamics of Porter's model to health care, this competition is destined to grow only more fierce.

Because all business activity proceeds, ultimately, along an endless food chain of buyers and sellers, Porter's model can and should be expanded outward in either direction. This allows for a more comprehensive view of the competitive forces at work across the entire spectrum of the health care industry. Moving up the chain, the provider is a supplier of health care services to the payer, who is a supplier of health insurance services to the employer, who is the supplier of products and services to the rest of the economy. Moving back down the chain, the provider is a buyer of health care products from medical suppliers, who are buyers of raw materials from manufacturers, and so on. These relationships are illustrated in the expanded version of Porter's model, as applied to the health care industry, in Figure II–2.

Embodied in this expanded version of Porter's model is one of the more fascinating aspects of health care: how easily entire links of the chain can be skipped. Health care suppliers can and do market their products directly to health care payers and consumers; health care providers can and do market themselves directly to employers; and so on. In fact, the ease of leapfrogging your customer in this model—or engaging in what is commonly referred to as "forward integration"—is the source of much of the complexity and confusion

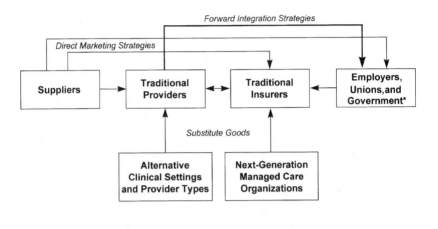

Figure II–2 Expanded Model of Competitive Forces in the Health Care Industry.

in the current health care system today as it transforms from an inefficient community of not-for-profit organizations into an industry of competing firms. The temptations posed by the competitive fluidity inherent in this model grow only greater as competition intensifies. *Forward and backward integration is a viable strategic move for every major player in the health care system.* The potential for such threats and opportunities contributes significantly to the simultaneous consolidations of each class of players in this model (e.g., MCO consolidation), particularly the rapid consolidation among provider organizations.

As the health care industry sorts itself into the competitive model pictured in Figure II–2, one key theme emerges, a theme confirmed almost daily in the health care trade journals and general business media: consolidation begets consolidation begets consolidation. This has come to so dominate the health care system in the 1990s that it comprises a consolidation domino theory of sorts:

- employers join into coalitions to exert their buying leverage on health care payers with the goal of reducing per employee health care costs;
- payers consolidate to respond to that leverage and lower per member administrative costs, while exerting leverage on *their* suppliers—the health care providers—to lower their medical costs;
- providers in turn consolidate to respond to the growing leverage of payers and to lower administrative costs, while exerting leverage on the suppliers of medical products to lower operating costs; and
- suppliers in turn consolidate to shore up their own bargaining position with the providers and lower their own administrative costs.

In addition to the pure chain-reaction nature of these consolidations, another driver of consolidation is the sudden emergence and eventual domination of health care's new currency: risk-assumption. As detailed in the previous chapter, *in the new century's health care system, the only transactions left will be the transfer and assumption of medical/financial risk.* The one constant in the economics of risk-assumption is the law of large numbers: larger risk pools can better absorb large losses. Adverse medical events are much less damaging statistically when they can be dissipated across greater populations. Bigger is thus less risky and ultimately more predictable. The global insurance industry has evolved based on this very principle: with its safety chain of insurance underwriting, underwriting syndication, reinsurance, and re-reinsurance, almost all insurance risk around the world ultimately rolls up to a handful of enormous multinational corporations to diversify risk across continents, populations, and risk products.

The consolidation of health care providers and MCOs into ever larger organizations is the result of the same economics in miniature. As providers shoulder the risk for covered populations, they need to cover ever larger populations. The attainment of critical mass through such consolidation helps risk-assuming providers attenuate the economic consequences of unexpectedly high disease incidence, protecting them from one bad year on an otherwise good multiyear contract. Because it safeguards the process of risk-assumption, consolidation allows providers to assume risk more aggressively from payers and, more importantly, paves the road to forward integration: it allows providers to assume *all* insurance risk for a population, and thus market around the consolidating payers to contract directly with employers and consumers.

A COMMUNITY HMO FOR ALL TIME ZONES

Fed up with double-digit increases in premiums throughout the 1980s, the nation's employers finally reached their breaking point. "Fix it!" they told the HMOs. "And if you don't, we'll put our dollars together and take them to somebody who will!"

Such is the consolidation of buying power as employers over the past decade finally began to exert their leverage in purchasing health care benefits. Through increasingly aggressive contracting, they transferred the financial risk for the medical care of their covered employees and dependents over to the MCOs, which serve as a collectivization of the employers' medical care buying power. Those employers too small to exert sufficient pressure on the MCOs formed health care "purchasing coalitions."

In direct reaction to this sudden mobilization of buying leverage, MCOs and other payers have moved rapidly to consolidate. This allows them to bargain more effectively upstream with employers and exert more leverage downstream with their own suppliers, the health care providers. The years 1995 through 1997 have witnessed a sweep of major mergers, acquisitions, and joint operating agreements across the payer community, the most significant of which follow:

	Total *Enrollment*[5] *(millions of lives)*
Aetna/US Healthcare	14.1
United Healthcare/MetraHealth	13.5
Cigna/HealthSource	12.3
United Healthcare/Humana	10.4
Kaiser/Group Health of Puget Sound	8.0
Foundation/HSI	4.9
PacifiCare/FHP International	3.9
WellPoint/Mass Mutual's group health	3.8
Aetna/NYLCare	2.2

These deals directly affect 73.1 million Americans, or nearly 30 percent of the U.S. population. Some represent the consolidation of pure MCOs; others represent the combination of MCOs and traditional indemnity insurers. The latter type of combination is a key factor in accelerating the spread of managed care across the industry as entire populations are pushed toward managed care models. They represent a telling admission by many organizations, Aetna's purchase of US Healthcare being the most obvious example: to create a managed care system and populate it with large, captive groups is no easy task, given how deeply entrenched the old values, old guard, and old reward systems can be in the typical large payer's organization and culture. Such deals by well-capitalized but immobile organizations point out that "buying your way into managed care" is often an easier route to this brave new world than fighting your way there.

The struggle attendant to payer consolidation is nowhere more evident—nor more tumultuous—than in the seemingly overnight reinvention of the nation's dozens of "Blues" plans. Among the Blue Cross and Blue Shield plans across the United States, three interdependent trends have arisen:

1. consolidation of plans across market boundaries that were created decades ago;
2. the rapid introduction of managed care products to fend off market share loss to MCOs; and
3. the creation of for-profit subsidiaries or outright conversion to for-profit status to raise sufficient capital to fund the consolidation and managed care product development.

Mergers completed or initiated in 1996 include Blues plans from Illinois and Texas; Blue Cross of Pennsylvania and Blue Shield of Western Pennsylvania; Blue Cross of Northeastern Pennsylvania and Capital Blue Cross.[6] Most aggressive among the Blues plans has been the Indiana plan, which changed its name to "Anthem" and went on an eating binge, gobbling up plans in Kentucky, Ohio, and Connecticut.[7]

The boldest consolidation move by the Blues plans as a class—a move that has yet to bear fruit as of this writing, but that reveals much of the strategic dilemma of the Blues plans—is the creation of "HMO-USA," a national network of MCOs owned by 59 of the 62 Blues plans across the country.[8] HMO-USA is an attempt by the Blues plans to replicate the national marketing presence and practices of the major MCOs. As with the individual plans' rapid consolidations, managed care product development, and for-profit conversions, this move is essentially a defensive one; it is meant to counter rapid consolidation and direct competition from the for-profit managed care industry. Initially a substitute good thrust into the sleepy market for indemnity insurance, MCOs' products have emerged as fierce competitors to the blank-check indemnity coverage traditionally offered by the Blues plans.

In their rush to consolidate, both the national MCOs and Blues plans are introducing significant leverage to their relationship with health care providers. As such, they are following Porter's dictum to the letter:

A buyer group is powerful if the following circumstances hold true: It is concentrated or purchases large volumes relative to seller sales. [Consolidation of payers in a market is designed specifically to have this effect on a provider's business.]

The products it purchases from the industry represent a significant fraction of the buyer's costs or purchases. [Provider costs usually represent 70 to 80 percent of a payer's total costs.]

The products it purchases from the industry are standard or undifferentiated. [Providers believe passionately that there are quality differences among themselves, but payers pay little heed to these differences, according to numerous industry sources and as detailed throughout George Anders' *Health against Wealth*.[9]]

It faces few switching costs. [Buyers can switch provider contracts with the stroke of a pen and printing of a new provider directory.]

The buyer has full information. [Payers have information about all providers due to claims payments over the years, whereas many providers have only their own or published rate information.][10]

All of these forces clearly reward the consolidation of payers.

There are obvious and significant economies of scale associated with purchasing health services from providers, another factor aided significantly by payer consolidation. Such economies govern information systems, liability insurance, "stop-loss" or reinsurance to protect against large medical losses; and the development of "guidelines" and other proprietary medical management protocols. There are even more significant economies of scale associated with marketing the health plans to employers and consumers. The enlightened MCOs are currently striving to consummate these economies at a furious pace.

Why? Because such economies are their only structural competitive advantages against the fundamental economic challenges posed by the forward integration of providers.

WELCOME TO McHOSPITAL, MAY I TAKE YOUR ORDER?

Health care providers, long burdened with overcapacity, had little incentive to correct the problem until consolidating MCOs threatened to bargain them out of their shirts. In direct reaction to the suddenly muscular buying power of consolidating payers, health care providers have moved just as rapidly to consolidate. The goals of such consolidation are many and varied:

- eliminate excess capacity, which reduces fixed costs and increases margins;
- shore up collapsing prices for commercially insured patients, which had been artificially high all through the 1980s so as to subsidize losses on Medicare patients;[11]
- stave off the strenuous bargaining power of the MCOs; and
- amass the capital, develop the infrastructure, and attain the "market-mass" necessary to assume medical/financial risk and forward-integrate past the MCOs, i.e., direct-contract with employers, the government, and consumers.

Such consolidations among providers take a variety of forms: stand-alone hospitals consolidate into multihospital "systems" or sell out to national hospital chains; freestanding medical facilities join local systems or sell out to national chains; fragmented physician group practices consolidate into ever larger group practices, or sell out to national "physician practice management companies." In 1996, a total of 768 hospitals were involved in mergers, acquisitions, or M&A-like alliances, up from 735 in 1995 and 650 in 1994.[12] In this three-year period, two out of every five U.S. hospitals were involved in a deal of this type.[13] The sum total of all this consolidation is the closure of nearly 10 percent of all U.S. hospitals in one decade, from 5,678 acute care facilities in 1986, to 5,194 in 1995.[14]

The most visible and controversial driving force behind all the deal making has been the sudden rise of the national for-profit hospital chains. Even the scandal that beset the largest, Columbia/HCA

Healthcare Corporation, has not slowed the pace of consolidation; even as Columbia/HCA was embroiled in federal and state investigations, new for-profit hospital systems were successfully launching themselves from Wall Street to Main Street, flush with cash and eager to buy up not-for-profit hospitals. Before its new management chose to appease the government and divest assets in the wake of the investigations, Columbia owned 344 hospitals, 135 surgery centers, and 550 home health facilities,[15] which brought in nearly $20 billion in patient revenues in 1996.[16]

Columbia's strategy of buying into, consolidating, and developing critical mass within a local health care market has been replicated in nearly every one of its markets by one or another of several national for-profit or not-for-profit hospital systems. In late 1996 the second largest chain, Tenet Healthcare, purchased the third largest chain, OrNda, bringing its ownership or control to 127 hospitals nationwide.[17] In third place in the hospital consolidation derby is Community Health Systems, purchased in 1996 by the buyout firm, Forstmann Little, with the express purpose of financing an acceleration of Community's own consolidation. "We plan on doubling the size of the company," Linda Horbach, general partner at Forstmann Little, told *Modern Healthcare* in early 1997. At the time, Community owned and operated 40 hospitals, which the buyout firm plans to grow to include 75 to 80 hospitals within five years.[18]

Such hospital corporations are not a new phenomenon. They existed for years at the fringe of the industry, in geographic areas that were legally and financially amenable to their presence. Only through the blitzkrieg-style acquisition strategies of Columbia, Tenet, and half a dozen other systems have they emerged as a force worthy of public scrutiny.

"Hospital corporations were born in the 1960s, then went through a retrenchment and restructuring period in the mid-1980s after Medicare introduced a new prospective payment system," Lutz and Gee write in *The For-Profit Healthcare Revolution*. "Then, during the early 1990s, they entered a period of resurgence."[19] This resurgence is the direct result of the pricing and overcapacity pressure in individual markets created by the sudden buying power of consolidating payers. In 1994, some 650 hospitals—"more than 10 percent of all U.S. hospitals—were caught up in merger and acquisition deals."[20]

The payers' buying leverage that has driven this consolidation affects even the rural hospitals, where managed care and other forces of industry transformation supposedly have less direct impact. Why? Because payers contract for the delivery of services to populations spread over entire regions, not just in local markets. As a result, rural facilities are swept up into the same market dynamics. As Lutz and Gee point out, "with purchaser coalitions being formed in large areas as well as small, the need for extensive geographic diversity is high and increasing. Consequently, the smaller hospitals in the United States (even those located in rural locations) will round out the network for many regional systems."[21] Underscoring how clearly this trend affects rural hospitals are the aggressive plans to grow through acquisition, as cited above, of Community Health Systems, which is focused almost exclusively on rural and nonurban markets.

The consolidation of hospital capacity by the for-profit chains is forcing similar action by groups of religious-affiliated hospitals around the United States. Hospitals related through their religious orders are undergoing the same rationalization. Catholic Healthcare West is in the process of assembling a chain of 41 hospitals across the West and Southwest, with annual revenues that will approach $5 billion when its merger with the 6 hospitals of Samaritan Health Systems of Phoenix is completed.[22] This merger makes the system of formerly stand-alone Catholic hospitals one of the five largest groups in the United States. Even so, it still lags the number three system, Daughters of Charity, with 49 hospitals nationwide.[23] Of course, the rankings change weekly: both systems will be trumped when Catholic Health Initiatives completes its merger with Sisters of Charity of Nazareth Health System, for a total of 61 hospitals.[24] Not to be outdone by the sisters in the West, 1998 saw the creation of

Catholic Healthcare East, a combination of three smaller systems into one 25-hospital regional system.[25]

A report on Catholic Healthcare West in the *Wall Street Journal* underscores the dynamics of consolidation: "Like their rivals, Catholic hospitals realize that growth may be a matter of survival. MCOs increasingly control where patients are treated, and only large hospital groups have the clout to contract with them."[26]

Such market-driven consolidations affect all other providers, not just hospitals. As the national systems "roll up" hundreds of stand-alone hospitals across the United States, freestanding outpatient surgery, rehab and home health facilities across the United States have been purchased by Wall Street–financed firms like HealthSouth and Integrated Health Services. HealthSouth grows especially fast by acquiring the smaller acquirers: in 1995, it paid $1.1 billion for Surgical Care Affiliates, turning the aggressive marketer of rehab services into the largest provider of outpatient surgery in the country; it followed in early 1997 with the purchase of its largest competitor in the rehab business, Horizon/CMS, for $1.6 billion.[27] To shore up the deal, HealthSouth then turned around and sold the subacute and nursing home portion of Horizon/CMS to Integrated Health Services, or IHS, which is moving in parallel with HealthSouth to consolidate this clinically adjacent segment of the industry.[28]

A report on HealthSouth's acquisition strategy cites Health-South's ability to provide a "predictable product at a predictable cost," a factor considered "very attractive to consolidating payors." Following this spate of deals, HealthSouth as of mid-1997 served nearly 2,000 MCOs and employers.[29] These third-party payers contribute approximately two-thirds of its $4.3 billion in *pro forma* annual revenues.[30]

As HealthSouth has "rolled up" the rehab and outpatient surgery business, so too have other nonhospital providers rapidly consolidated the still nascent "subacute" industry. Subacute care involves inpatient-type rehab and recovery services for patients following major surgery, but in a less costly, nonhospital facility. Once a niche for hospitals and nursing homes seeking to convert unused capacity, the entire subacute industry—which scarcely existed a decade ago and is now a $15 billion-per-year industry—has been consolidated under three national companies, IHS, Genesis Health Ventures, and ManorCare Health Services.[31]

The goal of each segment's consolidation is a competitive response to consolidations upstream: companies like HealthSouth and IHS are positioning themselves to provide "one-stop shopping" for the national MCOs. Underlying these consolidations is a positive-sum game where everyone makes the same move, almost at the same time, but the entire system is better off. Why? Because a by-product of provider consolidation is an elimination of the excess capacity that has dogged the health care system since the early 1980s. This is nowhere more evident than in the rapid consolidation of hospitals in the 1990s—here, provider overcapacity was the greatest and, not coincidentally, its consolidation has been the most aggressive.

"LIKE HERDING CATS"

Ever try to herd cats? No one actually ever has; but given how frequently the analogy is used to describe attempts to manage doctors, you would think that herding cats was the latest fitness craze, with prime time coverage of this emerging sport on ESPN2.

The analogy is used so frequently because of all the consolidation occurring in health care, the least intuitive and most difficult to manage is the consolidation of physician practices into captive groups or loose contracting alliances known as independent practice associations, or IPAs. These groups are formed specifically to give physician groups—traditionally small, stand-alone firms with two to five professionals at their helm—at least a fighting chance in their dealings with MCOs. There are now an estimated 3,000 IPAs, and another 3,000 alliances joining physicians practices with hospitals, each of which represents several hundred physicians.[32] According to the American Medical Association, roughly half the nation's 600,000 physicians now negotiate through an IPA.[33]

Because these alliances do not have the full clout of a national organization bargaining on behalf of doctors, a new entity has arisen in the 1990s supposedly to level the playing field: the physician practice management firm (PPM). The PPM strives to create the same national purchasing and marketing clout for physician groups that Tenet or the Daughters of Charity bring to hospitals. As of early 1997,

- 8 percent of the 527,000 physicians in the United States were affiliated with a PPM, up from virtually none in 1990;
- at their current growth rate, PPMs are expected to capture up to one-half of all U.S. physicians by the year 2003; and
- the largest PPMs—the multispecialty groups PhyCor, MedPartners/Mullikin, and Coastal Physicians Group—had a combined market capitalization of $9.4 billion.[34]

PPMs sing a tune that physicians have been wanting to hear for a generation: no more paperwork. PPMs promise blanket relief from the administrative side of medicine. No more contract negotiations with MCOs, no more haggling with insurance companies over unpaid claims, no more overpriced malpractice insurance, no more hassles with practice management software that doesn't work, no more photocopier sales reps. It is a lot to promise from companies spending most of their time on Wall Street, raising money to sustain growth rates through the acquisition of still more physician practices.

As the health care system grinds through its historic transformation—goaded by ever more meddlesome managed care control systems and technologies—the necessary evil of coping with an explosion of conflicting rules, legacy payment systems, and new reimbursement schemes grows exponentially more time consuming and perplexing for physicians. PPMs, at least in theory, fix the problem by taking it away: they handle everything from selling the group's medical services to MCOs, to collecting from their nonpaying patients; they deal with the purchases of insurance, information systems, and medical equipment; they hire, train, manage, pay, and fire support staff. In the process, PPMs allow physicians to focus exclusively on managing their patients, their physician extenders, and other aspects of their purely clinical operation.

That's the theory. The reality has proven far more complicated, thanks to the execution problems, leadership problems, and financial engineering shenanigans of the PPMs. These mask broader strategic flaws in the PPM model that will be discussed at length in the "MD, MBA" chapter.

Regardless of what form physician consolidation takes, it is clearly a strategic necessity in *some* form. If for no other reason, risk-assumption demands that physicians pool their labor in order to pool patient medical/financial risk. In a study of physician capitation, the percentage of reimbursement derived from this method of payment was shown to increase dramatically with the size of the group practice.[35] The financial and operating rigors of functioning under at-risk contracts requires multiple specialists, the ability to spread risk over larger pools of patients, and capital. This of course is a gateway to forward integration by physicians to directly contract with employers and consumers.

But such strategies are high-risk and high-cost. As a report in *Modern Healthcare* on physician-owned health plans put it, "some plans raised millions from physicians and local medical societies, but that wasn't enough to compete with big HMOs."[36]

VENDOR-BENDERS

As payer consolidation begets provider consolidation, so too does the increasing buyer power of providers beget the consolidation of *their* suppliers: the manufacturers of high-tech equipment, drugs, medical devices and supplies, and information systems. In fact, pricing concessions won from suppliers often provides the *only* rationale for provider consolidation in the first place, at least in short-run financial terms. As Lutz and Gee point out, "profits for hospital management companies in the early 1990s came at the expense of medical supply and technology vendors. Hit by falling profits, the stock prices of those vendors in 1994 reflected the turmoil in the industry."[37]

The master of this strategy has been Columbia/HCA. As the largest provider organization, it enjoys tremendous negotiating leverage, which it did not hesitate to wield under founder Richard Scott. In the wake of its acquisition of several other chains, its supply expenses as a percentage of revenue decreased 1.2 percent in 1994, to 14.7 percent.[38] At the time, Columbia's supply expense figure ran 2 percent below its nearest competitor; the additional 1.2 point reduction represented a *one-year savings of more than $174 million in expenses.*

Columbia's buying power was not the only the pressure on health care suppliers to consolidate, just the most obvious and easiest to measure. In the early 1980s groups of stand-alone hospitals formed group purchasing organizations (GPOs) to purchase supplies at discounts, many along geographic or other lines of affiliation (i.e., religious affiliations, not-for-profit status, etc.). The GPOs were less than perfectly effective because hospitals typically belonged to more than one at the same time, and still exercised the option to purchase outside the GPO. As a result, GPO purchasing entailed a great deal of confusion about best prices and guaranteed volumes, effectively diminishing their overall impact on the supplier industry.

It was not until the mid-1990s that the GPOs themselves began consolidating—with their own existence challenged by the rise of the large hospital chains like Columbia. Because of such consolidation, in 1995 the 10 largest GPOs accounted for 60 cents of every dollar spent on hospital supplies in the United States, up from 49 cents only a year earlier. This represents purchasing of $31.7 billion in 1995.[39] Only through such consolidation—which eliminated much of the self-defeating "price competition" among GPOs to purchase on behalf of their member hospitals—have GPOs as a group been able to exert leverage on the supplier community sufficient to effect that community's own chain-reaction consolidation movement.

Despite this pricing pressure, much of the health care supplier industry remains largely intact and highly profitable. Most of this is due to factors identified by Porter with regard to supplier power:

A supplier group is powerful if it is dominated by a few companies and is more concentrated than the industry it sells to. [Except for niche players, some of whom are extremely well protected and others who are not protected well at all, the pharmaceutical and medical supply communities are highly concentrated and are becoming even more so as a direct reaction to the latest GPO and hospital consolidations.]

It is not obliged to contend with other substitute products for sale to the industry. [Because of heavy regulation by the federal government, much—but not all—of the health care supplier community is well protected by patent law that impedes substitution.]

The suppliers' product is an important input to the buyer's business. [For all health care supplies, this importance is self-evident.]

The supplier group's products are differentiated. [Some supplies are extremely well differentiated; other are highly undifferentiated and are rapidly cannibalized by the market.][40]

The varying degree to which this last factor applies to two types of suppliers has directly determined their fate: most pharmaceutical manufacturers have fared well, while many medical/surgical device and supply companies have not.

Regardless, both types of suppliers have responded to the consolidation of health care providers upstream—and of health care payers farther upstream—by consolidating themselves. Indeed, there is a direct relationship between the competitive defensibility of the products marketed by a segment of suppliers and the concentration of that segment. At one extreme are the behemoths of disposable hospital supplies, the IV solutions, nutrition products, disposables, bandages, syringes, gowns, and such, which are manufactured and distributed by only three extremely large companies: Owens Minor; the Hospital Products Division of Abbott Laboratories; and Allegiance, the hospital supply spin-off of Baxter International, a company once so large it was barely capable of functioning. At the other extreme are niche companies like biotech's Amgen and heart valve manufacturer St. Jude Medical. These and others who develop high-tech, research and development (R&D) intensive, high-priced products are so highly differentiated, critical to the medical mission, and protected by patents that they can conceivably operate profitably on their own for the foreseeable future.

Much of the health care supplier community falls in the middle of these two extremes—precisely where most of the chain-reaction consolidations are occurring. There has been a rapid concentration in the pharmaceutical industry since 1993, including a number of major mergers between Glaxo and Burroughs Wellcome (now Glaxo Wellcome), Sandoz and Ciba-Geigy (now Novartis), Hoechst Roussel and Marion Merrill Dow (now Hoechst Marion), and Pharmacia & Upjohn. This advent of "Big Pharma" follows a similar wave in the late 1980s that witnessed the creation of SmithKline Beecham, Bristol-Myers Squibb, and others. Perhaps because of that earlier flurry of mergers, consolidation this time around has been less noteworthy than the major and unprecedented consolidations upstream in the health care payer and provider communities. If nothing else, the fact that concentration is business as usual for suppliers may help explain their continually high margins—and provider claims that high supplier prices are a major motivation for *their* consolidation.

BIG PHARMA'S RISK DIVERSIFICATION

There are stronger arguments for the consolidation of "Big Pharma" than increasing concentration up the food chain. The latest round of drug company mergers is driven by a combination of im-proving microeconomics and better R&D risk management.

New drug discovery has always entailed enormous fixed costs. The average new drug takes 9.4 years to go from initial screened compound to launched product, at an average cost of $359 million.[41] The infrastructure and overhead required to support this gauntlet from test tube to marketplace makes achieving economies of scale a critical success factor for every major drug company. The stakes as-sociated with this grow exponentially higher as the average cost to develop a new drug increases as a percentage of sales. With fixed costs rising, margins can only decrease if the cost of manufacturing, marketing, and/or administration is not reduced. The first is almost impossible to cut; the next unlikely culturally, and usually only through natural attrition following a merger; only the third is left to cut as an offset to increases in R&D expenses. Hence, one of the stated goals of the 1996 merger of Ciba-Geigy and Sandoz into Novartis was an 8 percent reduction in overhead by 1999.[42] The combined company has annual sales of $27.3 billion in 1996; based on continued gross margins of 40 percent and current operating mar-gins of 15 percent, this figure amounts to a total reduction in over-head of $545 million per year. Together with savings attributable to combining and streamlining their R&D operations, the merged en-tity has promised Wall Street annual total savings of $1.5 billion.[43]

Beyond the need to shrink overhead relative to R&D expenses, there is another rationale for drug company consolidation: risk-di-versification. For every drug that is eventually approved and mar-keted, another 10,000 attempts fail. Odds like this mirror those af-fecting the economics of insurance, but with the desired outcome reversed: you *want* flukes in a "population" of drug candidates—and the way you get a stable crop of them is to increase the total size of the population. Like disease incidence within pools of insured people, the best way to achieve reliable statistical occurrences is to pool large numbers of molecules. Drug companies consolidate spe-cifically to pool more attempts—and thereby increase the chances that their labs will perform at the industry's average or better.

Though serendipity is a major factor in new drug discoveries, the idea that the process is subject to the principles of probability are embodied in a confluence of new technologies currently revolutionizing the basic discovery process. The 1990s have witnessed the emergence of significant alternatives to basic drug research, driven by core breakthroughs in microbiology and information technology. The first, combinatorial chemistry, is a computer-generated matching of molecular agents and biologic targets that expedites the hit-or-miss labors of traditional drug design. The second, genome-based development, flows from the current mapping of the human genome, which involves codifying every genetic mutation at the root of human disease.

Both processes greatly accelerate the number of potential new drug candidates; both reward bulking up a drug company's total R&D capacity to maximize the likelihood that those candidates produce a sufficient number of winners. As an example of how drastically these technologies have changed the process, consider Genentech's recent reengineering of its R&D operation: it has broken down its vertically integrated discovery process—one small research team per series of compounds from start to finish—into a series of horizontally arranged, assembly-line processes.[44] Nearly 25 percent of Genentech's research staff is engaged in these processes, analyzing enormous databases of gene sequencing information, looking for potential keys to either replicating or inhibiting natural processes. Or consider the big bucks paid for a company with minimal revenue but a lock on the technology: Glaxo Wellcome shelled out $533 million in cash for five-year-old Affymax, the leading "pure technology" company in the arena of combinatorial chemistry.[45]

These are the real economic reasons behind consolidation in the drug industry. For Big Pharma, diversity is everything: this is how Bristol-Myers Squibb took over the number one spot in 1998 as the biggest drug seller in the United States.[46] While none of its major drugs are leaders in any of their therapeutic classes, it is a broad portfolio of midrange performers that pushed the company past

Glaxo Wellcome, which had held the spot for several years because of revenue from a small number of top-selling drugs.

A breadth of product, and R&D to keep that product coming, is the source of the drug industry's profits and staying power. Market leverage is less of a factor, given the collective value—galvanized by economic leverage and protected by medical malpractice liability—that leading edge drugs bring to the health care system. (These concepts will be explored at length in "Panaceas R Us.")

AND THIS NUMBER OF BEDS IS JUST RIGHT

Much of the consolidation among providers is driven by a desire to eliminate excess capacity, to "rightsize" the U.S. hospital industry relative to the number and types of patients requiring inpatient treatment every year. This consolidation of capacity is occurring only now—more than a decade and a half after it first emerged as a major problem—because of the fundamental fixes occurring to the health care system in the 1990s. Prior to the initiation of this fix, with the health care system plagued by the dysfunctional economics described earlier, overcapacity was simply absorbed by the system, through a misallocation and overutilization of resources, and through price inflation. Among the many paradoxes of the health care industry, none has been more perplexing than the one affecting the law of inpatient supply and demand. Under the faulty market economics of health care, the greater the supply of hospital beds, the higher the total costs. This inversion is based on the perverse collective clinical behavior in a health care market known as "Roemer's Law," which states that hospital beds will be used as long as they are available.

Without rational marketplace checks on demand (i.e., the price-discriminating behavior embodied in both managed care and consumerism), the availability of supply dictates demand. This problem applies not only to hospital beds, but to the presence of high technology, larger concentrations of specialists, and other big-dollar resources. It also gives rise to what many refer to as the "medical arms race" within local health care markets across the country. One hospital purchases an MRI; as a competitive response, so do all the other hospitals of its size in the market; suddenly there is a concerted effort across the market to cover the enormous fixed costs of all the machines by using them. Without marketplace checks, hospital competition serves only to make the situation worse; more supply induces still more demand. As Nguyen and Derrick note in *Integrated Health Care Delivery*, "increased hospital competition [in traditional fee-for-service markets] is associated with higher costs, lower occupancy rates, reduced efficiency, and more service offerings."[47]

The problem of hospital overcapacity was created by the government, borne of its attempt in the 1940s to alleviate an acute shortage of hospital beds with federal medicine—a shortsighted cure that created a chronic disorder far more destructive than the one it was meant to correct. In response to the perception that the United States had too *few* hospitals, the government bankrolled the Hill-Burton program in 1947, meant as a temporary boost to sagging capacity in selected areas of the country. Like most things involving government money, what was supposed to be extraordinary became expected; the medicine designed to relieve spotty symptoms became an addictive drug to empire-building state health officials and hospital administrators. The law aimed to set a "ceiling" on hospitals beds per 1,000 people at 4.5, which was higher than most states at the time; this ceiling eventually came to serve as the standard.[48]

Excessive expansion of hospital capacity development under the Hill-Burton program persisted until it was finally supplanted by an even greater aggravation to the problem: the introduction of Medicare in the mid-1960s. To win the support of the hospital lobby, part of reimbursement under the federal Medicare program included capital reimbursement for new hospital construction. This involved millions of dollars in new government spending on inpatient construction, and distorted what would almost certainly have been the marketplace's preference for the development of lower cost, outpatient capacity.[49] While government subsidies are typically at the root of any industry's overcapacity and resource misallocation—ranging from agricultural price supports, to antiquated mining rights laws, to defense contracting—health care seems particularly prone to detrimental government market meddling. The end result of decades of Hill-Burton—and faulty Medicare reimbursement schemes, which persist to this day—is a nation of 5,000 hospitals, half of which sit idle, subsidized by the artificially high prices charged for the patients in the other half.[50]

One of the most deliberate goals and immediate benefits of provider consolidation is the trimming of this excess capacity from individual markets. Doing so lowers the aggregate fixed costs associated with total provider capacity in a market and, most importantly, reduces the unnecessary admissions and lengthier stays that excess capacity generates under fee-for-service reimbursement. As pointed out earlier, Roemer's law holds that the law of supply and demand in health care is antithetical to classic economic analysis: more supply creates more demand and prices thus do not fall to find a new equilibrium point or drive excess capacity out of the market. If this is true, so too must be its inverse. A concerted effort to reduce supply by consolidators—a *de facto* collusion of sorts—will actually *lower* aggregate costs for an entire market. Such efforts of course do not occur out of the desire of hospital administrators to shrink their own turf; they occur because of marketplace pressures that administrators feel from consolidating payers.

This consolidation is a long overdue corrective to Roemer's law, a corrective that has generally been administered for the past decade through blunt and reluctant pricing concessions by hospitals and ever more intrusive forms of utilization management by payers. Responding to this first-ever concerted buying pressure in the history of their institutions, providers have been forced to consolidate, if only to preclude a continuing downward spiral in prices that would ultimately prove self-immolating, i.e., where marginal revenue dips below marginal cost. Such pricing wars are characteristic of all firms with high fixed costs and excess capacity; the cyclical pricing wars of the airline industry are a textbook case. Hospitals are little different, as it is turning out.

Through consolidation, providers are finally forced to coordinate assets, rather than simply deploy them with little regard for market need. This is something that regulators attempted to do for decades through "certificate of need" programs. But typical of a government program, "getting the C-O-N" from a state for more beds, an expanded cardiac cath lab, or a new MRI rapidly devolved into a rote exercise for hospitals: spin the numbers, churn the paperwork, and lobby the right bureaucrats; hardly the discipline of a market. Consolidation is forcing providers—market by market—to make hard choices about which beds to keep open, which cardiac cath lab to expand, and which MRI to continue operating.

Thus, in one short decade, the provider system is attempting to fix a problem that has been over a century in the making. "That there were too many small hospitals in America was a complaint already being heard soon after 1900," writes Paul Starr in *The Social Transformation of American Medicine*, "and it became a steady part of criticism of the hospital system."[51] It took almost a hundred years for the market to grow sick enough with the symptoms of overcapacity to address the underlying disorder. In this regard, the closure of nearly 10 percent of all U.S. hospitals in the past decade may merely prove to be a preview of coming attractions in the next.

OF ALLIANCES HOLY, UNHOLY, AND PURELY SECULAR

One of the more interesting aspects of consolidation is how readily it has brought together institutions whose cultural origins had previously kept them fully segregated. Like funeral homes and bowling leagues, U.S. hospitals have been "self-ghettoized" by religious affiliation or, in the absence of any religious affiliation (other than fealty to the almighty dollar), their tax status. As Starr notes, "cultural heterogeneity has been one of the chief factors inhibiting consolidation of hospitals in a state-run system. Ethnic and religious groups have wanted to protect their own separate interests."[52] This factor is not unique to the U.S. system. Medical sociologist and historian William Glaser notes that around the world, "the greater the number of religions in a society, the more diffused the ownership and management of hospitals and the smaller their average size."[53]

As the most heterogeneous of the world's major nations, the United States simply suffers from the worst diffusion and complexity of hospital ownership and management. This historic truism about our cultural diversity does much to explain the U.S. health care system's enormous fragmentation in comparison to the rest of the world. In this sense, the consolidation of the provider community, with little regard for religious or other affiliation, is a long overdue correction to an accident of our social history.

This correction is occurring, seemingly overnight, as a direct consequence of the rapid consolidation of payers *and* the rapid consolidation of hospitals into national systems. Markets with a dozen stand-alone hospitals in 1990 are currently dividing up into two to four "networks" or "health systems." Each is constructed from a variety of legal bricks and mortar, ranging from outright asset mergers to joint operating corporations to purely contractual alliances. Markets vary considerably from region to region, depending on history and regulatory factors, but if a typical market can be described, it would consist of the following:

- one or two for-profit hospitals, one or both of which is usually owned by a national chain;
- one or two not-for-profit hospitals owned or operated by a national religious system like Daughters of Charity or Sisters of Mercy;
- a hybrid for-profit/not-for-profit system of midsized community hospitals, often with a minor teaching hospital at its helm; or
- a not-for-profit system of community hospitals with a major academic medical center (AMC) at its helm (or, in the case of Boston and New York, two AMCs at its helm).

Again, there are endless variations from market to market, and no two markets look exactly alike. The one commonality is how thoroughly they have broken with the past. Numerous consolidations cross traditional barriers, resulting in a hospital with the unlikely name of "Barnes Jewish Christian" (St. Louis); the existence of what, a few short years ago, would have been an oxymoron: a for-profit teaching hospital (New Orleans, Wichita, Chicago); and the unholiest of alliances, two for-profit hospitals mixed in with five Catholic hospitals (the central valley of California).

Such consolidations have been driven by the market panic created by the national systems—both for-profit and not-for-profit—which seek to create critical mass within a local market while bringing to bear the cost advantages of membership in a national organization. The chains have the capital, focus, management discipline, and merger and acquisition (M&A) apparatus in place to purchase, manage, rationalize, and aggressively market a bloc of hospital capacity in a given market. Thus, in each market the chains have what Porter calls the "first-mover advantage," and all others are forced to scramble to catch up. As Porter argues, specifically as it pertains to hospital administration, "a first mover can lock in later sales if switching costs are present. In hospital management contracts, the pioneer that signed up hospitals first gained a significant edge in contract renewals because of the substantial costs to the hospital of changing management firms. Switching would result in disruption caused by a new administrator, a new computer system, and other changes."[54]

Such incumbency can be particularly important in health care, given the simultaneously high levels of uncertainty, risk, and dollars at stake in a rapidly transforming market. The first mover often wins if only because—in a marketplace where the old rules not only do not apply but actually mislead—the only teachers are the most recent experience and the data closest to real-time. A lack of both in the first round of innovation (e.g., the introduction of risk-assumption via full provider capitation to a market) locks out the hesitant competitor long after the initial hesitation is regretted. The first to innovate (e.g., the first to offer full capitation) may often hold a lead position long after all others have matched its innovation strategically. This is fully consistent with a key Porter dictum: "Pioneering may lead to a variety of potential first-mover advantages in cost or differentiation that remain after its technological lead is gone."[55]

THE QUESTIONABLE ECONOMICS OF PURE CONSOLIDATION

There is a rub to consolidation, especially of the national variety practiced by the big systems. Classic management theory, plus key research on newly consolidated hospital markets, both indicate that economies of scale associated with horizontal integration are *eventually* offset by diseconomies of size.[56] Aggregate hospital data indicate that the industry has yet to reach this point: they show that for system-affiliated hospitals, administrative expenses as a percentage of total operating expenses have been falling continuously, from 35.7 percent in 1991, to 33.9 percent in 1995.[57]

Specific examples of this trend are embodied in the experiences of the bigger systems: for-profit Tenet slashed corporate overhead in half as a percentage of revenues after it combined the hospitals of National Medical Enterprises and AMI;[58] not-for-profit consolidator Sutter Health System cut 25 percent of total overhead costs as a percentage of total expenses after merging with California Health System.[59] Given the continued fragmentation of the U.S. hospital industry, the data on the economics of consolidation clearly indicate the existence of an optimization point at which the economies and diseconomies of consolidation balance out.

While this point has not been reached by the industry as a whole, it clearly exists at the level of the individual corporation. In stark contrast to Tenet's experience, pure horizontal consolidations into national companies are rife with downside risk in terms of financial, management, and marketplace performance. Numerous health care companies, including the first generation of for-profit hospital chains, a number of physician practice management (PPM) companies, a major home health provider, and several others have stumbled badly, all after growing to a certain size that could not be easily managed centrally. In every case, the consolidator had failed to focus on matching local capacities to local market needs, instead using a one-size-fits-all strategy that inevitably does not work across heterogeneous markets.

After rolling up a number of troubled regional home health care providers into Coram Healthcare, James Sweeney, the original architect of the home health care concept, watched Coram suffer under mounting losses, management struggles, and $450 million in debt, one short year after its creation.[60] As in almost any industry, massive consolidation of far-flung enterprises are extremely difficult to manage from headquarters, a lesson lost on Coram. Any cost synergies in this type of consolidation can easily be offset by managerial inefficiencies, slowness to adapt to local market conditions, and the inability to seize idiosyncratic market opportunities.

Precisely the same dynamic has unfolded in the physician practice management community. Coastal Healthcare Corporation, also the pioneering firm in its industry, ran into trouble trying to control several thousand physicians scattered across dozens of markets. Once the darling of Wall Street, by mid-1996 the historically profitable PPM company was consistently losing money in all of its businesses, with a market capitalization down to $150 million from a peak of $900 million a few years prior.[61] Coastal simply proved too large an enterprise, was involved in too many varied markets, and faced the special challenge of trying to "herd cats." According to a report in the *Wall Street Journal*, "some doctors took [Coastal's founder and CEO] at his word that they would run the show, and they balked if they didn't like an order from headquarters. More important was the problem of market leverage."[62] Because a critical mass of physicians in a market still does not link those physicians to the rest of the system, any PPM is still subject to a buyer's power if that buyer has the same or more critical mass—which MCOs do. Again, according to the *Wall Street Journal*, "it was becoming increasingly apparent that the power Dr. Scott believed groups of doctors would wield was no match for HMOs' growing strength…HMOs locked up huge numbers of patients, deploying them—and the revenue they brought—to doctors of their choice."[63]

This disconnection of one vertical segment of the health care system from the rest—regardless of how fully consolidated it is horizontally—may well prove to be a doomed strategy over the long haul. Nonetheless, dozens of well-capitalized hospital systems, home health providers, nursing home chains, and PPMs continue to barrel down this road. The missteps of Coastal, Coram, and the others are important strategic lessons for these companies.

Alongside these strategic failures, there have been occasional outbreaks of panic that the economics of pure consolidation will ultimately prove more fantasy than reality. One such panic arose in the wake of a landmark study by the Healthcare Advisory Board in 1995 arguing that "unexpectedly, horizontal integration in the long run will probably not produce the desired cost savings nor strategic advantage."[64] These findings are frequently borne out by recent experience, the most extreme versions of which make for good contrarian copy in trade journals, including the following from a 1996 edition of *Health Care Strategic Management:* "While everybody talks about reducing their costs, the reality is that the average hospital in a multi-hospital system actually costs more to operate than stand-alone hospitals. On a case mix–adjusted basis, the average cost per discharge in a multihospital system is 15 percent higher than the average cost for the same case in a stand-alone hospital."[65] Typical of the mixed messages signaling across the health care system, however, the very same journal publishes just as much evidence to the contrary. Three months later, according to *Health Care Strategic Management,* "hospitals pursuing affiliations rather than mergers or acquisitions are opting for a low risk/low reward collaborative system…the most successful collaborative strategy is merger and acquisition…'You're pursuing penny savings of the affiliation side, whereas you're getting dollar savings on the mergers and acquisitions side.'"[66]

The persistently mixed news regarding the economics of consolidation is attributable to both the newness and unpleasantness of the
phenomenon. Many merged or allied hospitals have yet to face the
difficult cost cutting that true consolidation entails. In many cases,
merged or allied hospitals result in *more* bureaucracy, i.e., more administrators per bed, not fewer. Such are the struggles of melding the
entrenched managements of multiple hospitals. It took decades to
overbuild and overbureaucratize the hospital community. Though
the market *seems* to be moving overnight, it cannot clean up the entire mess in the same time frame.

CONSOLIDATION AS A STEPPING-STONE

The biggest danger of negative studies and journal commentary
on consolidation's economics, regardless of their relevance while
the system is in transition, is their potential to create a backlash to
the historic correction of overcapacity the system desperately needs.
Consolidation is a necessity for the long-term macroeconomic
soundness of the U.S. health care system; it is also a short-term strategic necessity for a system of local hospitals. The buying power of
consolidating payers and self-insured employers will not go away.
The revolution has begun. Consolidation is a painful, requisite first
step to surviving that revolution. As Lutz and Gee put it, "the stand-
alone hospital will not stand alone long. It will either choose to affili-
ate or (eventually) to disintegrate."[67] Why? Because risk-assumption
requires mass, and consolidation is the only way to build and sustain
such mass.

A fascinating study into this issue involved multispecialty group
practices. The study, published in 1996 in the *Journal of Ambulatory
Care Management*, found no economies in the consolidation of
multispecialty practices, either of scale or scope.[68] Any reductions in
per unit cost due to shared infrastructure proved to be offset by the
added costs associated with managing far-flung physicians. The
economic advantages the study *did* find constitute critical strategic

opportunities for consolidating group practices: *the studied groups were better able to enter at-risk contracts, integrate the delivery of at-risk care, and generally share risk with payers.* Typical of advanced forms of physician reimbursement, the merged practices had lower total costs—due to lower utilization of inpatient services. This occurred not for medical reasons but because lower inpatient utilization *always* occurs under full risk-assumption, and larger multispecialty groups are more able and thus more likely to assume medical risk.

Risk-assumption also requires vertical integration. This helps explain why the Advisory Board study, which found no economies in consolidation, recommended it nonetheless, specifically because it provides a stepping-stone to integration. It also explains why, beyond the hospital community, the best managed provider firms among the national horizontal consolidators are finding vertical integration a necessary next step. After the economies of provider consolidation are worked through the system, the buying power of consolidating payers will exert pressure on profitability elsewhere in the treatment continuum. Why else would Integrated Health Services, the largest and most successful subacute care company in the industry, move so quickly through acquisition to add vertical layers of services, including home health, rehab care, and assisted living care? It did so for the express purpose of building a continuum of care to be operated and marketed in conjunction with its subacute facilities.[69]

These moves are all smart business. They recognize that to cure the underlying ills of the nation's health care system, consolidation will prove to be only one therapy in a cure that requires several, all administered together.

REFERENCES

1. M. Flitter, *Judith's Pavilion: The Haunting Memories of a Neurosurgeon* (South Royalton, VT: Steerforth Press, 1997), 40.

2. Calculations developed later in this chapter, based on industry trade reports of HMO and insurance mergers and acquisitions.

3. Calculations developed later in this chapter, based on industry trade reports of hospital mergers, acquisitions, and equity conversions.

4. Based on revenue figures included in the annual reports for the five largest drug companies in 1997 and the 25 largest drug companies in 1987.

5. Compiled from reports of each transaction in the *Wall Street Journal* and *Modern Healthcare*.

6. L. Kertesz, "This Is Not Your Father's Blues Plan," *Modern Healthcare*, 14 October, 1996, 64.

7. K. Pallarito, "Anthem Sings Blues," *Modern Healthcare*, 30 June, 1997, 44.

8. Kertesz, *Modern Healthcare*, 66.

9. G. Anders, *Health against Wealth* (New York: Houghton Mifflin, 1996): throughout.

10. Adapted and reprinted with the permission of The Free Press, a Division of Simon & Schuster from *COMPETITIVE STRATEGY: Techniques for Analyzing Industries and Competitors* by Michael E. Porter. Copyright © 1980 by The Free Press, p. 24–26.

11. U. Reinhardt, "Columbia/HCA: Villain or Victim?" *Health Affairs* 17, no. 1 (1998): 32.

12. B. Japsen, "Another Record Year for Dealmaking," *Modern Healthcare*, 23–30 December 1996, 37.

13. Japsen, *Modern Healthcare*, 37.

14. American Hospital Association statistics, as reported in "The State of Hospitals," *Modern Healthcare*, 17 February, 1997, 56.

15. R. Tomsho, "Columbia/HCA Agrees To Acquire Value Health Inc.," *Wall Street Journal*, 16 January, 1997.

16. 1996 revenues $19.9 billion, as reported in Letter to Shareholders, Richard L. Scott, President and CEO, Columbia/HCA Healthcare Corporation.

17. J. Greene, "Does Integration Really Cut Costs?" *Modern Healthcare*, 10 February, 1997, 40.

18. B. Japsen, "System's Buyer Thinking Big," *Modern Healthcare*, 17 February, 1997, 146.

19. S. Lutz and E.P. Gee, *The For-Profit Healthcare Revolution* (Chicago: Irwin Professional Publishing, 1995), 3.

20. Lutz and Gee, *The For-Profit Healthcare Revolution*, 2.

21. Lutz and Gee, *The For-Profit Healthcare Revolution*, 50.

22. R. Rundle, "Catholic Hospitals, in Big Merger Drive, Battle Industry Giants," *Wall Street Journal*, 12 March, 1997.

23. Greene, *Modern Healthcare*, 34.

24. L. Scott, "Catholic Health Initiatives Plans to Add Kentucky System," *Modern Healthcare*, 19 May, 1997, 5.

25. L. Scott, "Catholics Form East Coast Powerhouse," *Modern Healthcare*, 2 June, 1997, 8.

26. R. Rundle, "Catholic Hospitals, in Big Merger Drive, Battle Industry Giants," *Wall Street Journal,* 12 March, 1997.

27. C. Snow, "HealthSouth's New Horizons," *Modern Healthcare*, 24 February, 1997, 20.

28. A. Sharpe, "Integrated Health To Pay 1.15 Billion for Package of HealthSouth Businesses," *Wall Street Journal,* 4 November, 1997.

29. A. Sharpe, "Medical Entrepreneur Aims To Turn Clinics into National Brand," *Wall Street Journal*, 14 December, 1996.

30. The $4.3 billion in revenues for HealthSouth is based on $2.5 billion in revenue, pre-Horizon/CMS, plus 1996 revenues for Horizon of $1.8 billion, as reported by C. Snow in "HealthSouth's New Horizons," *Modern Healthcare,* 24 February, 1997, 20.

31. C. Snow, "One-Stop Shopping," *Modern Healthcare*, 25 November, 1996.

32. American Medical Association survey data, as reported by M. Jaklevic in "Outgunned," *Modern Healthcare*, 17 November, 1997, 38.

33. Jaklevic, *Modern Healthcare*, 38.

34. A. Bianco, "Doctors Inc.," *Business Week*, 24 March, 1997, 204.

35. C. Simon and D. Emmons, "Physician Earnings at Risk: An Examination of Capitated Contracts," *Health Affairs* 16, no. 3 (1997): 124.

36. M. Jaklevic, "Doc-Owned Health Plans Struggle To Go It Alone," *Modern Healthcare*, 12 May, 1997, 3.

37. Lutz and Gee, *The For-Profit Healthcare Revolution*, 130.

38. Data included in a research report on the acute care hospital industry by Alex. Brown & Sons, 1 August, 1995, 34.

39. L. Scott, "Purchasing Groups Add to Their Bulk," *Modern Healthcare*, 23 September, 1996, 54.

40. Adapted and reprinted with the permission of The Free Press, a Division of Simon & Schuster from *COMPETITIVE STRATEGY: Techniques for Analyzing Industries and Competitors* by Michael E. Porter. Copyright © 1980 by The Free Press. p. 27–28.

41. New drug development cost, in 1990 dollars, from "The Contribution of Pharmaceutical Companies," The Boston Consulting Group, September, 1993, 93.

42. S. Moore, "Novartis Jumps Last Regulatory Hurdle To Create Global Drug-Industry Giant," *Wall Street Journal*, 18 December, 1996.

43. S. Moore, "Success of Ciba-Sandoz Merger Will Be Tested in the Lab," *Wall Street Journal*, 30 July, 1996.

44. R. King, untitled article on Genentech in the *Wall Street Journal*, 12 March, 1998, Interactive edition.

45. M. Schrage, "Drugmakers Need To Find New Ways To Make Their Voyages of Discovery," *Washington Post*. 3 February, 1995.

46. D. Morrow, "New Ranking on Drug Sales," *New York Times*, 27 February, 1998, Interactive edition.

47. N. Nguyen and F. Derrick, "Hospital Markets and Competition: Implications for Antitrust Policy," in *Integrated Health Care Delivery: Theory, Practice, Evaluation, and Prognosis,* ed. M. Brown (Gaithersburg, MD: Aspen Publishers, 1996), 219.

48. P. Starr, *The Social Transformation of American Medicine* (New York: Basic Books/HarperCollins, 1982), 349.

49. Starr, *The Social Transformation of American Medicine*, 376.

50. Based on 49 percent occupancy rate for the median, acute care, nonfederal U.S. hospital, as detailed in *The Comparative Performance of U.S. Hospitals: The Sourcebook 1996*, an annual study published by HCIA Inc., Baltimore.

51. Starr, *The Social Transformation of American Medicine*, 176.

52. Starr, *The Social Transformation of American Medicine*, 176.

53. Starr, *The Social Transformation of American Medicine*, 176, citing Glaser, *Social Settings and Medical Organization* (New York: Atherton, 1970).

54. Adapted and reprinted with the permission of The Free Press, a Division of Simon & Schuster from *COMPETITIVE ADVANTAGE: Creating and Sustaining Superior Performance* by Michael E. Porter. Copyright © 1985 by Michael E. Porter. p. 187.

55. Adapted and reprinted with the permission of The Free Press, a Division of Simon & Schuster from *COMPETITIVE ADVANTAGE: Creating and Sustaining Superior Performance* by Michael E. Porter. Copyright © 1985 by Michael E. Porter. p. 172.

56. This is a central theme of A. Chandler, *Visible Hand: The Managerial Revolution in American Business* (Cambridge: Harvard University Press, 1977).

57. *The Comparative Performance of U.S. Hospitals: The Sourcebook 1996*, an annual study published by HCIA Inc., Baltimore.

58. J. Greene, "Does Integration Really Cut Costs?" *Modern Healthcare*, 10 February, 1997, 35.

59. Greene, *Modern Healthcare*, 35.

60. R. Tomsho, "Fledgling Healthcare Provider Now Battling for Its Life," *Wall Street Journal*, 18 October, 1995.

61. N. Deogun, "Network of Doctors Touted as Panacea, Develops Big Problem," *Wall Street Journal*, 26 September, 1996.

62. Deogun, *Wall Street Journal*.

63. Deogun, *Wall Street Journal*.

64. Discussion of "Hospital Networking: Merger Acquisitions and Affiliations," published by the Advisory Board Company in 1995, included in Lutz and Gee, *The For-Profit Healthcare Revolution, 68.*

65. "Consultant's Corner," *Health Care Strategic Management,* March, 1996, 9.

66. S. Campbell, "Collaborative Strategies," *Health Care Strategic Management,* June 1996, 14.

67. Lutz and Gee, *The For-Profit Healthcare Revolution*, 50.

68. "Economics of Multispecialty Group Practice," *The Journal of Ambulatory Care Management*, July 1996.

69. C. Snow, "One-Stop Shopping," *Modern Healthcare*, 25 November, 1996.

4

INTEGRATION

Patients reporting problems with "continuity and transition"—28.7 percent

Highest response rate to survey of hospital patient problems, conducted by the American Hospital Association in 1996[1]

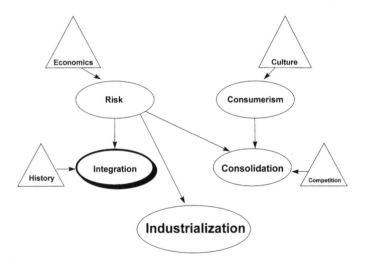

The one aspect of American medicine more literally incredible than the genius behind its mind-bending technologies is the stupidity of how those technologies are deployed for the average patient. For all our advances in medical science and practice, our providers' abilities to manage the delivery of care over time and geographic space are crude at best, nonexistent in the norm, and borderline negligent at their worst.

This disaster of inefficiency is a legacy of the history of American medicine, based on a simple but, until only recently, wholly unalterable clinical apartheid: physicians practice autonomously from facilities. This arrangement makes running a hospital extremely complex: those decisions with the greatest impact on the institution's costs and profits—and its quality and reputation—are made by a class of people usually not employed by that institution.

This clinical apartheid arose, strangely enough, because of the imbalance of power between physicians and hospitals at the turn of the century, and the fact that hospitals have almost always been at the mercy of doctors for referrals and thus their entire revenue base.[2] Physicians galvanized this power through hedging, exploiting of their prerogative to refer patients to more than one hospital in a community. Around this anachronistic arrangement, the entire system evolved; the separation of doctor and facility persisted as new care sites were introduced, including most types of outpatient clinics. The situation has been complicated further by federal "anti–self-referral" laws. These rules, which forbid physicians from referring patients to facilities in which they have a financial interest, are designed to protect Medicare and Medicaid patients from induced or excessive service; they are a legacy of the fee-for-service world and stand as a significant impediment to correcting a historic structural flaw in the U.S. health care system.

The disconnection between physician and facility has spawned a number of distorted features that have foiled efforts at integrating patient care. Methods for reimbursing physicians and facilities have developed along separate tracks, served by different coding systems for classifying patient diagnoses and treatments. Because the primary purpose of health care information systems has always been to manage reimbursement, these systems merely absorbed and perpetuated this problem, creating an information management nightmare, a Tower of Babel that makes the analysis of treatment or outcomes for a single hospital patient nearly impossible without major manual effort. This explains why one hospitalization typically generates a seemingly endless torrent of billing documents.

Provider information systems and their resident databases—which should serve as the nervous system of an integrated system of medical care—are thus woefully inadequate. As a symptom of this problem, to date there exists no commonly accepted classification system for grouping a patient's disease or injury-related records over time into a clinically coherent diagnostic group, despite multiple generations of systems for describing surgeries, grouping inpatients, classifying outpatient procedures, and recording physician visits and other ambulatory services. This underscores a central defect of the U.S. health care system: it did not evolve to treat people; rather, it evolved to deliver line-item, billable medical services to patients. Such a system cannot possibly be efficient. It relies too heavily on manual effort and human memory to avoid daily catastrophe, giving short shrift to the clinical miracles the system works daily. The economics of such a system are a disaster in slow motion.

While there is a legitimate debate in most industries about the benefits of true vertical integration, in medicine it should be a foregone conclusion. In fact, it is only because of an accident of history that we are forced even to wonder: Should doctors and hospitals be part of the same economic and operating entity? Would anyone ask that about Microsoft and its product managers? GM and its engineers? The *New York Times* and its editors? If decision making by one class of professionals controls up to 90 percent of a business' operating costs, it stands to reason that they ought to be captive to that business, accountable to it, and see their fortunes rise and fall with it. Yet, in health care, it is still up for debate: *to integrate or not?*

Common sense would dictate that as the maintenance of health, resolution of illness, and management of disease ought to be, from a clinical perspective, a highly interrelated, seamless process, so too should be the assemblage of care delivery resources. While the question brewing at industry conferences so often is "should we vertically integrate care?" it ought to be "why have we tolerated *dis*-integrated care for so long? How can it be that more than *one-fourth* of nearly 33 million annual customers report problems with 'continuity and transition?' Would this be tolerated from the aftermarket service of a car dealer, real estate agent, or computer store?"

The long overdue integration of medical delivery, introduced by the original MCO model and pursued in variously modified forms by the most progressive MCOs and provider networks, is central to the transformation of the U.S. health care system. It is a belated corrective to the artificial, wasteful, and dangerous fragmentation of care delivery that has presided over the U.S. system for the past century. The issues attendant to the nature, extent, and business structuring of this corrective is the subject of this chapter.

INTEGRATION'S "VALUE-ADDS"

Regardless of the legal form that vertical integration ultimately should take, it is an indisputable fact that a baseline level of integration is critical to fixing much of the inefficiency of the U.S. health care system. This notion acknowledges something so obvious to the casual observer that it seems rarely to occur to those people immersed in health care itself: the real product of health care is *not* the aggregation of doctor visits, hospitalizations, prescriptions, etc.; it is the management of health risks, disease, and injury in the most clinically and financially optimal way possible. Such optimization requires the coordination and measurement of all possible treatment alternatives across all possible care options, settings, and pathways. The more enlightened MCOs like Kaiser and provider networks like the Henry Ford Health System in Detroit recognize and exploit this fact: there is a competitive advantage embodied simply in the integration of care sites. As Michael Porter points out in *Competitive Advantage*, such an advantage "frequently derives from linkages among activities just as it does from the individual activities themselves."[3]

There is an element of natural industrial evolution embedded in the idea that the health care system's greatest gains can be won from seeking to improve the fluidity and functioning of the delivery system's whole, rather than from a fine-tuning of its individual parts.

Moving into the new century, the most important "breakthroughs" in medicine may well come in the form of clinical process improvement, rather than clinical product improvement, from coordinating the best of today's medical technologies rather than pushing the curve on new, isolated technologies. Indeed, as health care's technology curves flatten—due as much to diminishing technical returns for treating many disorders like heart disease and cancer as to increasing economic pressures—the development of protocols for delivering and tracking patient care across health care settings and over time may constitute the next big generation of health care innovations.

Figure II–3 illustrates the continuum of medical care that such innovations will by necessity span. They will add value not by changing *how* care is delivered within each site, but by optimizing how that care is timed, sequenced, and responded to by patients across all sites. The concepts and individual components of this continuum represent the full array of medical resources subject to our discussion of vertical integration; they will also be referenced for the remainder of this book.

For the integration and subsequent optimization to work, two things need to happen. First, reimbursement must change. Global

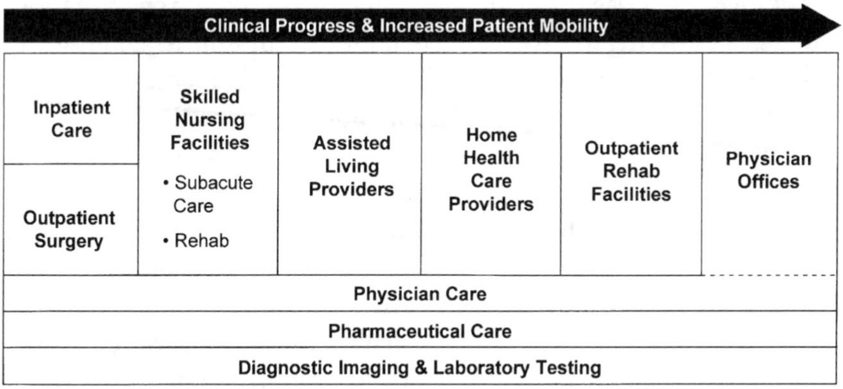

Clinical Progress & Increased Patient Mobility					
Inpatient Care	Skilled Nursing Facilities	Assisted Living Providers	Home Health Care Providers	Outpatient Rehab Facilities	Physician Offices
Outpatient Surgery	• Subacute Care • Rehab				
Physician Care					
Pharmaceutical Care					
Diagnostic Imaging & Laboratory Testing					

Figure II–3 The Continuum of Medical Care.

capitation needs to gain critical mass in a market to reverse the fee-for-service incentives for the operators of each type of care site to shift from maximization of patient traffic at that site to optimization across all sites. While numerous companies like HealthSouth and Integrated Health Services are rapidly assembling the continuum, they are still running them as distinct businesses, with separate accounting and separate accountability. One of the many reasons Columbia/HCA got into trouble with the federal government was its haste to build the continuum, and integrate its cost accounting and financial accountability—years ahead of the government's ability to contract directly with private provider networks on a capitated basis. It was inevitable that the company would run afoul of the government's rules about self-referrals and cost reimbursement from site to site.

Other companies have proven more prudent in assembling the continuum and running its components inside the Chinese boxes that fee-for-service reimbursement not only demands, but perversely rewards. At the same time, these companies are already functioning within—and thus bolstering their positioning for—the emerging world of global capitation. The innovations that can arise from the assembly and management of the entire continuum of care are a key driver of a major strategy shift by Integrated Health Services, the industry's largest provider of subacute services in 1996. That year, IHS moved aggressively into the home health care, rehabilitation, and assisted-living businesses, spending $1 billion to acquire the dominant players in each care niche. Overnight, IHS emerged as one of the country's largest providers of home care, offering services through more than 1,000 sites in 47 states.[4] In the process, the company assembled under one corporate roof every major type of care "downstream" from the hospital, transforming itself from the most aggressive consolidator of subacute care facilities into the most aggressive consolidator of the entire postdischarge continuum of care.

IHS's move was paralleled by HealthSouth's acquisition of the outpatient surgical chain, Surgical Care Affiliates, for $1.1 billion,[5] and the nursing home chain, Horizon/CMS, for $1.6 billion.[6] The deals combined to create the nation's largest provider of outpatient surgery and rehabilitation services. The theory behind them? HealthSouth is now uniquely able to provide seamless patient movement from the surgical suite to the rehab facility, under one roof and ultimately one contract, across much of the United States. While this strategy positions the company well for contracting with MCOs and other third-party payers, it also allows the company to cultivate the consumer market. By early 1998, HealthSouth was announcing its development of "plazas" that combine all of the company's services into one geographical location: surgery, rehab, and diagnostic imaging. It is to consumer medical purchasing what the mall is to retail shopping.

As a report on IHS's integration strategy in *Modern Healthcare* points out, "the more services an entity controls, the greater potential it has to save money by eliminating duplication and feeding its own services with referrals."[7] This is consistent with conclusions in the previous chapter, which argued that the surest economic gains flow not from horizontal consolidation, but from linking together those horizontal layers of care. Such conclusions are shared by Scott MacStravic in *Health Care Strategic Management*: "cost reductions may well be achieved through system improvements across the continuum of care, rather than within individual hospitals or physician practices...Through owning or otherwise managing other parts of the continuum of care, cost savings may be achievable to make up for price reductions."[8] In this sense, integration is viewed as a defensive strategy against profit erosion in a provider's core business, due to pricing pressure from consolidating payers.

This is borne out by numerous empirical analyses of the economics of integration. Typical among them is a report in *Health Care Strategic Management* that found for hospitals in integrated systems:

- higher occupancy rates averaging 52.1 percent versus 49.4 percent for non-system hospitals (a better match between hospital capacity and the population's needs);

- average lengths of stay of 5.5 days, 9.8 percent lower than nonsystem hospitals (longer stays indicate sicker patients and thus a more reactive and less focused use of the hospitals); and
- 190 hospital days per 1,000 MCO members in the system, versus 279 for MCOs not in the system (lower overall hospitalization for the population means lower total costs).[9]

Dean Coddington and his colleagues, in their study of various integrated systems, *Making Integrated Health Care Work,* draw the same conclusion: "Left to set their own course, integrated systems have not lowered their *unit* costs. None of the case study organizations are providing care of significantly lower unit cost than their competitors. However, integrated systems are finding numerous ways to cut *total* costs, primarily through lower utilization and other operating efficiencies. When both unit costs and utilization are considered, integrated health care has the potential to lower overall health care costs."[10]

Armed with this aggregate economic advantage, integration strategies can be used on the offensive. By controlling the entire continuum of care—meaning controlling where and how patients move within it—an integrated organization can better predict and control total costs and thus bid more aggressively on at-risk contracts. This approach provides the integrated health care organization with clear structural and competitive advantages against the traditional "disintegrated" approach, whereby the payer contracts with independent providers, adds up the costs associated with line-item services, and hopes for the best.

Finally, and if for no other reason, integration always wins because of reduced paperwork.

FIRST STEPS TOWARD INTEGRATION: GLOBAL PACKAGE PRICING

Many of the ideas in this book are driven by an underlying theory of economic determinism. One of its central themes argues that meaningful market-based reform of the health care system flows from reform in the system's methods of reimbursing providers. Indeed, as the archipelago of care settings was created by isolated reimbursement systems tied to different care settings, so too do sufficient changes in reimbursement have the ability to drive the system back together into a coherent, integrated whole.

The first step in this process is "package" or "global" pricing. Such a payment scheme bundles what it should cost to deliver *all* the care associated with a coherent medical or surgical episode, and pays this lump sum to a combined group of physicians and facilities. Such reimbursement represents an enormous improvement, if only because of its inherent simplification. Under the traditional system, a coronary bypass surgery generates separate fee-for-service reimbursements for

1. all the preadmission tests
2. all the preadmission and postdischarge visits to the cardiologist
3. the admitting physician
4. the cardiac surgeon, anesthesiologist, and perfusionists
5. the hospital to cover the costs of the surgery suite, supplies, staff, and stay
6. the cardiac rehab center for restoring the patient to health

Under global package pricing, there is one reimbursement for coronary bypass surgery.

Global pricing was introduced in the most advanced managed care markets on the West Coast in the late 1980s. Typical of historic reimbursement dynamics, what has proven viable in the market has been adopted by the federal government in its attempts to cope with ever-escalating Medicare costs. In a demonstration project initiated in 1996, the Health Care Financing Administration (HCFA) introduced global pricing to its "Centers of Excellence" or elite teaching hospitals, paying one prenegotiated price to each of seven participating hospitals for all aspects of open-heart surgery. The price covered all services rendered by the hospital, its anesthesiologists, the admitting cardiologist and treating cardiac surgeons, and all other consulting physicians.[11] HCFA is currently expanding the program nationwide, for open-heart surgery and for numerous other high-dollar, high-volume procedures.

According to a report in *Health Care Strategic Management,* "if all hospitals in the United States were eligible to participate in these new demonstration programs, one in every 13 Medicare hospitalizations would be affected. More than 900,000 Medicare beneficiaries are discharged from hospitals annually for these conditions, including nearly 600,000 annually for the selected cardiovascular conditions and more than 300,000 annually for the selected orthopedic conditions."[12] The many benefits associated with the global pricing project cited in the report include "increased coordination of care" as "providers utilize technology and personnel more efficiently…improved communications and collaboration among staff, thus allowing hospitals to channel resources more efficiently…and increased patient satisfaction. Surveys show that patients are clearly more satisfied with simplified billing because of less paperwork and fewer claim settlement problems."[13] Health care organizations that have successfully introduced global package pricing for selected cases for HCFA or other payers have wrestled to the ground generations of dysfunctionality, establishing the framework for integration that can be applied to the remainder of their business.

As with all economic changes underpinning an industry's revolution, the cost advantages of an integrated operating structure—once introduced into a market—are proliferated by competitive forces. The market dynamics associated with this process are hardly unique to health care. As Porter points out in *Competitive Strategy,* the integrated firm has a clear "competitive advantage over the unintegrated firm, in the form of higher prices, lower costs, or lower risk. Thus the unintegrated firm must integrate or face a disadvantage, and the new entrant into the business is forced to enter as an integrated firm or bear the same consequences."[14] If this principle holds in health care—which many suspect it does, judging by the often lemming like rush to integrate behind a market leader—then vertical integration is destined to shift rapidly from a bold and revolutionary move in the mid-1990s, to a competitive contingency by the turn of the century.

Trends by HCFA and other payers to move toward a global pricing model are met on the supply side by the more aggressive national provider organizations. Systems like Tenet and the not-for-profit Catholics on the inpatient side—and companies like IHS and HealthSouth on the outpatient side—are effecting market-by-market provider integrations designed specifically to accept global-type payments from payers. In fact, it was a premature rush to implement precisely this strategy that helped bring down Columbia/HCA. From the outset the company sought to integrate markets vertically, as quickly as it moved to consolidate them horizontally, under the direction of a local market manager.[15] While this was a sound approach to where the market was heading, Columbia pursued it too quickly—years before the Centers of Excellence program was launched—and it used financial incentives too freely, thus incurring the wrath of the federal government. To align the success of local physicians with the success of its local hospitals, Columbia offered them private equity, rather than fully encompassing, formal captive employment/ownership deals or *ad hoc*, contract-specific financial performance incentives. This practice ran afoul of federal self-referral laws and, along with its too aggressive manipulation of Medicare accounting and reimbursement rules, got the company in trouble. But regardless of that unhappy outcome, Columbia's strategy to align itself with physicians on a market-by-market basis has been emulated in principle by other national hospital systems, in particular, Tenet, through its alliance with MedPartners, the nation's largest physician practice management company.[16]

The key organizational design flowing from this strategy involves market-specific scaling of the franchise; strategically (and legally) appropriate integration of physicians and hospitals; and centralization of authority under a market manager endorsed by all parties within the integrated unit. All three ingredients are critical to an organization's ability to thrive under package pricing and survive under eventual full risk-assumption. The establishment of a clear governing authority is often missing from otherwise sound attempts at integration, even the most highly elaborate. This may not be the only flaw built into these attempts, but it is almost always a fatal one.

NEXT STEP TOWARD INTEGRATION: FULL RISK-ASSUMPTION

Global or package pricing helps accomplish the first goal of integration: it joins physicians and hospitals as co-contractors in the same transaction with purchasers, breaking down a century-old barrier to coordinated care. It also forces providers to confront the watershed behavioral and cultural changes demanded by success under shared risk-assumption, if only on the individual case. For the at-risk case that represents a fixed amount of revenue for both physicians and hospitals, the onus is placed on the integrated provider to optimize clinical resources and bear financial responsibility for adverse acute outcomes. But package pricing still focuses on *pricing*. It does not deal with the appropriateness question, nor the aggregation of appropriateness for an entire population, i.e., total utilization of a given surgical procedure. It does not address total medical costs, reward aggressive health risk identification and intervention, or encourage longitudinal management of the total health of an insured group of people. Under global pricing, the traditional incentive to overtreat the individual case, once presented, is finally reversed; but it has done nothing to reward providers for helping to keep healthy people from becoming cases in the first place.

Such risk isolation explains why package pricing tends to focus only on clearly definable cases that are acute in origin (e.g., a hip replacement surgery), and on high-cost, high-volume, inpatient intensive services. While these cases constitute a significant portion of total health care dollars, they represent only a minority of all the medical activities that need to be coordinated and rationalized for a population. This underscores why true integration of the health care delivery system requires the wholesale shifting of risk for entire populations, not just for selected acute subsets. Such shifting, embodied in capitation payments to a single provider entity, compels far more meaningful organizational reform on the part of all the providers represented by that entity; it also constitutes the only meaningful and sustainable way to control total costs and improve quality over the long term.

INTEGRATION REALIZED: THE EMERGING HEALTH CARE ORGANIZATION

As there is a seeming pestilence of terms and acronyms that attempt to describe these integrated entities generally (IDS, IDN, IHO, PSO), for purposes of our discussion it cannot hurt to add one more: the emerging health care organization (EHO). The use of the term "emerging" is an attempt to hedge; a recognition that the ultimate manifestation of the integrated provider system or network in the new century will surely incorporate mechanisms and elements well beyond those anticipated in this book.

EHOs represent the most evolved and elegant form of managed care. They are fully vertically integrated systems under which hospitals, physicians, and other facilities and providers gain the muscle and the critical mass to accept global risk contracts from MCOs, traditional insurers, and directly from self-insured employers, groups of employers, and consumers. Two things define an EHO:

1. the certainty of their existence, based on the health care market's insistence that providers ultimately bear the financial responsibility associated with delivering medical care, which necessitates vertical integration of some shape or form; and
2. the uncertainty of their shape or form, as EHOs truly are emerging, works-in-progress, organizations struggling for models that will function effectively, and identities that will market effectively.

EHOs represent the most progressive and appropriate alignment of financial incentives for the provision of care with those charged to provide it, and a fundamental correction of the health care system's historic fee-for-service dysfunctionality. The use of EHOs both to insure and deliver health care removes all the mistrust, antagonism, and costly, cumbersome nature of the relationship between providers and the traditional MCOs. Such contracting pushes financial risk and its associated responsibility away from employer groups and consumers, past the MCOs, and directly on to the providers of care, who are best equipped to balance financial incentives and clinical needs.

Those entities least fit to compete with EHOs, not coincidentally, are the chief critics of all the federal and state legislation designed to enable their formation, namely the traditional MCOs. They have opposed legislation on streamlined licensing and solvency requirements for EHOs because they clearly recognize the competitive advantage of a provider-driven—rather than insurer-owned—system for assuming risk and delivering medical services. In their attempts to obstruct EHO formation, MCOs in particular are acknowledging the inevitable: over the years they have pushed financial risk down to their provider-contractors through global pricing, capitation, and other risk-sharing arrangements, to align incentives and control the utilization of services. In the process, they have rewritten the health care economic playbook, trained providers in the new rules of risk-assumption, and created the very competition that, in the end, now threatens to destroy them.

This is the real power of full risk-assumption: it can change the economics of entire health care markets overnight. Full risk-assumption creates a competitive snowballing in a local market, with the new, much more competitive pricing model rapidly emerging as the norm. The only obstacles to the overnight transformation of every market in the United States are institutional as providers struggle with the many organizational design problems, cultural impediments, and uncertainty presented by EHO creation and management.

FORM AND FUNCTION: VERTICAL VERSUS VIRTUAL

The first step toward full risk-assumption embodied in global package pricing inspired the creation of organizational structures that have proven to be similarly rudimentary in terms of their transformational capacities. To enter into global pricing contracts, the market introduced a number of contracting vehicles, in particular the physician-hospital organization (PHO), under which an independent group of physicians and a hospital join into a legal entity, generally governed and financed through a 50/50 split, to provide purchasers with "single-signature" authority.[17] The market has also introduced a variety of PHO-like organizations too numerous, nuanced in structural variation, and ultimately transitory to justify lengthy descriptions within the scope of this discussion.

The PHO and these variants work well for package pricing, but they are distant antecedents of true EHOs. They suffer from problems in execution: meaningful and lasting clinical integration of facilities and physicians is extremely difficult to achieve for entities that are "integrated" only through legal and financial obligation but not in any real organizational, operational, or cultural sense. PHOs generally also do not integrate the total continuum of care necessary for full risk-assumption, only the hospital and physician components. As a result, Donald Johnson, writing in *Health Care Strategic Management,* argues that PHOs "have to be viewed as transitional structures…to an organization that includes all aspects of care under one system of payment, delivery, and information. In other words, integration. Unfortunately, the intended goal and what has occurred don't necessarily match. Instead, the industry has developed a legal structure for contracting purposes."[18]

Successful execution of full risk-assumption contracts—under which physicians, hospitals, and others agree to deliver all care to a population for a per capita fee or capitation rate—requires a truly integrated organizational design, i.e., the formation of a full-blown EHO. The efforts to create such an entity are no small undertaking; they typically generate enormous trepidation from physicians and hospital managers; and they have been, at least well into the mid-1990s, characterized less by their success stories than by numerous false starts, bad industry press, and mixed reactions from the managed care and traditional health insurance community. MCOs generally encourage full risk taking by providers—but only when they can control the terms and guarantee their position as the middlemen in what are essentially straightforward, currency-for-risk transactions between capitated provider groups and the ultimate purchasers.

As a result, the degree of true organizational integration is in flux, and highly variable from market to market across the United States. In a study published in *Health Care Strategic Management*, 58 percent of all provider organizations within highly integrated systems had contracts with their systems, while only 42 percent were wholly or partially owned by their systems.[19] As will be explored momentarily, the debate over ownership versus more informal types of integration has raged on through the 1990s; here the national data show an almost even split between these two markedly different approaches to the same problem. Such a clean split is illustrative of the arbitrariness and uncertainty attendant to EHO development, and the raw heterogeneity of different health care markets.

If one considers the structure of the following three markets, it is not difficult to imagine how little commonality there is in their comparative EHO formations:

- Minneapolis-St. Paul has five major integrated systems, which include 57.1 percent of the market's 35 hospitals, 73.1 percent of its discharges, and 1 of its 4 MCOs.
- Los Angeles-Long Beach has four major integrated systems, but they include only 13.1 percent of the market's 122 acute care hospitals, 18.1 percent of its discharges, and 2 of 19 MCOs.
- Worcester, MA has two major integrated systems that include *all* three of the market's hospitals and 1 of its 2 MCOs.[20]

While these markets are far-flung regionally, the divergence in their structuring is still striking, given another fact: *they are nearly identical in terms of managed care penetration and thus market evolution.* The sharp contrasts among these markets underscores the effects of historic market structure, and points to a fundamental ambivalence at work within the health care system as it transforms itself through the integration of care delivery.

There is an even greater ambivalence surrounding the obvious next step in this transformation: the nature and degree to which an

EHO should forward-integrate to include the financing and under-writing functions of the Mcos and traditional insurers. The forma-tion of fully "MCO-like" EHOs for the express purpose of contract-ing directly with employers represents health care vertical integration taken to its logical conclusion. Because it is rife with risk, uncertainty, and bad precedent, the question of full forward in-tegration is one of the most hotly debated strategies in health care today. The remainder of this chapter explores the arguments on both sides of each debate: outright ownership versus alternative align-ments of providers and physician groups by EHOs; and the forward integration of EHOs into the underwriting function.

INTEGRATION PATH I: THE CASE AGAINST OWNERSHIP

Because skepticism sells more newspapers in a world suspicious of threats to the *status quo*—and because most experiments fail sev-eral times on the pathway to perfecting a formula—there has emerged a highly visible body of evidence that EHOs involving out-right ownership are unworkable. A trio of authors write in *Inte-grated Health Care Delivery* that "almost all findings suggest nega-tive effects of owned integration on performance."[21] Their conclusion is based on hard evidence that "owned, vertically inte-grated arrangements do not appear to significantly reduce organiza-tional costs or yield other efficiencies. On the contrary, research sug-gests higher production cost and exit barriers and, when unstable demand exists, higher administrative costs as well."[22]

These findings seem to embody Porter's observation that "vertical integration increases the proportion of a firm's costs that are fixed...Thus, integration increases the operating leverage of the firm, exposing it to greater cyclical swings in earnings."[23] This is precisely what has happened in numerous health care markets as EHOs have formed amidst chaotic marketplace changes. While there is no holding of variables constant for the sake of scientific experimentation in the real world, few experiments are subjected to more confounding variables than those conducted in health care markets. The very emergence of the EHO itself is a confounder: it factionalizes the physician and hospital community; emboldens self-insured employers to consider direct contracting; and puts all the local MCOs on competitive red alert.

Based on their analysis, the trio of authors cited above recommend a phased approach under which "managers should first seek contractual, non-owned mechanisms to accomplish their objectives and avoid the increased bureaucratic costs of ownership."[24] This is consistent with Porter's observation that "when facing considerable uncertainty, firms tend to select strategies that preserve flexibility, despite the costs in terms of required resources or diminished competitive position."[25] Such an approach is also much more culturally palatable for health care organizations with substantial numbers of stakeholders who may resist outright asset mergers, which would be interpreted as a threat to both jobs and institutional values.

The medical schools and hospitals associated with Columbia and Cornell Universities, both located in New York City, are creating an alliance among 2,800 of their physicians to "negotiate jointly with managed care companies and insurers, and to develop joint practices sites throughout metropolitan New York City. The medical schools and research programs will maintain separate identities." As reported in *Health Care Strategic Management,* as Herbert Pardes, dean of Columbia's College of Physicians and Surgeons, for the alliance said, "The merger of medical schools is a complicated business. We felt we needed to move in a more timely way. The schools are looking for ways to become more competitive in the marketplace for managed care contracts. It will be much easier to create a system to combine the schools' physicians than to merge."[26] This approach is a begrudging recognition that certain types of health care organizations are large bureaucracies. Getting them to move forward on an initiative as bold and threatening as an outright merger is often not a viable option, either in principle or, more importantly, in execution.

Even in the absence of the "urge to merge" created by health care transformation, there are compelling strategic reasons for merger-type alliances. As Porter points out, "interconnections through joint ventures or joint participations can promote stability in an industry through fostering a cooperative orientation and exposing the players to fairly complete information about each other. Full information is usually stabilizing because it helps firms avoid mistaken reactions and keeps them from attempting ill-advised strategic initiatives."[27] While this smacks of a recommendation to collude, it more importantly anticipates a critical initiative among providers and physician groups as they develop into nonownership models of vertical integration; such models are often termed "virtual integration" among health care's *cognoscenti*. Such integration allows for a historic first in many health care markets: it forces providers with excess capacity to measure, compare, and coordinate their expensive medical resources, rather than blindly continue to grow their clinical assets and run up utilization to amortize the fixed costs of that growth.

As of this writing, this appears to be the strategy of choice for most architects of EHOs. Many in the health care industry clearly prefer to hedge, using the general uncertainty of health care transformation as their stated rationale. Such a rationale is more often rationalization, a convenient cover story for what is really behind the hedging: organizational resistance and cultural paralysis. The builders of these new and untested organizations also recognize the cost-expediency of letting others bring down the experience curve. As Porter points out, "experience may accumulate more rapidly for the second and third firms in the market than it did for the pioneer because followers can observe some aspects of the pioneer's operations."[28]

But there are glaring exceptions to this hedge-and-see strategy, embodied in virtual versus actual vertical integration of provider types. These exceptions are the large national chains like IHS and HealthSouth, both of whom clearly favor outright ownership strategies. Such companies prefer to purchase providers of other pieces of the continuum of care, and then move rapidly to integrate these into their own vertical market development efforts. While the evidence may argue against such moves, and while there are clear "second-and third-mover" advantages, the strategic acumen and market successes of both these firms provides a cautionary tale to those who would proceed with too much caution.

INTEGRATION PATH II: THE CASE FOR OWNERSHIP

The most significant problem with virtual versus actual vertical integration is execution and control, which begs a number of unpleasant questions:

- Can an EHO with financial responsibility for delivering on a full-risk contract effectively manage "its" people—i.e., one hospital's nurses, another outpatient rehab center's physical therapists, and a separate group of physicians—if that EHO is not perceived as "the boss?"
- Can accountability be established and managed?
- Is it really wise for the "virtually" integrated EHO to create yet another governing body and management layer on top of the layers of management still in place in the distinct organizations?

There are strong and convincing opinions that the answer to all of these questions is clearly "no." A realistic observer would also have a strong intuitive sense—crystallized through the hard experience of navigating through the typical health care organization—that more layers of decision makers, turf fighters, and naysayers is the last thing that any health care organization needs.

One of the clearest voices on the subject is Douglas Cave. Writing in *Integrated Health Care Delivery,* the same collection that also includes essays favoring virtual versus owned integration, Cave argues categorically that an EHO "should have one controlling entity with a defined mission statement. Only the staff and equity models [both ownership models] support a health system with a single governance structure."[29] Cave arrives at this conclusion after rigorously tracing the incentives and control issues associated with numerous models of virtual versus actual vertical integration. He also points out that ownership is important from an investment and development perspective. "Health systems need to grow their PCP [primary care physician] networks to succeed under full-risk capitation. The IRS and Medicare require that health systems purchase all physician assets before infusing capital into the PCP network. Systems based on [ownership] models are exempt from incremental restrictions and fraud and abuse regulations. Other models cannot legally invest in PCP network growth."[30]

But perhaps the most convincing argument for ownership comes not from a specific analysis of integrated health care organizations, but from Porter's analysis of integrated organizations in general. He points out that managing across the boundaries of integration is particularly challenging, more so than managing the individual components of integration. "Managing linkages is a more complex organizational task than managing value activities themselves," he writes in *Competitive Advantage*. "Given the difficulty of recognizing and managing linkages, the ability to do so often yields a sustainable force of competitive advantage."[31] This difficulty in "linkage management" is particularly problematic in the development and operation of an integrated health care delivery system, given the fierce autonomy of physicians and decentralized nature of an EHO's operations. Acknowledgment of precisely this difficulty is central to Cave's conclusions that integration works only when physician incentives and behaviors are aligned through equity participation (i.e., through an ownership interest) in the EHO.

The strategic superiority of ownership is confirmed by a perspective that encompasses a historic viewpoint. The move to vertically integrate health care services in every market in the United States is a one-time event, a brief moment of transformation in a century's worth of industrial history; hesitation now will spell failure in the coming years as markets sort into exclusive, owned, fully vertical players. This is consistent with Porter's analysis of the economies of vertical integration: "a type of economies of scale entry barrier occurs when there are economies to vertical integration, that is, operating in successive stages of production or distribution. Here the entrant must enter integrated or face a cost disadvantage, as well as possible foreclosure of inputs or markets for its product if most established competitors are integrated."[32] In health care markets, this means that hospitals and physician groups that hedge too long on choosing partners may find themselves excluded from the dance.

EATING AT THE ENEMY'S TABLE: FORWARD INTEGRATION AND THE SUPER EHO

The debate over ownership versus alliance-based vertical integration is downright courtly in comparison to the acrimony between the schools of opinion over the full forward integration of the EHO. Should such an organization bypass the MCOs and other types of insurers and bid directly for an employer's and consumer's business? The very existence of operating margins for the typical MCO makes a compelling case for doing so; such margins are unnecessary for EHOs, which already have their margins built into what the MCOs pay them for medical services.

An even more compelling case resonates in the typical provider's view of the typical MCO. The view ranges from, at best, benign indifference toward this necessary evil of a marketing vehicle to, at worst, unvarnished contempt for this usurious middleman who contributes nothing to the delivery of medicine but complexity, antagonism, and confusion. In the most evolved markets, providers generally recognize that the typical MCO is nothing more than a marketing and financing conduit that assumes full financial/medical risk from employers and consumers and then hands it off immediately to the EHO, after skimming off 20 percent for its marketing, administration, and shareholders.

While the temptation to forward-integrate is borne of years spent tangled up and trying to cope with managed care systems, the decision is ultimately strategic in nature. Porter has propounded guidelines for all industries regarding forward integration and, like much of his work, these guidelines apply readily to health care as it converts into a more normalized industry prone to such analysis. "If a firm [the EHO] is dealing with customers [MCOs] who wield significant bargaining power and reap returns on investments in excess of the opportunity cost of capital, it pays for the firm to integrate even if there are no other savings from integration."[33] In most markets, payers have significant bargaining power over providers, but only through the incumbency of their financial infrastructures. MCOs were first to establish systems that isolated the financial risk associated with health care benefits for employers. They have used this entrenchment to stand between providers and these purchasers, even as these same MCOs now push more and more of that risk down to their provider-contractors.

A cursory examination of MCO economics makes a strong case for forward integration by EHOs:

> Assume that an MCO spends 75 cents of every premium dollar on medical costs and 15 cents on SG&A [sales, general, and administrative functions]. This leaves 10 cents for operating margins.[34]

> Given that EHOs have their own margins built into the 75 cents passed down from the MCOs, forward integration then returns to the EHO an additional operating profit margin of 40 percent (10 cents' operating margin on 25 cents' marginal revenue) on the activity associated with forward integration.

> Excluding the cost of capital, if the EHO is a taxable entity and we assume a tax rate of 35 percent, the net profit is 6.5 cents on the 25 cents in marginal revenue, *for a total net margin of 26 percent!*

Twenty-six percent is several times the cost of capital for any viable organization. And if the EHO is *not* a taxable entity, it can theoretically eliminate the operating margins from its pricing, reducing premiums by 10 percent. Thus, it quickly becomes clear that the opportunity cost of capital is trivial compared to the potential returns, given the leverage of the 25 cents of the premium dollar absorbed by the MCO middlemen.

The economic case for forward integration by EHOs is galvanized further by additional intangible savings associated with bypassing the payers and contracting directly with employers and consumers. As Porter points out, "offsetting bargaining power through integration may allow the firm [the EHO] to operate more efficiently by eliminating otherwise valueless practices used to cope with the powerful suppliers or customers."[35] Under traditional managed health care, examples of such "valueless practices" abound, bogging down physicians and hospitals with everything from up-front wrangling over contracts and guidelines, to extensive administrative paperwork, to continuous battles with utilization managers over patients and procedures.

While the medical delivery side of the EHO saves significant money as these practices are streamlined and integrated into the development and operation of the organization, the forward-integrated EHO saves these costs nearly in duplicate: valueless practices are a two-way street; the MCO's share of the expense associated with perpetuating such practices is drawn from its own administrative budget of 15 cents of every premium dollar. George Anders translates this wastefulness into human terms in his stinging critique of managed care, *Health against Wealth*: "at each stage middlemen who never see patients skim off their share. By the time Dr. Greenberg presses a stethoscope to a baby's chest or asks a mother if her child is eating properly, only a sliver of the original premium is left."[36]

Despite the clear economic and psychic rationale for ridding the system of the noise created by today's MCOs, there are substantial obstacles and objections to forward integration by an EHO:

- the problem of competitive strategy—"Is it wise to initiate competition against your current sources of patients for an employer's business?"
- the problem of cultural resistance—"Managed care is the enemy!"
- the problem of both resource and market incumbency—"MCOs have the technologies in place to manage populations and the relationships with employers to market their services."

The first objection is the most complex, and will be addressed momentarily. The second objection is emotional, irrational, and ultimately indefensible; those who cling to it despite the opportunity that forward integration offers to trump it, do not understand the historic and economic necessity of the initial intrusions of managed care, nor the transience of its first wave; those who cling to it after an explanation in so many words should be offered early retirement packages. The third objection is becoming increasingly less relevant as the market evolves, and thus is proving to be nothing more than a guise for the second objection, and is therefore the easiest to address directly.

The *resource incumbency* of managed care is undergoing a self-cannibalization. The tools and technologies that MCOs have developed to capture and manage populations—primarily sales forces, provider relations staffs, information systems, utilization management programs, and stop-loss insurance—are proving more intellectual property than tangible assets. Such resources are highly portable to an EHO; an EHO can readily replicate them in-house or purchase them commercially. Which begs the obvious question: do these resources really justify 25 cents of every premium dollar, especially if the MCO is really spending only 15 cents on them?

The *market incumbency* of managed care is undergoing a similar self-cannibalization by the MCOs themselves. They have been forced by the advent of consumerism to broaden their provider networks (i.e., expanded "point-of-service" options) in order to compete for market share; the result has been an almost chaotic consumer mobility—characterized by the constant annual churning of enrolled populations—in the typical health care market today. From the employer's or consumer's perspective, an MCO is devolving into a premium-collecting and claims-paying channel for accessing a network of providers. Any "value-add" is specious, and clearly not worth the sacrifice in provider choice. What is driving the consumer's decision making is not the presence of the MCO; it is the presence of the providers on the other side of the MCO, which is forced to give way, or risk losing market share.

HUMANA: THANKS FOR THE BAD MEMORIES

A much more compelling argument against forward integration is the strategic problems that arise when an EHO competes against its payer customers for the business of employers and the government. This biting of the hand that feeds you is a structural fact of health care's long transitional period to full consummation of forward integration strategies across whole markets. Many in the industry cite as the embodiment of this problem the failure of Humana in the 1980s to run a fully integrated MCO and national hospital chain. Because Humana as an MCO exerted the usual managed care pressure on physicians, they in turn boycotted Humana hospitals, choosing to admit their non-Humana patients elsewhere. The result was a substantial loss of business and eventual spin-off of the hospitals to the public and then to Columbia/HCA.

But it is important to note that what is written off as a classic version of the forward-integration problem did not derive from boycotts by Humana hospitals' payer customers or other MCOs. Rather, it was inflicted on the company from their *faux* "customers," the admitting physicians who, back in the 1980s, had the luxury of remaining fully independent from Humana and any other organization that attempted to build an EHO-like organization. They maintained numerous other sources of fee-for-service and managed care patients, could admit to any of the dozens of then stand-alone hospitals in Humana's markets, and thus had leverage over Humana as a chain of hospitals *and* health plan. This is a legacy problem, one quickly growing immaterial. It stems from the fact that physicians are not the natural "customers" of a hospital, and yet they have been able to behave as such only because of their historic autonomy. This anachronistic separation is irrelevant to a strategic analysis of today's EHO, which has as its core premise the *a priori* alignment of physicians and facilities.

The real problem with Humana, then, was the prematurity of its vision. It recognized the economic and strategic value of full forward integration, but was unable to integrate into its strategy a key constituency. As Lutz and Gee point out in *The For-Profit Healthcare Revolution,* Humana's "vision was marred when the changes foretold didn't come nearly as fast and comprehensively as predicted. It's one thing to set off on a voyage with certain provisions to sustain you until you reach your destination. Still, all the vision in the world doesn't help when the destination keeps stretching beyond your reach. In Humana's case, the timing was off by about five years."[37] As the lingering memories of Humana's failure continues to plague discussions of forward integration by providers and their EHOs, it has emerged as an object lesson less about health care integration and more about a universal business pathology identified by Porter. "The memory of past failures," he writes in *Competitive Strategy*, "and the impediments to further moves in those areas they bring, can be very lasting and given disproportionate weight. This is particularly true in generally successful organizations."[38]

As Lutz and Gee point out, there are more important lessons regarding forward integration in the Humana episode. Even though the development of Humana's managed care business was "unprofitable in the early years, it would eventually prove more financially viable than the hospital business...Ironically, the move to diversify eventually led to divestiture of Humana's core business: hospitals."[39] Humana's foray into forward integration indeed has proven prescient, if premature. It occurred when health care was still highly fragmented and physicians were mobile, autonomous, and still enjoyed for the most part full discretionary power over where and how patients moved about in the system. Now, with consolidation occurring at breakneck speed and markets dividing up into two to four competing systems, Humana's strategy is not only relevant; in many markets, it is strategically necessary. As Lutz and Gee conclude, "where Humana was once chided for its seeming folly, hospitals now scurry to obtain the mechanism to accept risk and capitated contracts."[40] This scurrying is consistent with the broader strategic principle developed in the chapter on risk-assumption: *in the new century's health care system, the only transactions left will be the transfer and assumption of medical/financial risk.* The organization that controls the premiums will control everything downstream from them, including provider resources, referrals, and physician activities.

This algorithm embodies what little incumbency is still left to the MCOs: they control premium dollars, if only because they have controlled them for years. More importantly, they have access to the data associated with how those premium dollars historically are spent. This control of information is key to the MCO's continuing ability to exert and maintain bargaining power over both providers and purchasers (employers *and* consumers). Up the purchasing chain from the MCO, the control of information limits an employer's understanding of the real economics of a given health care market; back down the chain, it limits a provider's understanding of the real economics of health benefits design and delivery.

But even the most tentative, limited flirtation with forward integration breaks the spell of this incumbency. In fact, gaining access to previously unattainable information, gleaned from experience as a forward-integrated EHO, may be sufficient to justify whatever initial losses are generated by those first steps, providing insight into the economies of integration and the cost structures of the MCO customers. As Dean Coddington points out, "by owning a health plan, a health care system often develops a clear picture of customer needs. In addition, the data generated relative to physician practice patterns can be valuable in terms of further physician integration into the system."[41] This is consistent with Porter's observation that integration provides economies of information: "The fixed costs of monitoring the market and predicting supply, demand, and prices can be spread over all parts of the integrated firm, whereas they would have to be borne by each entity in an unintegrated firm. Market information may well flow more freely through an organization than through a series of independent parties. Integration may thus allow the firm to obtain faster and more accurate information about the marketplace."[42] Given the turbulence of most health care markets, the currency and accuracy of information may turn out to be the single most important advantage of integration.

This is consistent with experience in markets across the United States. "One of the errors we've made in the past was responding to what the insurers were telling us, because the insurer had that interface with the employer," Patrick Aberle, senior vice-president of managed care for Sutter/CHS, told a reporter for *Health Care Strategic Management.* "And typically the employer and insurer were separated by additional filters—brokers, PPO networks, or some marketing organization. I think it has been a key shortcoming of health care providers for many years."[43] This situation is changing as competition among MCOs grows more fierce, leading-edge EHOs market directly to employers, and a deeper and more sustained backlash against MCOs heats up in the popular media and on Capitol Hill in the late 1990s.

According to *Integrated Health Care Delivery,* "employers see the interplay of managed care and provider systems as potentially beneficial to them because of the promise of having price competition among providers. But when they see price cuts that fatten the bottom lines of managed care firms but don't reach them they look for other ways to break through the system to get more affordable care."[44] If this observation holds true over time and across enough health care markets, then the movement toward full forward integration may be driven not by the bold strategies of EHOs, but by the bold demands of the marketplace.

THE EHO AND DIRECT GOVERNMENT CONTRACTING

A relatively new and significant source of demand for forward integration by EHOs is the government purchaser, as federal and state agencies shift much of the Medicaid- and Medicare-eligible population into managed care systems. Nearly all viable proposals introduced between 1995 and 1998 to reform Medicare include "privatizing" the program's financing and delivery through the use of MCOs in one form or another, and include special provisions that encourage direct contracting with EHOs as a competitive alternative to those MCOs. ("Provider-sponsored organization" or PSO is the designation for provider-based networks that would contract directly with HCFA to service Medicare beneficiaries under full risk-assumption contracts.)

This inclusion of provider-based systems provides a substantial impetus for rapid development and proliferation of EHOs across the United States. However, the challenges facing these nascent organizations will be extremely difficult in this arena. Both the economics and competition associated with assuming risk and delivering care to Medicare beneficiaries will be brutal: the Medicare population is the highest cost and highest risk to insure, treat, and manage; and the traditional MCOs have targeted Medicare as the next major market to feed their growth.

The competitive pressures will be particularly strong for EHOs, given the incumbency problem. As Donald Johnson points out in *Health Care Strategic Management:*

> About 25 large national MCO chains control some 33 percent of the nation's more than 55 million MCO enrollees. They know what works and what doesn't. They have several years' head start on [EHOs], which means they know their costs, the cost of entering new markets, the time it takes to orient new providers and Medicare enrollees, and the investment required to expand their Medicare businesses. The advantage of a year's head start could be enormous, because, historically, once a Medicare beneficiary enrolls in an MCO, he or she is in for life.[45]

Despite the sternness of this cautionary message, it is essential that providers participate in this reform of Medicare through their development of EHOs. With more than 34 percent of all hospital patients and 50 percent of all hospital revenues derived from the Medicare population,[46] hospitals that do not seek to contract directly with Medicare will find that in short order, more than half their business will be controlled by either competitors or MCOs.

PROGRESS, SORT OF...

Beginning with Humana in the late 1980s and proceeding through the 1990s, efforts to fully integrate health care financing and delivery have followed the familiar pattern of two steps forward and one step back. The backward steps seem to garner more press, if only because bad news sells more trade journals. But the health care business as a whole is clearly transforming itself in the direction of full vertical integration. The economics of this integration are intuitively obvious on their own; add to that the steady progression toward full risk-assumption by providers, which makes dis-integrated care that much more costly and unworkable; and finally consider all the inefficiencies inherent in perpetuating distinct and ultimately adversarial provider versus insurer systems. It just does not make sense to maintain walls this thick anymore. *With a culture that will always demand the best medical care—but has at the same time grown intolerant of runaway health care costs—25 cents of every premium dollar is the obvious next target for a churning marketplace.*

There are also major motivations for full integration on the supply side, which are similarly steeped in culture. As Montague Brown observes in *Integrated Health Care Delivery,* "physicians who have owned managed care and sold it off seem to come back in other forms still wanting more control and more revenue than they had in earlier iterations of the agreements."[47] Providers yo-yo back and forth between forward-integrating into the insurance role and spinning back out because of a certain financial impatience, one that tends to trump the longer-term strategic importance of developing and maintaining forward integration. This financial impatience is triggered by the inevitable up-front losses associated with entering a new, risky, and complicated business. Sharon McEachern acknowledges this short-sightedness, and attempts to put it into an appropriate context: "expect to lose money the first time around, that first year of direct contracting between your hospital or health system and a self-insured, self-administered employer...Look at that first year the same as you would if you had to invest in a consulting firm that would give you theory, but not the implementation experience for which there's no substitute."[48]

McEachern's perspective is underscored by Porter, whose observation on the subject applies to the economics of horizontal consolidation as well as to those associated with vertical integration. "Unwillingness to accept lower profits during the transition can be seriously short-sighted if economies of scale will be significant in the mature industry. A period of lower profits may be inevitable while industry rationalization occurs, and a cool head is necessary to avoid overreaction."[49] Health care is indeed in the most significant "transition" in its history; it is nothing if not an industry in the midst of a massive rationalization ultimately leading toward Porter's "maturity." A few years of financial struggle are a small price to pay for long-term survival and success.

The single best argument for full forward integration is the notion that it represents not so much an aberration or revolutionary change, but simply a belated curative for a century-long affliction to the health care system. As with the concept of integrating medical care across settings, perhaps the "super-EHO"—or the emergence of the provider as insurer—is more historic fix than futuristic innovation. In the early part of the 20th century, had contract medical practice (fixed fees for providing all medical care to a group of laborers) emerged as the norm instead of the fee-for-service system, then the insurance function would have been built into the U.S. health care delivery system from the outset. Viewed from this perspective, it is readily apparent that—as the assumption of medical risk emerges as the only real medical product bought and sold in the new century—full forward integration by providers into the insurance function is not only strategically likely, but historically inevitable.

THE PATH TO INDUSTRIALIZATION

A key competitive advantage of the vertically integrated health care firm is how readily it yields itself to meaningful operational measurement, analysis, and improvement. Unlike those trying to coordinate care across the archipelago of unrelated care settings under the old system, for the integrated firm the consequences of one set of clinical choices in one setting can be tracked, measured, and compared across all settings. This is the concept of optimization introduced earlier in this chapter, put into practice. *Total* costs and *final* patient outcomes are the end points for the integrated firm's self-analysis; this is a far cry from all the intermediate measures—length of stay, number of doctors visits, or the cost of prescriptions—used by insurers when analyzing all the isolated aspects of traditional care. The empirical analysis necessary for true optimization of care across health care settings is a bulwark in the "industrialization" of medicine—another major force of transformation in the health care industry and the subject of the next chapter.

As integration is the gateway to medicine's industrialization, there are additional indirect economic benefits associated with integration that go beyond the more obvious ones. Integrated systems lend themselves better to systemic rather than isolated study and process improvement, the kind central to Deming's principles of business transformation: "Here is a stable system for production of defective items," he writes in *Out of the Crisis*. "Any substantial improvement must come from action on the system, the responsibility of management. Wishing and pleading and begging the workers to do better was totally futile."[50] The traditional arrangement of medical care delivery has made all the clinicians in the system victims of this futility. MCOs and others can "wish, plead, and beg" individual clinicians in isolated care settings all they want; if they have any impact at all, it may actually be negative. Pushing for the earliest possible discharge from the hospital after cardiac surgery may actually end up causing postoperative infections or other complications that triple the readmissions rate, or drive twice as many patients back to the emergency department with residual chest pain. Switching a thousand depressed patients onto a cheaper class of antidepressants, to save a few hundred dollars a month, hardly pays for itself if one of those patients attempts suicide and ends up in the intensive care unit at a cost of $5,000 per day.

In the absence of true integration, the best time to discharge—or the most clinically effective and economically feasible antidepressant—will remain mysteries to both the providers and purchasers of medical care. And while they remain mysteries, providers and purchasers will continue to engage in discourse of little value: purchasers will "wish, plead, and beg" health care providers to perform better, a pointless exercise manifest in managed care's obsession with utilization management; providers will wait on hold for permission to provide. While this may help control costs in the short run, it is in Deming's phrase, "totally futile" from the standpoint of real reform of the system.

The traditional managed care practice of haranguing physicians and hospitals flies in the face of Deming's central principle that "the bulk of the causes of low quality and low productivity belong to the system and thus lie beyond the power of the work force."[51] Integration is therefore a necessary step to understanding total system dynamics, and stands on the critical path to medicine's industrialization and its most profound reforms of all.

REFERENCES

1. L. Lagnado, "AHA Survey on Hospital Patient Satisfaction," *Wall Street Journal*, 28 January, 1997.

2. P. Starr, *The Social Transformation of American Medicine* (New York: Basic Books/HarperCollins, 1982), 162.

3. Adapted and reprinted with the permission of The Free Press, a Division of Simon & Schuster from *COMPETITIVE ADVANTAGE: Creating and Sustaining Superior Performance* by Michael E. Porter. Copyright © 1985 by Michael E. Porter. p. 48.

4. C. Snow, "One-Stop Shopping," *Modern Healthcare*, 25 November, 1996.

5. D. Blackmon, "HealthSouth Agrees To Buy Surgical Care," *Wall Street Journal,* 14 December, 1995.

6. C. Snow, "HealthSouth's New Horizons," *Modern Healthcare*, 24 February, 1997, 20.

7. Snow, "One-Stop Shopping," *Modern Healthcare*.

8. S. MacStravic, "Price Wars Are No-Win Games for Health Care Systems," *Health Care Strategic Management,* May 1996, 20.

9. D. Johnson, "Digest: Integrated Systems Can Save," *Health Care Strategic Management,* September, 1996, 2.

10. D. Coddington et al., *Making Integrated Health Care Work* (Englewood, CO: Center for Research in Ambulatory Health Care Administration, 1996), 217–218.

11. W. Unger and R. Kraft, "Package Pricing Roils Cardiac, Orthopedic Services," *Health Care Strategic Management,* June 1996, 1–20.

12. Unger and Kraft, *Health Care Strategic Management,* 1–20.

13. Unger and Kraft, *Health Care Strategic Management,* 24.

14. Adapted and reprinted with the permission of The Free Press, a Division of Simon & Schuster from *COMPETITIVE STRATEGY: Techniques for Analyzing Industries and Competitors* by Michael E. Porter. Copyright © 1980 by The Free Press. p. 308.

15. S. Lutz and E.P. Gee, *The For-Profit Healthcare Revolution* (Chicago: Irwin Professional Publishing, 1995), 82.

16. R. Rundle, "Tenet and MedPartners Agree To Form Health Network in Southern California," *Wall Street Journal,* 10 April, 1997.

17. R. Rognehaugh, *The Managed Health Care Dictionary* (Gaithersburg, MD: Aspen Publishers, 1996), 150.

18. "Consultant's Corner," *Health Care Strategic Management,* November, 1995, 14.

19. D. Johnson, "Digest: Integrated Systems Can Save," *Health Care Strategic Management,* September 1996, 3.

20. Johnson, *Health Care Strategic Management,* 3.

21. S. Watson et al., "Owned Vertical Integration and Health Care: Promise and Performance," in *Integrated Health Care Delivery: Theory, Practice, Evaluation, and Prognosis*, ed. M. Brown (Gaithersburg, MD: Aspen Publishers, 1996), p. 75.

22. Watson et al., *Integrated Health Care Delivery: Theory, Practice, Evaluation, and Prognosis*, 75.

23. Adapted and reprinted with the permission of The Free Press, a Division of Simon & Schuster from *COMPETITIVE STRATEGY: Techniques for Analyzing Industries and Competitors* by Michael E. Porter. Copyright © 1980 by The Free Press. p. 310.

24. Watson et al., *Integrated Health Care Delivery: Theory, Practice, Evaluation, and Prognosis*, 75.

25. Adapted and reprinted with the permission of The Free Press, a Division of Simon & Schuster from *COMPETITIVE ADVANTAGE: Creating and Sustaining Superior Performance* by Michael E. Porter. Copyright © 1985 by Michael E. Porter. p. 446.

26. "Strategic Notes," *Health Care Strategic Management,* September 1996, 4.

27. Adapted and reprinted with the permission of The Free Press, a Division of Simon & Schuster from *COMPETITIVE STRATEGY: Techniques for Analyz-*

ing Industries and Competitors by Michael E. Porter. Copyright © 1980 by The Free Press. p. 91.

28. Adapted and reprinted with the permission of The Free Press, a Division of Simon & Schuster from *COMPETITIVE STRATEGY: Techniques for Analyzing Industries and Competitors* by Michael E. Porter. Copyright © 1980 by The Free Press. p. 16.

29. D. Cave, "Vertical Integration Models To Prepare Health Systems for Capitation," in *Integrated Health Care Delivery: Theory, Practice, Evaluation, and Prognosis*, ed. M. Brown (Gaithersburg, MD: Aspen Publishers, 1996), 167.

30. Cave, *Integrated Health Care Delivery: Theory, Practice, Evaluation, and Prognosis*, 169.

31. Adapted and reprinted with the permission of The Free Press, a Division of Simon & Schuster from *COMPETITIVE ADVANTAGE: Creating and Sustaining Superior Performance* by Michael E. Porter. Copyright © 1985 by Michael E. Porter. p. 50.

32. Adapted and reprinted with the permission of The Free Press, a Division of Simon & Schuster from *COMPETITIVE STRATEGY: Techniques for Analyzing Industries and Competitors* by Michael E. Porter. Copyright © 1980 by The Free Press. p. 9.

33. Adapted and reprinted with the permission of The Free Press, a Division of Simon & Schuster from *COMPETITIVE STRATEGY: Techniques for Analyzing Industries and Competitors* by Michael E. Porter. Copyright © 1980 by The Free Press. p. 307.

34. Premium revenue and medical loss ratio figures for the median U.S. MCO in 1995, published in the *1997 Guide to the Managed Care Industry* (Baltimore: HCIA Inc., 1996) .

35. Adapted and reprinted with the permission of The Free Press, a Division of Simon & Schuster from *COMPETITIVE STRATEGY: Techniques for Analyzing Industries and Competitors* by Michael E. Porter. Copyright © 1980 by The Free Press. p. 307.

36. G. Anders, *Health against Wealth* (New York: Houghton Mifflin, 1996), 85.

37. Lutz and Gee, *The For-Profit Healthcare Revolution*, 33–34.

38. Adapted and reprinted with the permission of The Free Press, a Division of Simon & Schuster from *COMPETITIVE STRATEGY: Techniques for Analyzing Industries and Competitors* by Michael E. Porter. Copyright © 1980 by The Free Press. p. 61.

39. Lutz and Gee, *The For-Profit Healthcare Revolution*, 37–38.

40. Lutz and Gee, *The For-Profit Healthcare Revolution*, 38.

41. D. Coddington et al., *Making Integrated Health Care Work* (Englewood, CO: Center for Research in Ambulatory Health Care Administration, 1996), 67.

42. Adapted and reprinted with the permission of The Free Press, a Division of Simon & Schuster from *COMPETITIVE STRATEGY: Techniques for Analyzing Industries and Competitors* by Michael E. Porter. Copyright © 1980 by The Free Press. p. 304.

43. S. McEachern, "Invest in Direct Contracting," *Health Care Strategic Management,* March 1996, 19.

44. M. Brown, "Where in networking and vertical integration are we?" *Integrated Health Care Delivery: Theory, Practice, Evaluation, and Prognosis,* ed. M. Brown (Gaithersburg, MD: Aspen Publishers), 274.

45. D. Johnson, "Provider-Sponsored Networks a Top Priority," *Health Care Strategic Management,* November 1995, 3.

46. From data on Medicare discharges and revenues as a percentage of total discharges and total revenues, included in *The Comparative Performance of U.S. Hospitals: The Sourcebook,* 1996 ed. (Baltimore: HCIA Inc.)

47. Brown, *Integrated Health Care Delivery: Theory, Practice, Evaluation, and Prognosis,* 273.

48. S. McEachern, "Invest in Direct Contracting," *Health Care Strategic Management,* March 1996, 1.

49. Adapted and reprinted with the permission of The Free Press, a Division of Simon & Schuster from *COMPETITIVE STRATEGY: Techniques for Analyzing Industries and Competitors* by Michael E. Porter. Copyright © 1980 by The Free Press. p. 248.

50. W. Deming, *Out of the Crisis* (Cambridge, MA: MIT Center for Advanced Engineering Study, 1986), 7.

51. Deming, *Out of the Crisis,* 24.

5

■

INDUSTRIALIZATION

A man who falls sick at home or abroad is liable to get heroic treatment, or nominal treatment, random treatment, or no treatment at all, according to the hands into which he happens to fall.

Jacob Bigelow, in a speech to the
Massachusetts Medical Society in 1835[1]

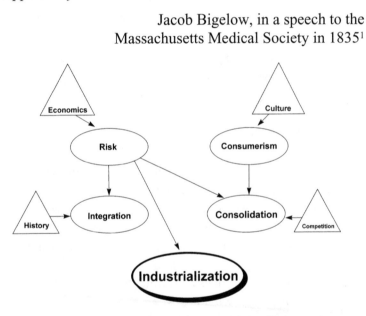

One of the most troublesome if least widely discussed symptoms of the U.S. health care system's chronic illness is its enormous, bewildering, and costly variability in clinical decision making. Such variations characterize nearly every aspect of medical delivery: surgery rates, hospital admission rates, hospital lengths of stay, invasive versus noninvasive treatments, diagnostic imaging and testing patterns, drug selection, *ad infinitum*. Such variations are financially and emotionally expensive; as described earlier with regard to

C-section and hysterectomy rates, they also often border on the scandalous.

As medical research is driven by science, its practical application should have similarly scientific underpinnings. Nonetheless, medical practice has evolved in the United States in a way that—until only recently—has isolated the delivery system and its practitioners from any scrutiny with the very scientific methods that medicine purports to represent. That isolation is finally coming to an end, driven by the concurrent rise over the past decade of managed care and the proliferation of empirical studies on variations in care patterns across the country. Such studies have served less to jar hospitals and physicians out of a complacency with regard to their fundamental clinical inconsistencies than to burn them from the studies' fanning of the managed care flame. With the utilization management tactics of MCOs serving as the main messenger of the problem, physicians have been put on the defensive; their inability or unwillingness to embrace this process and make it their own has only further emboldened MCOs.

The pioneering researcher in the field, John Wennberg, MD, of the Dartmouth Medical School, warned of precisely this phenomenon back in 1986, in a clarion call essay in the *New England Journal of Medicine* that still reverberates today: "Unless the medical profession accepts responsibility for the question of 'which rate [of medical or surgical utilization] is right' and addresses these issues within the current cost-containment context, others will see to it that the 'least is always best' theory dominates by default. After all, if physicians can't agree on what is best, why do more?"[2] This warning has turned out to be not only prescient; it could serve as the tacit mission statement for many of today's utilization managers.

As Stoline and Weiner note, "Wennberg and other investigators have found that some surgical procedures, including hysterectomy, tonsillectomy, and prostatectomy have consistently shown high variation in incidence (up to 6-fold) across populations or regions...Significant variation has also been shown in the treatment of several medical conditions, such as congestive heart failure."[3] In the years since the widespread publicization of Wennberg's work, his methods have been quickly absorbed—often times with necessary methodological rigor and other times with almost none—into the health care industry as it seeks to identify and eliminate variances in medical decision making.

That wide variations in care exist is hardly a surprise, after a century of fee-for-service medicine. Before MCOs put themselves at financial risk for covered populations—and well before they transferred any of that risk to physicians and hospitals—incentives under fee-for-service were backwards. The system rewarded inconsistency, inefficiency, and resource maximization. As Figure II–4 illustrates, the broader the variations in care across a population, the greater the total volume of services inevitably delivered to that population. (Because there is a rate at which not performing a service constitutes medical malpractice, greater variability around a normative mean rate—assuming a normal distribution—will in-

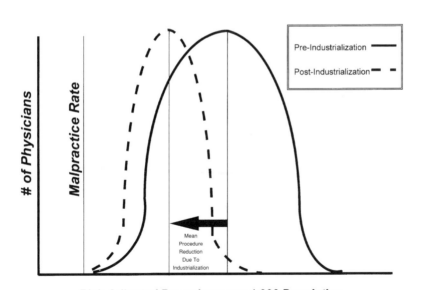

Risk-Adjusted Procedures per 1,000 Population

Figure II–4 Practice Pattern Distribution and Mean Procedure Rates.

crease that mean rate to accommodate the wider, lower end of the distribution.)

Unlike every other industry, whereby efficiency results in lower prices, more market share, and greater profits, efficiency in the traditional health care system actually *penalized* providers. Any effort to find a more efficient way of getting the same medical result for lower cost was rewarded with less revenue and less profit. Under this dysfunctional system, physicians delivered care in a vacuum, devoid of feedback except for the most extreme (medical malpractice, again). Improvements in clinical practice and process were self-directed and occurred at random, subject to the vagaries of individual training, clinical experience, continuing education, journal articles, and the marketing efforts of drug and device manufacturers. What this self-rewarding myopia across the medical delivery system has wrought is an enormous, complex, and expensive industry bereft of the practices that characterize even the most primitive industries. This is unfair to doctors, who are trained through an apprenticeship model and then cut loose to practice in the manner of folk artisans, semi-isolated professionals without the benefit of quantitative feedback about their practices in comparison with best practice standards. It is also unfair to patients, who are receiving their medical care from apprentices and folk artisans who may or may not be delivering the best possible medicine.

All this has changed in a few short years, under the sudden glare of managed care's harsh half-light. MCOs have imposed upon the health care system a task-master's accountability, one that continually dwells on cost, but is ultimately driven by excessive variability in clinical decision making. Such variability afflicts not only the broader decisions about what type of medical care to provide: Should we operate? Try drugs first? Do both now? It also characterizes the entire process of how the delivery of that care proceeds: *Which* drugs? *Which* surgical technique? In what setting? How much rehab for optimal recovery? Until only recently, variabilities that affect each and every macro and micro clinical decision were zealously, consciously guarded by the medical profession, in its efforts to protect its hegemony, autonomy, and professional self-determination. Thus sequestered, the process of delivering care has indeed been practiced like a folk art, an alchemy impenetrable to patients, their family members, their insurers, and anyone else outside the sacred society of medicine.

But regardless of how or why the sudden scrutiny of clinical variability occurred, two things are clear. First, it *needed* to occur: too many billions of dollars—and too many millions of lives—are at stake. Second, why it occurred is less important than the inevitable end result: *for the first time in its hundred years of modern history, medicine is finally undergoing the process of true industrialization.*

What exactly does the "industrialization of health care" really mean? It means that the system is finally adapting the tools and techniques of classic and contemporary operations research to the delivery of medicine. These range from the use of traditional statistical process control methods, driven by aggregations of patient data to analyze variations in care delivered by physician, hospital, and disease; to the application of the principles of total quality management, manifested in health care as "continuous quality improvement"; to the development, adoption, and monitoring of processes empirically demonstrated to produce superior outcomes.

What does this mean in practice and what's the payoff? As noted earlier, one of the areas of widest variation uncovered in Wennberg's research was congestive heart failure (CHF) patients. CHF is a complex illness, and often involves related diseases like hypertension and diabetes. Drug choices and other treatment options are many, varied, and often conflicting; patient compliance, education, and monitoring are critical factors in treatment success but have traditionally received short shrift. Why? Because when physicians are not at risk for the total cost of the illness, they have little motivation to invest resources in these activities. Patient education and monitoring do not pay the way high technology procedures and traditional physician-based office visits have always paid.

Against a tradition of high-tech, high-variability treatment of CHF, one physician organization's success with managing the disease provides a sterling example of how the introduction of a few elements of industrialization can reduce variations in treatment, improve outcomes, and lower cost. Vivra Heart Services, a network of 400 cardiologists, developed standardized protocols for medicating, educating, and tracking patients with the disease, including pathways for ongoing risk assessment, drug compliance monitoring, and resolution of acute events. Within six months of launching the program for a covered population in Florida, patients in the program had 90 percent fewer emergency department visits and 30 percent fewer hospital admissions than in the previous same year period.[4]

Such industrialization is a critical force behind the transformation of the U.S. health care system. And like all five forces described in this book, it is highly interrelated to the other four. Why? Because industrialization directly addresses and corrects much of the dysfunctionality of health care as a functioning marketplace. As Stoline and Weiner point out in *The New Medical Marketplace,* "classical economic theories base their assumptions on the consistent nature of the product that is supplied, but medical services are heterogeneous."[5] Health care industrialization seeks to neutralize this heterogeneity, standardizing how we measure and compare patient care processes, with the goal of quantification. Industrialization helps physicians, researchers, and management determine what works, at what cost, and what does not, regardless of cost. Such industrialization is thus an enabling process, eliminating generations of subterfuge about pricing, utilization, and soft-headed notions of "quality," and opening the gateway to true value estimation, cost benefit analysis, and individual performance assessment.

All of these activities are critical to provider organizations as they assume financial/medical risk for covered populations. Such risk-assumption finally reverses the perverse economic incentives of traditional medical delivery. With revenue fixed on a per case, per disease, or per capita basis, the objective for providers seeking to maximize their own income becomes cost minimization—rather than revenue maximization—for the same medical outcome. In the brave new world of at-risk reimbursement, physicians and hospitals literally have vested interests in efficiency. As a consequence, they begin for the first time to act like all other producers in a normal, functioning marketplace. Systems, tools, and processes that help promote efficiency are financial allies, not threats.

In markets where risk-assumption has been fully consummated, such systems become competitive necessities. Competition among providers for covered lives and capitation dollars compels the adoption of any recourse to reduce clinical variability and thus lower total medical costs. Industrializing the process of care standardizes that care, makes costs more manageable, and helps make outcomes more predictable. This is critical as the ability to manage cost becomes *the* critical success factor in a health care system where risk-assumption is the only product bought and sold.

One of the loftier goals bandied about in health care today—and one generally classifiable as part of health care's movement toward industrialization—is the improvement in quality. While many give lip service to this goal, hard experience in the industry teaches that, with a corporate benefits-purchasing community obsessed with premium dollars and intense competition, quality is a poor second cousin to cost. As Lutz and Gee point out in *The For-Profit Healthcare Revolution,* "the one with the lowest cost gets the covered lives and the one with the most covered lives wins."[6] Many have attempted to resolve the conflict by arguing that higher quality does indeed translate into lower cost, and for acute outcome measures like postoperative infections, that is certainly the case. Regardless of the outcome of the debate, either candidate ultimately will push the same agenda: industrialization has long been missing from the health care system and its introduction can only make it work better.

THE CONFLUENCE OF FACTORS DRIVING HEALTH CARE INDUSTRIALIZATION

There are a number of forces at work in health care—some coincidental, others interrelated—that are compelling its industrialization.

The movement toward rationalizing the delivery of care is promoted heavily by employers, who recognize not only the cost consequences, but also the quality shortfalls associated with wide variability in clinical decision making. Even with all of its risk for medical costs pushed down to insurers, MCOs, or directly to providers, a self-insured employer knows that substandard clinical performance has far-reaching, if indirect economic ramifications. Poor choices about surgeries, drugs, and other medical interventions will increase

- the amount of paid time off required for recovery;
- the costs of absenteeism;
- total disability costs; and
- the costs associated with substandard job performance for employees who receive less than optimal medical care.

Larger manufacturers in particular have a natural interest in rationalizing the medical delivery system, if only because their corporate cultures expect nothing less of their own operations and organizational behavior. An excellent example is the intensive involvement by General Motors in the health care delivered to its employees. The largest private purchaser of medical services in the United States, GM spent $3.6 billion on health care in 1995.[7] Because this amounts to more than $1,200 per car (versus $500 for steel for the same car), GM views health care no differently than it views any other factor of production. As a result, it focuses on the cost and quality of health care services delivered to its employees the same way it focuses on the cost and quality of the steel, glass, rubber, and other components of its cars.[8] GM has deployed productivity teams—precisely the same type of work force reconfiguration that turned around the entire American auto industry in the late 1980s—to work directly with its health care providers to "reengineer" the way medical services are delivered to GM employees. "Look at what GM did with Saturn," remarked the president of Genesys Health Care System, a Flint, Michigan, provider system assisted by the GM team. "An entirely new concept of building a car. We decided that health care must also change."[9]

Another major factor driving the push toward health care industrialization is the shift to lower cost treatment settings. Lower cost settings have, literally, less margin for error. As a report in *Health Care Strategic Management* observes, "you have much less opportunity to be efficient in outpatient procedures—there is less money, making efficiency more vital. Standardization is particularly important under these circumstances."[10] As most of the procedures that can shift to outpatient settings have already done so over the past decade, the macro–cost savings associated with the shift itself have already been worked through the system. What is left? The myriad micro–cost savings that industrialization of the outpatient delivery system will yield.

Another factor driving the push toward health care industrialization is the emergence of consumerism. As Richard Scrushy, founder and chairman of HealthSouth, the largest operator of outpatient surgery centers in the United States points out, "it's time for health care standardized protocol and treatment. If people like to go to Holiday Inns because they like the quality, that's fine. That's what we're doing."[11] Scrushy's belief stems from the American consumer's recurrent market preference for predictability, stability, and quality control, hence the success of franchised food outlets.

Such preferences represent a compact between producer and consumer, one that accepts a certain blandness in taste for the elimination of the symmetrical extremes associated with taking risks. The approach may not be that breathtaking, but it quite literally reduces the likelihood of either extraordinary successes or spectacular failures. This principle of the consumer market's preference for driving everything toward the mean is readily applied to medicine. Jonathan Harding, in his discussion in *Physician Executive* of the use of "clinical guidelines," a key manifestation of health care industrialization, observes that "most patients will choose a proven recipe over risking an experiment that *could* result in a better outcome, but is more likely to result in a worse one."[12] The typical consumer's general discomfort with science, combined with the notorious remoteness of physicians, does much to ensure a preference for predictability in the delivery of medical services.

Still another factor driving the push toward health care industrialization is the rapid introduction—but highly uneven adoption—of new medical technology. Stoline and Weiner identify one of the major flaws in the system for working new medical breakthroughs into the health care delivery system. "No standardized process for the evaluation and incorporation of new technology into medical practice exists: it usually occurs in an unscientific, unplanned way. All too often, new medical technologies are applied before their cost, safety, and usefulness are adequately considered."[13] While this is a problem in and of itself, it is particularly problematic in the context of Porter's views on innovation as an industry matures: "The relative importance of process innovations usually increases in maturity, as does the payoff for designing the product and its delivery system to facilitate lower-cost manufacturing and control."[14] This is a *de facto* formula for describing the impetus behind the wholesale industrialization of health care—the quintessence of which can be described as full-scale "process innovations"—as we move into the new century.

ANALOG DOCS IN A DIGITAL WORLD

The industrialization of health care is enabled by the sudden proliferation of tools and technologies for analyzing large repositories of patient data. The growing availability and reliability of such resources are the keys to Wennberg's work; they allowed him and his colleagues to look both broadly and incisively at medical practice patterns around the United States. Payers work extensively with databases in an effort to control costs by identifying "outlier" providers, i.e., those whose medical, surgical, and other utilization patterns vary from empirically derived norms or targets. As Stoline and Weiner argue, "in the era of cost consciousness, variation in clinical decision making is not well tolerated by payers. It supports to some extent the contention that some practice patterns cost too much and that costs can be reduced by identifying efficient practice patterns as well as adequate (though not excessive) levels of care."[15] While payers have the clearest vested interest in moving quickly to mobilize the information resources central to health care industrialization, these resources are every bit as useful—and are becoming every bit as business-critical—to health care providers as well.

As risk is shifted to providers, so too do the economics associated with identifying and eliminating excessive utilization and variability. Providers' use of such resources resembles many of the efforts of payers, but generally in much greater clinical detail. *This is the result of the superior richness of the underlying operations-level data streams available to providers—an important strategic advantage for providers, given that payers generally have access to only financial-level (claims) data.* At a given point in time, the degree to which a provider organization engages in such activity reflects almost precisely where that provider sits on the continuum of reimbursement reform. Under global package pricing, the provider seeks only to minimize variability of costs per case; under full capitation, the provider seeks to minimize total disease incidence and total costs per person. As the logical end-point of reimbursement reform is full risk-assumption under capitation, it clearly offers the greatest financial incentives for reducing total variability. Under capitation, providers are motivated to manage a population's health, not just treat its illnesses.

As Deming would be quick to observe, the variations that flourish across the health care industry—and are only now coming to light through emerging information resources—are *not* the "fault" of physicians. Rather, they are the fault of a system that, until recently, did not have the incentives to discover these problems—and thus had not created a viable marketplace for the tools and technologies required to mobilize these resources. Yes, physicians have been working in a vacuum of the health care industry's own making. But how quickly they choose to leave that vacuum is their decision, or at least the decision of the organizations in which they participate.

Unfortunately, many in the medical profession have not been quick to embrace the great leap of progress for the industry embodied in the development and use of databases and statistical methods for identifying variations in practice patterns. It would be easy to attribute this reaction as part of providers' general disdain for the source of the "digitized" scrutiny, i.e., the MCOs, whose use of these valuable analytical tools can readily be viewed, fairly or not, as so many more bludgeons of utilization management and care denial. It would also be easy to write off this resistance to bad timing: these tools and technologies are emerging amidst a broader professional crisis imposed upon many physicians by myriad and growing pressures of an industry undergoing transformation. But there is historic precedent for this reaction, this perception by physicians that empirical analysis of their clinical practice patterns is a threat, an unprompted criticism. In the past, reactions to such efforts have often been swift and unpleasant.

The earliest attempt to rationalize and standardize care dates back to the turn of the century, to the work of Ernest Avery Codman, a Boston surgeon and professor at Harvard Medical School. Codman proposed the development of a system for tracking the outcomes of surgical patients, one that correlated treatment choices and approaches to patient functional status at subsequent points in time.[16] While precisely this type of system underlies nearly all of the now-emerging medical outcomes measurement methodologies, for proposing such a system in 1910 Codman was ostracized, professionally and socially. His idea was so threatening to the unassailability and hallowedness of his fellow medical professionals that he was forced out of Harvard Medical School and Massachusetts General Hospital. He finally resorted to opening his own fledgling hospital as a laboratory for his idea, only to be derailed permanently by a combination of debts and service in World War I.[17]

Many physicians are just as incensed today about the tracking of their outcomes. As with the thrust of Codman's work, the very activity implies variability not only in decision making, but also in skill level. Luckily, many more physicians today embrace what is one of the most profound of all health care reforms: the introduction of empirical analysis to every physician's practice. (My personal experiences educating physicians in the tools and technologies that facilitate empirical measures of individual clinical behavior is illuminating: physician acceptance of the movement tends to vary inversely with age, income, discomfort with information technology, and insecurity with clinical performance.)

Regardless of the motives and reactions of physicians, the industrialization of medicine is reversing decades of professional self-determination. Starr points out that as American medicine evolved, "physicians maintained the integrity of their craft and control of the division of labor. While medicine itself became highly specialized, the division of labor among physicians was negotiated by doctors themselves instead of being hierarchically imposed upon them by owners, managers, or engineers."[18] But such impositions are inevitable as health care transforms itself from a cloistered folk art to a hard-headed, professionally managed business. Physicians who oppose the many and varied strains of health care industrialization resent the "intrusion" into their artisanship, quibble over its methods, and actively dispute whether any empirical analysis of medical decision making is even possible.

But the very difficulty of conducting meaningful, standardized analysis only serves to underscore the necessity of doing so, at least according to a broader principle developed by Porter: "The benefits of a standard of comparison are most important in industries where accepted standards for product quality and service are not apparent, where a wide range of cost/quality tradeoffs are possible, and where buyers would be more prone to price sensitivity in the absence of perceived differentiation."[19] One of the reasons industrialization has been promoted most aggressively by payers is the desire to standardize quality measures, neutralize the perception of differentiation, and thus focus the industry on price, all for the ultimate goal of reducing health care costs. While perhaps inadvertent, resistance to such efforts by physicians to this end is a good instinct, while price-driven payer organizations remain in control of the purchasing market.

Such resistance to efforts at standardization is not helped by physicians' clinical training, which for the most part dictates caution, skepticism, and circumspection. As Stoline and Weiner observe, "clinicians are strongly attached to a traditional method even when the superiority of a new technique or approach is clearly demonstrated. Staying with the known practice and its known properties seems safer than taking the risks that accompany change, yet the costs that result from such inertia can be high."[20] This inertia has been broken by the economics of managed care, which does not tolerate high costs of any kind. Managed care's cure for this inertia has been swift and severe: take the patients elsewhere.

Once again, we have economic determinism working its charms, making the industrialization of health care both visible and inevitable. As every type of health care organization, including all those on both the for-profit and not-for-profit side of the aisle, begin to act more businesslike in their battles over premiums and patients in a dynamic marketplace, industrialization is a cultural inevitability. Studies have shown that leaders of investor-owned hospital systems rely more heavily than the community systems on hard numbers: complications rates, patient satisfaction scores, outcomes, etc.[21] As established earlier, the behaviors of these leaders sets the tone for entire markets, and the health care business in general evolves into a more "business-like" culture. And there is nothing a "business-like culture" craves more than predictability of operations, costs, and outputs. The strenuousness of physician resistance to health care's industrialization—which cannot prove but futile in the end—merely underscores the belatedness of the movement itself.

THE NUMBERS GAME

One of the key elements of health care industrialization is *quantification*. A central tenet of Deming's teachings on quality, productivity, and industry development is that "productivity does indeed improve as variation is reduced."[22] The application of Deming's principles to health care is extremely complex, and involves a multitude of academic and professional disciplines: medicine, biostatistics, industrial engineering, microeconomics, epidemiology (the analysis of disease patterns), nosology (the analysis of disease, procedure, and patient classification systems), and actuarial science (the analysis of the costs of disease and procedures). The goal of these efforts is to bring Deming-style production methods, which seek to find the most statistically reliable and cost-efficient way to produce any good, to health care.

While many take issue with—indeed, are often offended by—the notion that industrial production methods can be applied to the delivery of medicine, Deming himself would probably not be shy in applying his views to the industry. He would refer to excessive surgical utilization, unusually high-cost cases, or substandard outcomes as "production defects." And, as he points out, "defects are not free. Somebody makes them, and gets paid for making them."[23] Regardless of clinician sentiment, those leading the managed care revolution would consider any variability in medical delivery as just such "defects." Every utilization management tool and technique introduced by MCOs in the past decade originates from this core idea.

This idea first manifested itself as utilization review, the ongoing analysis of past physician and hospital activity that drives much of utilization management going forward. Utilization review involves the search for what Deming would probably describe as "medical performance outside the boundaries of statistical control." For medicine, this means that for a normalized population (i.e., a population adjusted for age, income, race, and clinical and physiologic conditions), there are hospital admissions, surgeries, complications and deaths from surgeries, total costs, and other measures that diverge from norms in ways that are both measurable and statistically significant. Utilization review mobilized these analyses in their crudest form. As Stoline and Weiner point out, "to the extent that feedback from utilization review induces outlying or non-conforming physicians to modify their clinical decisions, it can be used as a mechanism for quality assurance as well...however, by stiffening criteria and disallowing reimbursements when established standards are not met, utilization review becomes a cost-control measure."[24] Regardless of the nobility of its origins and usefulness of its other applications, utilization review has proven to be an outdated and cumbersome system. It is commonly and often correctly perceived as punitive and adversarial, as nothing more than a tool for identifying "bad" doctors and "bad" hospitals.

If utilization review were a true tool of Deming-style methods, it would seek out *under*utilization as vigorously as it does *over*utilization. Variability is a symmetrically negative phenomenon: falling *below* statistical norms for care delivery indicates a great, if not greater, failure of the system; it means that a population is not receiving adequate care—not enough preventive, curative, palliative, or rehabilitative services—a situation that may prove even more costly in the long run. Unfortunately, with 20 percent of their memberships turning over every year, few MCOs are motivated to invest in systems that improve care over the long run.

There is another key failing specific to medical utilization review that Deming himself unwittingly describes when discussing the failing of quality assurance generally: "Unfortunately, the function of quality assurance in many companies is too often to provide hindsight, to keep the management informed about the amount of defective product produced week by week. What management needs are charts to show whether the system has reached a stable state (in which case management must take on the chief role for improvement), or if it is still infested with special causes."[25] The most progressive forms of utilization review have evolved to precisely this level: they automate much of the surveillance of providers, seeking only the true statistical outliers in the aggregate rather than micromanaging every provider and every case. But such systems are still the exception rather than the rule; and their development is slowing rather than accelerating as utilization review becomes less relevant in an industry converting to risk-assumption, leaving the payer with little financial incentive to conduct such surveillance.

In general, such legacy utilization review is ultimately fruitless because it violates one of Deming's key principles about individual versus systemic reform. "The aim of leadership is not merely to find and record the failures of men, but to remove the causes of failure; to help people to do a better job with less effort."[26] Though this should describe the essence of the relationship between utilization reviewer and clinician, it is a far cry from the current antagonisms that characterize the process. As Stoline and Weiner observe, "most payers will continue to consider low users as their point of reference, arguing that high users should conform unless they can make a strong case to the contrary."[27] This approach is confrontational and ultimately self-defeating, and represents only a crude first step on the long road to the industrialization of health care.

It is not the recognition of the ham-fisted quality of utilization review, but rather the emergence of risk-assumption—with its emphasis on *total* per member costs—that is compelling the shift in health care industrialization from management of all medical services to the management of population-based patterns of care. The more enlightened MCOs and their risk-sharing providers have displaced line-item utilization review with tools for controlling variation, adverse outcomes, and high costs in the aggregate, across the full treatment system. They do so through the introduction of aggressive prevention and intervention strategies, the use of protocols and treatment guidelines, and the development of epidemiological-based analyses of care delivery. This next generation of industrialization is perfectly consistent with Deming: "The type of action required to reduce special causes of variation is totally different from the action required to reduce variation and faults from the system itself."[28]

BEST DEMONSTRATED PRACTICES

Consciously or not, health care has absorbed Deming and deployed his methods in ways that are at once consistent with his views and unique to medicine. A core element in current health care industrialization is the use of empirical benchmarks known as "best demonstrated practices." These represent statistically correlated clinical choices and results that are superior in terms of cost and outcomes to statistical norms; at the same time, they are still readily achievable, generally defined by standard deviations above the mean result or percentile breakpoints above the median result. Best demonstrated practices become the benchmarks against which all clinicians are measured and toward which all should strive. "Anyone out of control on the good side is there for reasons that need study," Deming writes in *Out of the Crisis*. "He may use methods or motions that other people could learn and thereby improve their performances...Discover which people if any are out of control with respect to the group. If anyone is out of control on the side of poor performance, investigate the circumstances—his eyesight, tools, training—and take any remedial action indicated."[29]

Deming's formulation for improving industry in general applies with elegant specificity to health care. Best demonstrated practices can be identified; then communicated through the information tools that are the key drivers of health care industrialization; then in turn emulated throughout the medical delivery system. As described by Kenneth Ackerman in *Integrated Health Care Delivery:*

> Well-defined standardized care protocols and clinical indicators may begin to be developed for systemwide use. Thus, physicians will be better equipped to monitor the performance of their peers and, as a result, take corrective action when necessary. This will undoubtedly result in real economies of scale. In addition, it may prove to be even more beneficial if the system owns its own managed care program, which enables it to do its own quality review, its own utilization review, and ultimately develop its own protocols.[30]

This whole process, as Ackerman makes clear, is facilitated best by provider systems that are fully vertically integrated. This is one more argument for ownership, rather than looser forms of integration. As Stoline and Weiner point out, "the involvement of practicing clinicians in this process [of protocol development and variance measurement] is critical, because they have technical knowledge to contribute and also because they will be the ones to implement any resulting decisions."[31] And what better way is there to engage the physicians than through ownership stakes in the EHO?

As protocol proliferation and measurement is automated and distributed through the EHO, only specific variations in care are triggered for inquiry. This is a far cry from the enormous duplicative efforts of managed care's inquiry into every encounter between provider and patient. It also describes the very industrial maturity that Deming idealized in anticipation of the full consummation of his methods:

> In the state of statistical control, all special causes so far detected have been removed. The remaining variation must be left to chance—that is, to common causes—unless a new special cause turns up and is removed. This does not mean to do nothing in the state of statistical control; it means do not take action on the remaining ups and downs, as to do so would create additional variation and more trouble...The next step is to improve the process, with never-ending effort. Improvement of the process can be pushed effectively, once statistical control is achieved and maintained.[32]

This statement embodies the theoretical underpinning of the total quality management movement that grew out of Deming's work. As applied to health care, it perfectly describes the process of continuous quality improvement.

An interesting side note: Deming wrote next to nothing about the health care industry specifically, focusing most of his research and writing on manufacturing. Nonetheless, he accurately foresaw the value of industrializing health care, a wholly inconceivable notion in 1982 when he wrote that "construct[ing] operational definitions of special causes of unfortunate results from medical interventions of various kinds...is a huge task, and a never-ending one, but until it is brought to a usable stage, physicians in the United States, and their insurance companies, will continue to fight off unjustified accusations of carelessness and will live a life liable to legal tangles."[33] Remember that in 1982, the most pressing issue in health care was not cost, access, or managed care: it was medical malpractice litigation. Then as now, standardization of care—perceived as a threat by many physicians today—is paradoxically a physician's best defense against the unreasonable expectations of the hopelessly ill patient.

A "GOOD MEDICAL OUTCOME" BY ANY OTHER NAME

One of the more significant impediments to the industrialization of health care is that of semantics. Few in the industry can agree on numerous key concepts, even the most simple: what is "quality" in health care? What is a patient "outcome?" Deming himself has pointed out the contingent nature of an industry's agreement on standards before reform of that industry's practices can proceed. "An operational definition of safe, round, reliable, or any other quality must be communicable, with the same meaning to vendor as to purchaser, the same meaning yesterday and today to the production worker."[34]

While this difficulty is hardly insurmountable, those most vigorously opposed to the forces of industrialization readily use it to invalidate those forces. Instead of focusing on the task of improving health care delivery, they thwart all the critical discussions, analyses, and conclusions to be gained through industrialization over these simple ground rules. Indeed, it will take 5 to 10 years for the various disciplines that are essential to the process of health care industrialization simply to reach a full agreement on definitions of what is measured and how. If this seems like too excruciating a wait, we need to recall that most of the industry has been struggling with these definitions in earnest for only the past 5 to 10 years.

There are similar problems associated with methodologies. Much of the analyses described above are, of necessity, drawn from retrospective or existing streams of patient data, most of which are gathered for reasons other than to analyze clinical decision making (e.g., for financial analysis, inventory control, or other purposes). Such data clearly do not have the scientific or statistical purity of data gathered specifically and prospectively for the purposes of isolating and studying clinical decisions, i.e., the types of data captured to support a regulated drug or device clinical trial. In the current first wave of industrialization, retrospective data are being leveraged for the process of studying physician practice patterns and patient outcomes, a practice rife with the potential for statistical problems. There are numerous methods designed to cope with these problems, with hugely variable effectiveness and credibility. This too is an issue identified by Deming: "Change the method of sampling or the method of test and you will get a new count of defectives in a lot, and a new process average. There is thus no true value for the number of defective items in a given lot, and no true value for the process average."[35] As with the problem of semantics, many use this issue as the spoiler for the entire movement, thus hoping to avoid the insights and accountability inherent in its conclusions.

The health care system is currently in the process of sorting through these and other problems associated with the nascent field of health care industrial analysis. A few key principles are, however, already emerging: as one example, the tools and technologies for analyzing retrospective medical data, though typically developed and distributed by private companies, clearly need to be made available to the academic and research community for peer review, for their confirmation and successful acceptance by the medical community. Medicine is a science, and the methods mobilized to improve its performance must be as rigorous as the science that has husbanded all of its progress to date.

Galvanizing these methods—e.g., standardizing their measures—is still very much a work in progress. Unfortunately, much of it is forced to proceed through manual fixes, while the standards evolve almost accidentally, often through attrition among the opposing voices. Deming has observed that "the framework of standardization provides greater clarity of expression between all the parties concerned and is much more flexible than the 'consultation' process of regulation-making, where the number of people that take part is strictly limited."[36] Consultation, however, like medical training in general, is still the primary mode for delivering and educating the medical community on industrialization's new methods and findings; it will remain so until standards are fully accepted and information technology is better integrated into the clinical setting.

These obstacles notwithstanding, the industrialization of health care will be the next wave of innovation in medicine. In *Competitive Advantage*, Porter argues that this is typical of any industry's natural evolution as it moves from "product innovation" to "process innovation":

> As an industry matures, product designs begin to change more slowly and mass production techniques are introduced. Process innovation takes over from product innovation as the primary form of technological activity, with the aim of reducing the cost of an increasingly standardized product...As product design stabilizes, increasingly automated production methods are employed, and process innovation takes over as the dominant innovative mode to lower costs.[37]

The industrialization of health care is the sum total of the tools and technologies that will drive its myriad process innovations moving forward. It will define the progress of the coming decades of medical breakthroughs—the same way that application of the principles of infectious disease ruled the first third of the 20th century, surgery the middle third, and new generations of breakthrough drugs the final third.

TAKE TWO ASPIRIN AND CALL THE 800 NUMBER IN THE MORNING

There is no more profound a "process innovation" in health care than the emergence of automated triage systems. Such systems route patients to the most appropriate level of care and, in many cases, actually resolve their acute but benign medical conditions. The late 1990s has witnessed the rise and rapid proliferation of "telephonic triage," which seeks to eliminate the unnecessary use of physicians and emergency departments for a host of ultimately "non-event" medical events. Such non-events include colds, simple fevers, allergy attacks, bone bruises, muscular strains, heart burn, and indigestion. Nonetheless, millions of patients with "disorders" no worse than these consume billions of health care dollars every year.

The economics of telephonic triage are self-evident: under the traditional system, a patient experiences symptoms and goes either to the emergency department, which diagnoses, treats, and admits or releases the patient; or the patient goes to his or her "primary care physician," who diagnoses and either treats or sends the patient on to a specialist. Both systems are highly inefficient: it has been estimated that 30 percent of patients who visit the emergency department every year could have gone to an outpatient physician office for the same diagnosis and treatment, and another 20 percent needed no medical attention at all.[38] This number is galvanized by separate estimates that, for many patient segments, telephonic triage systems will reduce emergency department visits by up to 50 percent.[39]

Telephonic triage systems began as medical education systems for the community, and were sold to providers as an outreach tool rather than to MCOs as a cost-reduction initiative. Patients could call a toll-free number and question nurses about their symptoms, receiving recommendations about self-care, and whether or not they should seek medical treatment. Repositioned as a managed care tool with the potential for drastically reducing medical utilization and costs, these systems quickly mutated into medically complex, aggressive technologies. Leveraging the growing sophistication in "expert-systems" and "decision-support" systems—two levels of computer-based tools that replicate the diagnostic path followed by clinicians—telephonic triage systems have evolved rapidly from simple medical advice tools to actual medical screening and diagnostic programs.[40]

Putting a rational, low-cost mechanism at the very front end of the treatment system dramatically reduces utilization. Such a mechanism for Colorado's Medicaid system allows Medicaid patients to avoid the emergency department—the traditional "clinic" for much of this population—while educating them about the managed care procedures necessary to seek care under the state's program. The adoption of such systems by both public payers and private MCOs has occurred in a few short years and is predicted to blanket the United States in another few.[41]

A premier example of such a program in place for an MCO is the "Fourth Generation" system, developed by Health Systems International, an MCO acquired in 1996 by Foundation Health Plans. Deployed throughout its networks, the Fourth Generation system

- uses sophisticated decision tree analysis of patient symptomology (e.g., "does the pain increase or decrease when you walk up the stairs?");
- integrates symptom assessment with on-line access to the patient's medical history, enrollment, and utilization information, primary care physician data, etc.; and
- routes the patient to the most appropriate care setting, which can range from primary care physician, directly to a specialist, to the emergency department, or simply to bed.[42]

This key element in the industrialization of health care delivery is flourishing so rapidly not because it is trendy and "tech-sexy," but because of the very clear return on investment associated with a technology solution that precludes billions of dollars in medical service consumption.

The goal of these systems is obvious: to minimize utilization of the second highest cost component of the health care system, the physician. (Hospitals are the highest.) With such systems in place, both telephonically and live within the medical clinic itself, according to Montague Brown, "managed care patients face even greater behavioral modification exercises. Such patients learn early on that an advice nurse intercedes to check things out initially. Past the advice nurse may be a nurse practitioner or physician assistant. Since most patients present themselves to physicians with self-correcting problems, this may be the primary contact with the system for many."[43] Such systems represent a key element of industrial rationalization across a vertically integrated system.

Full implementation of these systems will have a profound impact on health care costs in the long run. They will allow the MCO (and eventually the EHO) to staff less for every "patient-perceived need,"[44] and more for their true medical needs. As any physician who has treated patients in a busy emergency department will tell you, the difference between the two is significant.

INDUSTRIALIZATION'S BOTTOM LINE

The economics of industrialization are indisputable. If nothing else, the simple attainment of predictability brings its own financial rewards—especially in a world of fixed revenue and risk-assumption. This is proven nowhere more powerfully than in the inverse: medical costs under the old fee-for-service system were completely unpredictable for all but the largest populations, hence the cost problems for self-insured employers, which sought the quickest fix by handing risk over to the first generation of MCOs. As for those MCOs, the notion of predictability becomes particularly relevant as medical risk-assumption emerges as the only remaining medical product sold by providers.

But even in the absence of risk-assumption, as consolidating payers drive down prices and payments, managing costs becomes the critical success factor for the EHO. As Porter indicates, this is typical of any maturing industry: "a quantum improvement in the sophistication of product costing is necessary to allow pruning of unprofitable items from the line...The need to rationalize a product line sometimes creates the need to install computerized costing systems, which had not been of high priority during the industry's developing years."[45] This describes without qualification a key process at work in health care today, as providers seek to rationalize operations and costs that for decades evolved and expanded with little regard for long-term viability or sustainability.

In the continued absence of risk-assumption in a less evolved local health care market, the process of industrialization is less important for surviving current market conditions, but every bit as critical from the perspective of strategic sequencing. Adopting these methods now, in advance of the sea change that will occur under managed care's risk-assumption end-point, will prepare providers to advance to new stages of contracting. Indeed, it may give a provider in an unsophisticated managed care market an enviable first-mover advantage. As Scott MacStravic writes in *Health Care Strategic Management,* "to master price cutting, master cost cutting first. Where costs can be minimized well in advance of price cutting, providers can build up reserves that will help them survive price wars, particularly if their competitors have no such reserves."[46]

Of course, cost-cutting can often be an expensive proposition. Industrialization leverages the sudden ubiquitousness of information technology in health care and other industries, but such technologies are not cheap. Like the consolidation of health care facilities and physicians, the formation of integrated systems, and the assumption of medical risk, the process of industrialization described in this chapter requires substantial investment capital. And investment capital requires the promise of profitability. Thus, industrialization as a force compels still more consolidation, which is driven by the need to accumulate development capital; at the same time, it helps accelerate the emergence of a "business culture" within health care.

None of this is a coincidence. Technology, economic development, and cultural change have been interrelated phenomena since the invention of the plow. Stoline and Weiner describe the convergence of information technologies and health care industrialization most eloquently: "When the computer's ability to store and process vast amounts of information is added to human judgment, the best of technology can be combined with the best of the healer's art."[47] The "downside" of this observation, of course, is how easily technology accelerates competition, where little had existed because of problems of standardization and comparison. The more information people have, the faster they can act upon it, improve, profit, and leverage this competitive advantage—but so too can the competition, rendering such advantage painfully ephemeral.

As competition and industrialization are closely linked through the enabling power of information technology, so too does industrialization evolve, symbiotically, with the advent of full risk-assumption. Under risk-assumption—with providers rewarded financially for keeping patients healthy rather than treating them when they fall ill—the eventual acceptance and full embrace of many of the technical innovations described in this chapter will result in the greatest paradox of all: *physicians will be driven, by their own financial self-interest, to create and support systems that measure their own performance, reduce variability, and promote treatment paths where they themselves are the providers of last resort.*

Now *that's* health care reform.

REFERENCES

1. J. Bigelow's speech to the Massachusetts Medical Society in 1835, as cited in the Dartmouth Atlas of Health Care, American Hospital Association, 1996, 114.

2. J. Wennberg, "Which Rate Is Right?" *New England Journal of Medicine*, 30 January, 1986, 311.

3. A.M. Stoline and J.P. Weiner, *The New Medical Marketplace: A Physician's Guide to the Health Care System in the 1990s*, (Baltimore: The Johns Hopkins University Press, 1993), 144. © 1993. The Johns Hopkins University Press.

4. R. Pozen, "Companies in Action," *Managed Healthcare*, February 1998, 41.

5. Stoline and Weiner, *The New Medical Marketplace: A Physician's Guide to the Health Care System in the 1990s.* © 1993. The Johns Hopkins University Press.

6. S. Lutz and E.P. Gee, *The For-Profit Healthcare Revolution* (Chicago: Irwin Professional Publishing, 1995), 154.

7. R. Blumenstein, "Auto Makers Attack High Health-Care Bills with a New Approach," *Wall Street Journal*, 9 December, 1996.

8. Blumenstein, *Wall Street Journal.*

9. Blumenstein, *Wall Street Journal.*

10. S. McEachern, "Orthopedics One of the Easiest Product Lines To Integrate," *Health Care Strategic Management*, February 1996, 21.

11. A. Sharpe, "Medical Entrepreneur Aims To Turn Clinics into National Brand," *Wall Street Journal*, 14 December, 1996.

12. J. Harding, "Cookbook Medicine," *Physician Executive*, August, 1994.

13. Stoline and Weiner, *The New Medical Marketplace: A Physician's Guide to the Health Care System in the 1990s*, 147.

14. Adapted and reprinted with the permission of The Free Press, a Division of Simon & Schuster from *COMPETITIVE STRATEGY: Techniques for Analyzing Industries and Competitors* by Michael E. Porter. Copyright © 1980 by The Free Press. p. 243.

15. Stoline and Weiner, *The New Medical Marketplace: A Physician's Guide to the Health Care System in the 1990s*, 152–153. © 1993. The Johns Hopkins University Press.

16. A. Donabedian, "The End-Results of Health Care: Ernest Codman's Contribution To Quality Assessment and Beyond," *The Milbank Quarterly*, 22 June, 1989.

17. Donabedian, *The Milbank Quarterly*.

18. P. Starr, *The Social Transformation of American Medicine* (New York: Basic Books/HarperCollins, 1982), 220.

19. Adapted and reprinted with the permission of The Free Press, a Division of Simon & Schuster from *COMPETITIVE ADVANTAGE: Creating and Sustaining Superior Performance* by Michael E. Porter. Copyright © 1985 by Michael E. Porter. p. 204.

20. Stoline and Weiner, *The New Medical Marketplace: A Physician's Guide to the Health Care System in the 1990s*, 148. © 1993. The Johns Hopkins University Press.

21. Study of hospital governance practices conducted by the American Hospital Association and Ernst & Young, and reported in *Modern Healthcare*, 23 February, 1998, 44.

22. W.E. Deming, *Out of the Crisis* (Cambridge, MA: MIT Center for Advanced Engineering Study, 1986), 3.

23. Deming, *Out of the Crisis*, 11.

24. Stoline and Weiner, *The New Medical Marketplace: A Physician's Guide to the Health Care System in the 1990s*, 97. © 1993. The Johns Hopkins University Press.

25. Deming, *Out of the Crisis*, 134.

26. Deming, *Out of the Crisis*, 248.

27. Stoline and Weiner, *The New Medical Marketplace: A Physician's Guide to the Health Care System in the 1990s*, 167. © 1993. The Johns Hopkins University Press.

28. Deming, *Out of the Crisis*, 309.

29. Deming, *Out of the Crisis*, 251.

30. F. Ackerman, "The Movement toward Vertically Integrated Regional Health Systems," in *Integrated Health Care Delivery: Theory, Practice, Evaluation, and Prognosis,* ed. M. Brown (Gaithersburg, MD: Aspen Publishers, 1996), 39.

31. Stoline and Weiner, *The New Medical Marketplace: A Physician's Guide to the Health Care System in the 1990s*, 154. © 1993. The Johns Hopkins University Press.

32. Deming, *Out of the Crisis*, 321.

33. Deming, *Out of the Crisis*, 485.

34. Deming, *Out of the Crisis*, 277.

35. Deming, *Out of the Crisis*, 280.

36. Deming, *Out of the Crisis*, 299.

37. Adapted and reprinted with the permission of The Free Press, a Division of Simon & Schuster from *COMPETITIVE ADVANTAGE: Creating and Sustaining Superior Performance* by Michael E. Porter. Copyright © 1985 by Michael E. Porter. p. 194.

38. W. Bell, "Telephone-Based Demand Management," *Health Care Strategic Management*, February 1996, 6.

39. "Providing Telephone Advice from the Emergency Department," American College of Emergency Physicians, *Policy Resource and Education Paper*, 8 April, 1997.

40. Bell, *Health Care Strategic Management*, 6.

41. "Strategic Notes," *Health Care Strategic Management,* July 1996, 4.

42. From a research report on Health Systems International by Volpe, Welty & Company, 22 July, 1996, 20.

43. M. Brown, "Commentary: The Economic Era: Now to the Real Change," in *Integrated Health Care Delivery: Theory, Practice, Evaluation, and Prognosis*, ed. M. Brown (Gaithersburg, MD: Aspen Puiblishers) 53.

44. Brown, *Integrated Health Care Delivery: Theory, Practice, Evaluation, and Prognosis*, 53.

45. Adapted and reprinted with the permission of The Free Press, a Division of Simon & Schuster from *COMPETITIVE STRATEGY: Techniques for Analyzing Industries and Competitors* by Michael E. Porter. Copyright © 1980 by The Free Press. p. 42

46. S. MacStravic, "Price Wars Are No-Win Games for Health Care Systems," *Health Care Strategic Management,* May 1996, 20.

47. Stoline and Weiner, *The New Medical Marketplace: A Physician's Guide to the Health Care System in the 1990s*, 163. © 1993. The Johns Hopkins University Press.

PART III

PROGNOSIS

Charles Darwin's law of survival of the fittest, and that the unfit do not survive, holds in free enterprise as well as in natural selection. It is a cruel law, unrelenting.

W. Edwards Deming
Out of the Crisis[1]

What does all this equal? What will the typical health care market look like when the five forces of health care system transformation have finished coursing through its tissues?

Part III will attempt to figure out just that, by putting the five forces detailed in the previous chapters into the same analytical petri dish, stirring, and creating a coherent description of the U.S. health care system when the transformation is complete.

To many, the resulting vision will seem like an apocalypse of sorts: the end of a glorious age of modern medicine, borne of boundless optimism, fueled by once-unlimited money, and unchecked by the normal rules of the marketplace, let alone common sense. The sober new system left in its wake will seem an egregious and immoral encroachment on scientific and clinical hegemony by the mean-spirited, lower-order concerns of economics: a repeal—without the due process of public policy debate—of medicine's mandate to explore all scientific possibilities, free of any criticism of its methods, inefficiencies, or inequities. To others, this author among them, the foregoing vision describes a belated course correction of a fundamentally good system finally tripped up by its unsustainable idealism and self-indulgence, a system confronting for the first time the laws of economic finitude, reason, and restraint.

Regardless of the moral judgment we are all entitled to, the foregoing vision is the extrapolation of what I believe to be an awesome, invigorating moment in health care—as the most intimately human and critical 15 percent of the world's largest economy plays out precisely the same drama that has shaped most of the rest of that economy. As a culture that has endured and survived for the most part the caustic lessons of managed care, we are finally finding that most delicate of balances—how to mobilize the best medicine in the world, in the smartest possible way.

THE EMERGING HEALTH CARE ORGANIZATION

As introduced earlier, the end result of all the horizontal consolidation and vertical integration of health care providers will be the rationalization of previously fragmented local markets. What was characterized by dozens of unorganized, occasionally competing, but mostly coexisting players, is slowly coalescing into two to four unified business entities. Lutz and Gee predict that "by the end of 1998, there will be very few large markets with more than three systems. Even many of the midsize markets will have consolidated to only two or three competing networks."[2] Such "networks" will consist of physician/hospital/continuum alliances of varying degrees of formality that, for the remainder of this book, will continue to be described as "EHOs."

The term "EHO" is chosen not because it is more accurate than the slew of other acronyms meant to describe integrated health care systems. Rather, in a description of pure market evolution independent of any other agenda, the term seems to be the most politically neutral: it does not specify tax status, nor does it carry the already considerable baggage heaped on other acronyms of the moment like PSO, for "provider-sponsored organization," a hot button in recent Medicare reform debates. "EHO" is also pointedly neutral with regard to specific legal/capital/ownership structure, transcending all the legally nuanced distinctions among physician-hospital organizations (PHOs), independent practice associations (IPAs), MSOs, etc., that, in the end, are useful more for keeping lawyers employed than physicians productive. The market will surely sort out these early-stage models, and state and federal legislation will slowly bring some clarity to the various legal obfuscation currently afflicting decisions about ownership, conflicts of interest, and the like. Hence the use of the term "emerging." One structure—probably a hybrid of the service-fee–based MSO and equity-driven foundation—eventually will come to serve as the dominant model.

Great Leap Forward or Backward?

There is an argument that the dominant model EHO may simply be the staff model HMO—fully remodeled for the health care consumer generation. Because of capital and market incumbency, critical mass nationally (if not locally), and the sheer inertia of benefits purchasers, the EHOs developing in today's markets could all eventually be ensnared through the backward integration of today's health plans, rather than the forward integration into the insurance function by providers.

Luckily, common sense, current trends, and hard experience all indicate that such a possibility is highly unlikely. Because they represent the only truly manageable costs in the health care system, it is much easier for providers to forward-integrate into insurance, than it is for insurers and MCOs to backward-integrate into care provision, if only for cultural reasons. Kaiser has been attempting this all along and, as a result, has lagged its competitors in terms of enrollment growth during most of the years that total MCO enrollment grew the fastest. As a belated defensive strategy, Kaiser introduced an option that specifically broke with its backward-integration model: a point-of-service plan in 1996. This finally jump-started its growth and spared the MCO from further losses in terms of relative share. But it has signified the beginning of the end for all insurer-based, closed-model MCOs. (Humana suffered precisely the same problem in the late 1980s, though its problems were exacerbated by the fact that it was a minority player imposing fairly radical managed care changes on a mostly indemnity world.)

The general difficulty for payers in their effort to backward-integrate and assume the role of the EHO is part of a broader business phenomenon, described by Watson in *Integrated Health Care Delivery*: "Ownership and backwards integration create exit barriers that 'trap' firms in industries that may cause destructive competition and reduced profits."[3] In a typical health care market, it is extremely difficult for a traditional payer to manage providers "backwards"—particularly given all the other emerging options for physicians that offer far greater freedom, and cultural conscience, than becoming captive of an insurer-owned EHO.

Market Rationalization

In today's typical local market, the rudiments of EHOs are engaged in a bewildering variety of contracting situations: some are captives or near-captives of managed care operators; others contract with a plethora of MCOs, preferred provider organizations (PPOs), and traditional insurers; others contract directly with purchasers and the government under experimental Medicare and Medicaid programs. The result is a market free-for-all, a hodgepodge of relationships between purchasers and EHOs that not even the most vigilant of local executives can keep straight. While direct-contracting continues to struggle through an awkward adolescent stage, the primary market battles today consist of EHOs fighting for the lives still controlled by the MCOs. They do this primarily through hard selling to the MCOs and soft selling to consumers.

This utter proliferation of arrangements—and the fact that the EHO is, by definition, an emerging phenomenon—certainly explains the current chaos of the health care system, the befuddlement of physicians and patients, and the massive administrative burdens daunting everyone. But consolidation is slowly transforming markets into segments; it is sorting EHOs by cost structure and the cultural heritage of its most visible hospitals. The end result is a market positioning by each EHO relative to the three product-market segments described later in this chapter. This transformation will continue as

- markets firm up and consumers become aware of the emerging two-to-four party structure;
- the EHOs amass working capital, pick up market momentum, and mature organizationally; and
- the EHOs eventually gain the market leverage necessary to dictate price terms back at the national MCOs.

When this process is complete, each competing EHO will be defined by its unique market and price positioning. These factors will be either directly associated with, or affected by, the degree to which the local EHO is affiliated with one or more national organizations like Tenet, Daughters of Charity, Columbia, Catholic Healthcare West, PhyCor, MedPartners, Integrated Health Services, or

HealthSouth. Each individual EHO will be characterized by the origin of its flagship sponsoring institution:

- the heavily branded for-profit national hospital company;
- the low-cost national or regional religious hospital system;
- the community-engaged local not-for-profit hospital system; or
- the prestigious academic medical center.

Some markets will have one or more of each and every type; others will have one or more of some types and none of another. The ultimate structure depends on the unique histories and regulatory environments of the markets and their host states.

Inevitably, there will be an "upmarket" EHO built around the leading local academic medical center or institution of similar cache. This EHO will serve as a constant differentiation check to the price-positioners and will market heavily based on an association of its reputation and heritage with higher quality. Price-positioning against the upmarket EHO by the other EHOs will be underwritten by ownership or affiliation with a national corporation like Tenet or MedPartners. This association will give the midmarket and downmarket EHOs significant buying and selling power, prepackaged marketing programs, and the capital necessary to create infrastructures to compete against each other and against the upmarket quality-positioner.

This association will also provide what may prove to be the most critical success factor for the EHO in the new century's health care system: *the intellectual property that is the lifeblood of health care industrialization.* Such intellectual property will consist of all the industrialization elements discussed earlier in this book, including an understanding of how best to integrate and coordinate the delivery of care; methods of eliminating variations in clinical decision making; and all the medical "informatics" tools, control systems, and organizational designs necessary to support care delivery and optimize resource consumption under risk-assumption.

Each EHO will be integrated with all the insurance functions necessary to manage full medical risk-assumption. As risk-assumption emerges as the only medical service bought and sold, capitation rates will come to represent the only currency flowing from purchasers to providers—either directly from employers and consumers, or indirectly through the remains of the national insurers, MCOs, and other payers. To the bereavement of no one but their last generation of shareholders and middle managers, the MCOs will be systematically reduced in terms of scope and size to a combination of marketing and reinsurance vehicles. With their handful of real innovations in population and medical management fully woven into the fabric of health care financing and delivery across the United States, the MCOs' once lofty missions will be reduced to shuttling enrollees from national employers, small businesses, and individual households into local EHOs and paying via capitation. Medical risk management will play out at the provider level, insured against catastrophic losses for specific cases and in the aggregate by the MCOs themselves.

When reduced to reimbursing providers in lump-sum, capitation-based risk dollars instead of millions of discounted fee-for-service payments for tens of thousands of medical services, MCOs as organizations will be trimmed back to fit precisely the same role of the insurers of old. They will comprise a dull, bureaucratic oligopoly of financial management firms, their profits derived not from managing medicine but from managing investments. Their margins will be governed even more tightly by market conditions and the classic underwriting cycle than the old insurers ever were, given the constant presence and market alternative of direct contracting by EHOs at the local level.

Few physicians, hospital administrators, nurses, social workers, allied health care professionals, or researchers—not to mention patients—will mourn this turn of events.

THE CUSTOMER IS ALWAYS RIGHT

What drives the rationalized market described above are the needs, preferences, risk tolerances, and price sensitivities of consumers. How patients perceive, purchase, and consume medical products and services ultimately drives real reform of the health care system. This concept—still disturbingly new and radical to a trillion-dollar industry built on the premise of unlimited, undifferentiated third-party reimbursement by employers and the government— is critical to understanding the emergence of the new century's health care system.

The differentiation of individual EHOs within local markets, while following a classification established on the supply side of provider evolution, is enabled only by growing differentiation on the demand side, as consumers grow older, wiser, sicker, more skeptical about managed care, and more informed about their medical choices—and as they shoulder an increasing proportion of the financial burden associated with their health care. This differentiation has been creeping into benefit design and financing for a generation, with the emergence of "cafeteria" plans, copremiums, and flexible spending accounts. The health insurance function has served merely to match the demands of these designs and implement their differentiation most efficiently.

The end result of nearly any consumer differentiation movement is product-market segmentation—precisely the same phenomenon described in the rationalization of the local health care market. How will this segmentation play out? Given both the inexorable movement to convert the Medicare and Medicaid programs into privately managed systems, and the persistent preference for a pricier, less restrictive alternative to the traditional, access-control-driven MCO, segmentation will emerge and solidify as a three-tiered system. This system, which resembles much of the benefit-design tiering already in place, will be segmented as follows:

1. An upmarket EHO, which provides unlimited choice and mobility within the EHO's network (and access to "out-of-EHO" providers), and involves substantial direct-to-consumer marketing. This EHO's "plan" will serve as a major perquisite for employees—either across the board at high-end employers

who foot the entire bill and use this as a recruitment/retention strategy, or as a benefits-differentiator within organizations for higher-end employees.

2. A midmarket EHO, which allows for more choice regarding access to specialists, nonstandard procedures, preferred drugs, and other discretionary resources, at added out-of-pocket cost to beneficiaries, but which generally defaults to managed care–type controls and the EHO's network. In this plan, the onus for utilization review is placed on the patients, who will have to confront any nonstandard medical options with their own personal cost benefit—because they will be paying for it out-of-pocket. If they place sufficient value on truly discretionary medical treatment or the use of out-of-plan treatment options, they will have to pay for them. This will be the most popular alternative with most employees in insured groups, and will probably result in the largest EHO. Not coincidentally, it most resembles the financing and operation of today's popular point-of-service (POS) plan, with its ownership transferred from insurer to provider.

3. A downmarket EHO, which is driven by cost, is fully funded, and offers no treatment or physician choices. This plan will offer cut-rate premiums for standard coverage, feature the lowest payment scales for providers, and offer no out-of-network coverage.

All three options will be available to Medicare-eligible beneficiaries through Medicare risk-contracting. Passed into law in 1997 as part of more comprehensive Medicare privatization legislation, the government's new plan allows for beneficiaries to purchase full coverage directly from provider-based health plans, or PSOs. The plan allocates a fixed amount per beneficiary per month; the beneficiary is free to "buy up" from that coverage for better benefits and more expensive plans. This arrangement mirrors what occurs under an employer's "cafeteria" plan, with its floating contribution toward the health insurance premium that the employee can choose to enhance (though the sacrifice of other benefits or larger contributions) for richer coverage or not.

Similarly, larger employers and business purchasing coalitions will also offer all three plans. The lowest tier will comprise a baseline level of coverage; employees and their families will have the option to "buy up" from this baseline coverage. Smaller employers will offer the midmarket and downmarket options. Medicaid will offer only the downmarket option.

The lower and middle tiers will be cost driven and the source of intense competition. EHOs will be pitted against each other to win this business by minimizing total medical costs for purchasers and their national MCO middlemen. The highest tier will seek to differentiate itself, placing the most prestigious teaching hospital in town at its helm, tirelessly promoting its research and quality data, and recruiting elite physicians. The divergence of its costs will be held in check somewhat by its likelihood of remaining not-for-profit, and thus resembles the market positioning of the traditional Blue Cross/ Blue Shield plans.

THE FREEDOM TO (PAY TO) CHOOSE

The main differentiating currency in the market described above will be *choice,* not only of physicians—who become captive of each EHO and who therefore become the spearhead of segmentation— but of specific care choices available to a plan's members: longer hospital stays; access to nonroutine, investigative, or elective procedures; branded versus generic drugs; and other discretionary care choices. This luxury of choice, which follows naturally the way indemnity plans are now considered luxury plans, will be purchased at a premium

- directly by consumers for what they perceive as quality;
- by high-end employers who will offer this premium benefit as a major job "perk"; or
- for high-end employees at large firms seeking to differentiate compensation using benefit design strategies.

As a consequence, this emerging market will complete a movement, already underway since the late 1980s, from uniform benefit
plans and treatment access to differentiated benefits and access. Here,
the health care product market is segmented like any other offered up
in a consumer-driven market in a pluralistic economy. People will
approach health care purchasing like they approach buying cars:
some will have the money and inclination to drive a Mercedes; others
will be happy (or reluctant) to drive Fords; and still others will be
forced by frugality or economic misfortune to take the bus.

It isn't pretty—take it up with the economics professor who told
you capitalism was supposed to be. But it works, it is consistent with
our cultural preferences, and it guarantees, at bottom, the provision
of necessary medical coverage (for those inside the insurance system). It also illustrates what the MCOs have tried to point out for a
decade: freedom to choose any physician, of any specialty, for any
treatment you need (or think you need), is a luxury the system cannot
afford. If you really want this kind of premium access, then you are
going to have to pay for it yourself.

Within the cost-constraints set by this segmentation of benefit
funding, consumers will follow their physicians. As discussed earlier, people value their right to choose "their" personal physician
above all else. This then serves as the crucial differentiator for EHOs
in the market described above. As the MCOs quickly unravel and
allow members access to virtually all physicians in a community—
either through their growing POS plans or through a broadening of
their provider panels to the point of liquefaction—the managed care
industry systematically undoes one of its founding organizational
principles. This undoing of MCO control is a response to consumer
market demands, hence the proliferation of the terms "freedom" and
"choice" in numerous new MCO products. It is accelerated in the
direct marketing of the rudiments of EHOs, which typically promise
care by "its doctors and hospitals *regardless of who your insurer
is.*"[4] Such promises represent the triumph of the provider over the
payer—as consumers vote with their feet and force the plans to adapt
accordingly.

This is the road to a truly consumer-driven health care system, one in which patients follow their doctors, and the rest of the system falls in behind. Even after all the tools of industrialization and labor rationalization are in place at the EHOs—elements of care automation such as telephone triage, the use of physician assistants, etc., developed and disseminated by the MCOs—people will still pick the EHO plan that offers the physicians they want. *If* they can afford the luxury, that is. As physicians join one of the EHOs competing for patients within a market, so flow the capitation dollars associated with their patients' choices. These capitation dollars—continuously calculated by their physician's EHO to cover their likely medical needs—will echo back to those patients in the form of market prices.

Among many in health care who have lived through premature versions of this vision, the notion of a market divided along the fault lines of exclusive alignments between physicians and EHOs sounds like a bad idea all over again. Behind this reaction are numerous, well-publicized difficulties with—and outright failed attempts at—the creation and management of exclusive contractual relationships between hospitals and physicians in the late 1980s and early 1990s, through the "physician-hospital organization" or PHO model. But in contrast to the consummate EHO described in this book, the typical PHO sought to tie physicians up with stand-alone, predominantly inpatient facilities, long before the horizontal consolidation of hospitals and vertical integration of services within the PHO's host market had occurred. In evolutionary terms, the PHO model was an amphibian in a world still covered entirely by ocean. Unlike the hospitals at the helm of the early PHOs, EHOs consist of coordinated networks of stand-alone, system-affiliated, or chain-owned hospitals, all of whom by definition have already worked through the difficult process of rationalizing both horizontal capacity and vertical delivery.

With only two to four EHOs constituting a typical market, the exclusive alignment of physicians is not nearly as drastic or divisive as it sounds. In fact, it is really just a formalization of the traditional custom of "hospital privileges." Under the old system of privileges, the typical physician maintains a working relationship with only one-fourth to one-third of the hospitals in a market. Patients had their surgeries and delivered their babies at one of the hospitals where "their" physician maintained privileges. The sorting of physicians and hospitals embodied in this custom is fully echoed in the EHO's more formalistic structuring of the market. This structuring, however, does not occur in keeping with the traditions and politics associated with gaining hospital privileges, but rather along the market battlefield lines of consumer choices and price preferences.

MLR PLUS: THE EHO'S NICE PRICE

The prices that the fully realized EHOs present to the national HMOs, PPOs, indemnity insurers, and other third-party payers will constitute the medical loss ratio or "MLR" traditionally borne by these payers. (The MLR is the percentage of a covered group's total insurance premiums consumed by all the fees paid by the payer for medical services and products consumed by that group: physician fees, hospital charges, prescriptions, and other costs.) The prices that EHOs present directly to employers will be the same MLR they offer the national MCOs and other payers, plus additional costs for administering the integrated health plan: sales, enrollment management, stop-loss insurance, pharmacy benefit management (PBM), and other commodity-like plan administration services.

The EHOs can already buy these services with great ease and increasing bargaining power on the open market, often from the MCOs themselves. An example of this in an earlier incarnation was United Healthcare's Diversified Pharmaceutical Services—originally the PBM servant of its own MCO business—which it subsequently built into the third largest commercial vendor of PBM services before selling it to SmithKline Beecham for $2.3 billion in 1994.[5] An example of this today is the decision in 1998 by both PacifiCare and Humana to launch products that will help EHOs administer direct risk-contracts for Medicare beneficiaries. With competitors like this, who needs allies!

As incredible as it is to believe, MCOs have been and continue to be perfectly eager and willing to cannibalize their own future, by creating and vending services that merely empower EHOs to contract around them. Thus, it is useful to introduce another term, the Post-MCO (P-MCO). The P-MCO anticipates the devolution of the national managed care company into the next generation indemnity insurer described in the previous section. The P-MCO is what remains of a national MCO after relinquishing control of care delivery by pushing medical risk down to providers. The P-MCO is reduced to an organization that merely vends its sales, general, and administrative (SG&A) functions to EHOs organized from the ranks of its former medical contracting providers. SG&A represents the overhead or infrastructure costs included in an MCO's gross margins. The MCO uses this infrastructure to manage the MLR and the rest of its plan's packaging for employers and the government. These elements are essential to managing any population's health care financing and delivery.

Until the transformation of the health care industry is complete, the national MCOs will continue to compete against each other and the EHO direct contractors with their current insurance products. But the inevitable slowing of their growth through market saturation—and through market share gains by the "substitute good" offered by the direct-contracting EHOs—will force the managed care companies to search for new revenue sources. This search will inevitably and increasingly take the form of P-MCOs selling their SG&A, at ever more commodity-like prices, which in turn will exacerbate their competitive dilemma and accelerate the MCO industry's wholesale erosion toward P-MCO status.

In this context, the economics of the direct contracting EHO grow more and more compelling. The EHOs will find it ever easier to win business away from the MCOs because they can price at the same MLR they currently offer to those very MCOs, buy only bare-bones versions of the SG&A built into the MCOs' gross margins at competitive prices, and offer better final premiums to employers and the government. Why? Because the EHO's profit margins are already built into the MLR. Unlike the national MCOs, the EHOs do not need to mark up the SG&A to generate the operating and net margins that justify their existence as middlemen.

National MCOs can match the EHO's price only through significant buying power on the SG&A. What they take out in operating margins they must at least make up in cost advantage on the SG&A, making any price advantage between themselves and the direct-contracting EHO a wash. The inevitable result of this dynamic: the eventual market price or premium for a covered life will be driven down to the medical loss ratio plus reduced cost SG&A. Figure III–1 illustrates the comparative cost components of the direct-contracting EHO and the national MCO.

The pricing realignment in a health care market driven by these new dynamics (MLR plus commodity-priced SG&A, offered by EHOs directly or with MCO layers) represents the best possible out-

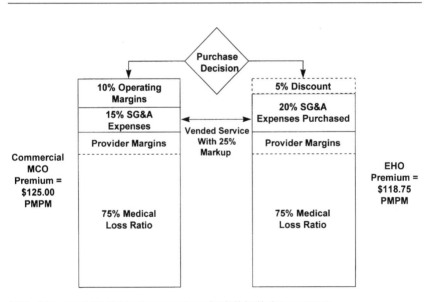

SG&A—Sales, general, and administration expenses associated with health plan management
PMPM—Per insured individual member per month
All data are hypothetical

Figure III–1 The Economics of MCO versus Direct Contracting.

come from the perspective of pure economic philosophy: *the process is market driven and results in no onerous profit-making.* Profits are kept in check by competition among two to four dominant EHOs—and between the EHOs and what is left of the MCOs. Insurance premiums will be a direct reflection of true medical costs, which in turn will accelerate the drive for continual innovation in meaningful cost reduction, process improvement, prevention (where it pays), and all the other elements of health care industrialization by large, well-funded, risk-bearing provider organizations.

This is consistent with the EHO's culturally derived focus on managing medicine by its provider-sponsors—a major reform from the MCO's obsessive focus on managing money. In the rationalized market described in this chapter, the only moving part in the machine is what gets delivered for the MLR. This is the mechanism by which the innate structure of a local health care market emerges in the new century's health care system—a structure based on segmentation by price, product differentiation, and customer satisfaction.

CHOOSY CUSTOMERS

In the new century's health care market, out of what has been a monolithic delivery system, will emerge a much more discretionary system, one segmented along a continuum of price and perceived quality. As described above, consumers will approach health care purchasing as they do other expensive goods.

The Mercedes model will resemble the positioning of the Blues indemnity and managed indemnity plans in today's markets. Traditionally, Blues plans have been open-ended with regard to physician selection and utilization. Members generally have not been required to pay coinsurance or deductibles for inpatient care. As a result, Blues policyholders have typically paid higher premiums.[6] These premiums would be still higher of course, if not for the unusual not-for-profit charter of the Blues plans, with all profits reinvested in the plan rather than paid out to shareholders. Blues plans are also well positioned because they have lower SG&A cost structures, spending only 11.2 percent of premiums on administrative expenses in 1995, versus 25 percent for the typical commercial insurer or MCO.[7] These advantages will continue to keep pricing for the Blues plans well within the tolerances of the high end of the market; unless the trend toward for-profit conversions turns out to be the rule rather than the exception and Blues plans, as a consequence, end up trading down their unique cost advantages for whatever broader competitiveness they believe they can win with the additional capitalization.

Because the richer plan design of the Blues goes hand in hand with the upmarket EHOs' positioning of clinical superiority, it is inevitable that these entities align themselves in the typical market. Such an alignment hearkens back to another historic precedent of provider-driven insurance plans. According to Starr, "the standard response of physicians in a community was to organize a more generous service-benefit plan...in order to compete more effectively with Kaiser."[8] This underscores an opportunity for a combined Blues plan/upmarket EHO to position itself above the pack and market itself not so much to purchasers, but to those consumers who will pay a premium above baseline for the perceived quality and prestige of these systems, in addition to the flexibility of an indemnity-like plan.

There are already numerous examples of this segmentation in action. Across the nation, Blues plans are taking advantage of the occupancy downdraft created at major teaching hospitals by low-cost–seeking MCOs. The plans are winning previously unthinkable discounts in exchange for patient volume at these name-brand hospitals. This helps to keep the hospitals afloat while offering Blues members access to the most prestigious facilities. In 1996, on the eve of hospital deregulation in New York state, Empire Blue Cross and Blue Shield entered into an exclusive deal with the renowned cancer center, Sloan-Kettering Memorial, a quick counterpunch to Salick Health Care's sudden entry into the New York market with its cut-rate prices for cancer care at St. Vincent's.[9] According to a report in the *Wall Street Journal,* "aligning itself with a premier medical institution that has a great cachet within the medical community gives [Empire Blue Cross] a new prestige."[10] This is a prototypical example of coming market differentiation: a high-end plan teams up with a prestigious teaching hospital; a price-cutting "carve-out" like Salick goes with the lowest-bidding community hospital.

Standing in sharp contrast to the positioning of the upmarket EHO (proposed marketing pitch: "because there is nothing more priceless than your family's health") will be the positioning of the midmarket and downmarket EHOs along the dimension of better value (proposed counterpitch: "quality health care you can afford"). The competition within and across segments will be extraordinarily complex, as the midmarket and downmarket EHOs compete with each other both for the business booked by national plans and directly with those plans for purchasers' business. Unwittingly, the national MCOs have created much of the momentum for this market differentiation, a trend they will accelerate through continual restrictions in care delivery choices—either overtly or through their familiar cycle of denials, dissatisfaction, and defections. As they attempt to drive down the MLR with lower capitation rates, the only EHOs willing and able to accept them will be the downmarket ones. As the Blues plans cleave to the upmarket EHO, the low cost MCOs go in the other direction.

The MCOs will patently avoid the high-end EHO, the cost of which will be prohibitive after factoring in the plan's SG&A. The high-end EHO thus is forced to market itself more quickly and aggressively to purchasers and consumers, its higher MLR offset by its lower SG&A and absence of net margins associated with that overhead. As the market develops, MCOs are thus pushed downmarket, forced by their SG&A expenses and margin requirements to work more exclusively with only the lowest cost EHOs, while competing with each other with diminishing value-added products. This merely accelerates their downward spiraling toward P-MCO status: as risk flows to the EHOs, along with ever greater cost pressure, the growing EHOs are emboldened (and eventually empowered and capitalized) to figure out a way around them. For the MCOs this will prove a transitory strategy as they push more lives toward the low-end EHO, and the middle-tier EHOs break from the pack to market directly. This will become increasingly easier as those EHOs connect with the national hospital systems and/or physician practice managements (PPMs).

As the MCOs mutate toward P-MCO status, their missions will shrink to marketing EHOs, processing their data, and providing them with reinsurance. The economics of these low-growth, low-margin activities will compel numerous business combinations among the already consolidating MCOs. At that point, such mergers will be more strategically defensive than offensive; the only products left for the former MCOs to sell will be commodity services, the profitability of which will rise and fall with the underwriting cycle.

As this process unfolds, the MCOs will be reduced to an echo of their formerly lofty ambitions to manage care. They will, early on in the new century's health care system, have devolved into businesses that closely resemble the indemnity plans they elbowed past only a short generation ago.

EVOLUTION OF A MARKET

Figure III–2 represents a market in the "Alpha" stage through which most major U.S. markets have already passed in the last few years. EHOs have yet to emerge among the market's still unorganized community of hospitals, physicians, and outpatient facilities. As a result, all of the providers' business flows haphazardly from a community of consolidating payers.

In the alpha stage market, the bargaining power of buyers is increasing. With no organized resistance from providers—who have yet to consolidate horizontally or integrate vertically—competition increases to the detriment of the providers. Most hospitals are still stand-alone, not-for-profits; with the exception of the teaching hospital and academic medical center, they have similar cost structures.

Figure III–3 represents the same market in the "Beta" stage. As a community progresses through this stage, the rudiments of EHOs

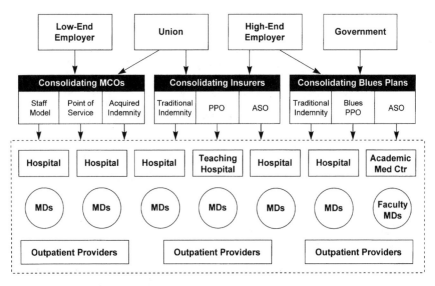

Figure III–2 Local Health Care Market—Alpha Stage.

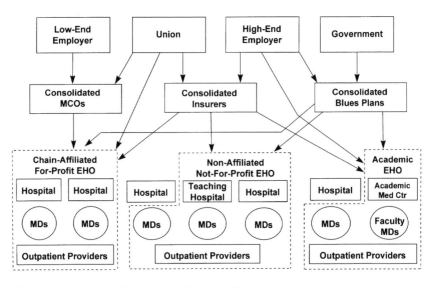

Figure III–3 Local Health Care Market—Beta Stage.

begin to form, and experiment with direct contracting. These still nascent "health systems" eventually fall in line with two of the three types of generic competitive strategies that Porter codifies in *Competitive Strategy*: cost versus differentiation.[11] The two hospitals remaining outside the EHOs will either close or be purchased by the EHOs and converted to outpatient and/or subacute facilities.

At this stage, which characterizes most urban markets around the United States as of this writing, EHO formation is accelerated by the entrance of a for-profit hospital chain and/or PPM. These chains have directly inspired—and indirectly spurred—rapid consolidation of the market's hospitals and the rudimentary integration of these with large numbers of physicians. While the cost economics associated with the national chains vary tremendously by individual market (hence numerous conflicting findings on the subject), in this particular market the national chain aligns with the lower-cost facilities and positions itself accordingly; in response, the not-for-profit EHO positions itself for the middle of the market. Armed with expertise from corporate headquarters, the chain-affiliated EHO enters into a direct contract with a handful of local unions.

Having been cut off from much of the commercial population due to the shuttling of patients to lower-cost hospitals by MCOs, the academic medical center forms its own EHO (academic-EHO, or A-EHO). Marketing its brand name to the high-end employers in town, it enters into a few direct contracts, as much to learn as to profit from them. Losses on these fledgling deals will represent cheap tuition for the A-EHO when the market moves onto the next phases. The A-EHO is also holding onto much of its Medicaid business, a legacy of its location in the inner city, which has yet to be converted to managed care.

Figure III–4 represents the market in the "Gamma" stage. The consolidation and streamlining of the payer and provider communities have allowed all employers and unions to greatly simplify their health care benefits of financing and purchasing. They provide baseline coverage and allow their employees to choose their coverage from a variety of MCO plans, from what remains of the tradi-

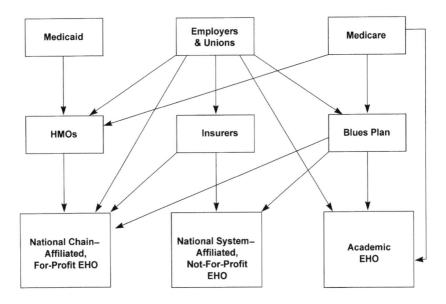

Figure III–4 Local Health Care Market—Gamma Stage.

tional insurers, or directly from plans sponsored by the downmarket, for-profit EHO or upmarket A-EHO.

Medicare is abandoning three decades of government control and now mimics private-employer financing and delivery, offering beneficiaries everything from traditional indemnity coverage through the Blues administrator, which provides access to all providers in the market, to a variety of much more affordable direct coverage plans from all three EHOs. The Medicaid population has been rolled into a managed care plan, representing a sizable revenue loss for the A-EHO for everything except emergencies.

The midmarket EHO has aligned with a national not-for-profit system. As a result, it enjoys numerous purchasing and marketing advantages that match those enjoyed by the low-end EHO through its inclusion in a for-profit chain, preparing it for direct marketing to employers.

MCOs and insurers both lose significant market share to the two direct contracting EHOs.

Figure III–5 represents the market in the final "Zeta" stage. Insurers have retreated from the market, along with most of the MCO capacity. Their more entrepreneurial managers have salvaged the best elements of their infrastructures, transforming themselves into vendors of informatics systems, medical management programs, and reinsurance services.

The not-for-profit system-affiliated EHO has finally entered into direct contracting with employers, based on its recent risk-contracting experience with, paradoxically, the much more difficult to manage Medicare population. As the new lowest cost producer in the absence of an external insurance layer, this formerly midmarket EHO begins growing market share at the expense of the for-profit EHO.

The Medicaid population now moves exclusively through the "social HMOs." These are the natural outgrowths of the not-for-profit MCOs of the same description that have been servicing Medicaid since the program first moved in to embrace managed care. These

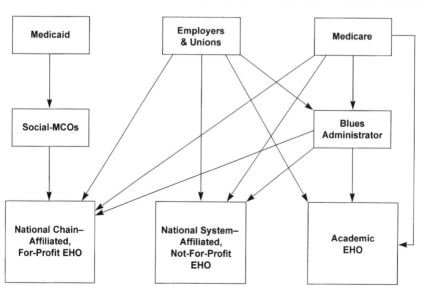

Note: Most HMOs and all traditional insurers have departed market; now service-vendors to EHOs.

Figure III–5 Local Health Care Market—Zeta Stage.

social HMOs will increasingly start to mimic quasi-public community health agencies; and they will continue to exist as they add social service components to the total medical care delivered to the Medicaid population.

In the unique case of this market, the for-profit chain is the recipient of the Medicaid population's business, even though it is not the lowest cost producer. It does so because the midmarket EHO is affiliated with a Catholic religious order, and thus cannot provide all the services needed by the Medicaid population. This is an accident of history for this market, and can easily be reversed by marketplace forces here and elsewhere.

A HAPPY (IF PARADOXICAL) ENDING

As the discussion on "MLR-plus" pricing revealed, in the fully realized health care market, MCO profits will disappear. Competing EHOs will earn only what economists refer to as economic "rents" for their efforts, defined as normalized rates of return that characterize competitive markets. As a consequence, the economics of health care markets will come to resemble the economics of public utility markets. As utility rates, until only recently, have been regulated by the government and the presence of substitute goods (i.e., natural gas, oil), so too the market for health care services will be regulated by direct government purchasing from the EHOs at the rate of the MLR plus SG&A and from the presence of substitute goods (i.e., the MCOs).

These profits or rents will be defined by the cost of capital—the same way nominal profits built into regulated utility rates were defined by interest costs and stable dividend payout ratios required to float the utilities' shares on Wall Street. *This is precisely the idealized market-based system envisioned by many of the more government-heavy reform proposals, in particular the infamous Clinton Plan of 1993–94.* The crucial difference is that the market evolved to this simple, elegant end point on its own, a feat that a bumper crop of new government planning probably would not have accomplished.

Even more paradoxically, the eventual utility-like nature of the typical health care market will inevitably drive away the bulk of the profit-seekers and entrepreneurs currently revolutionizing health care delivery as discussed in earlier chapters. Just as managed care—the once harsh medicine for a desperately ill system—is now destined to fade away when the cure is complete, so too the profit-seeking visionaries who introduced radical concepts in alternative site care delivery, information systems, telephonic triage, and medical management will see their window of opportunity slowly close.

Indeed, the profit-seekers whose "intrusions" into health care have prompted such scorn from those favoring a publicly run system will depart from a market-based system whipped into better shape than they found it—and in far better shape than any monstrosity borne of the central planners' imaginations.

REFERENCES

1. W.E. Deming, *Out of the Crisis* (Cambridge, MA: MIT Center for Advanced Engineering Study, 1986), 155.

2. S. Lutz and E.P. Gee, *The For-Profit Healthcare Revolution* (Chicago: Irwin Professional Publishing, 1995), 152.

3. S. Watson et al., "Owned Vertical Integration and Health Care: Promise and Performance," in *Integrated Health Care Delivery: Theory, Practice, Evaluation, and Prognosis*, ed. M. Brown (Gaithersburg, MD: Aspen Publishers, 1996), 75.

4. Television advertisement by Helix Health Care, Washington-Baltimore media market, March 1997 campaign.

5. E. Tanouye, "Value of Some Drug Firms' Acquisitions Is Questioned," *Wall Street Journal*, 11 November, 1996.

6. A.M. Stoline and J.P. Weiner, *The New Medical Marketplace: A Physician's Guide to the Health Care System in the 1990s* (Baltimore: The Johns Hopkins University Press, 1993), 63. © 1993. The Johns Hopkins University Press.

7. L. Kertesz, "This Is Not Your Father's Blues Plan," *Modern Healthcare*, 14 October, 1996, 68.

8. P. Starr, *The Social Transformation of American Medicine* (New York: Basic Books/HarperCollins, 1982), 324.

9. L. Lagnado, "Famed Cancer Center Gives In to Managed Care," *Wall Street Journal*, 25 October, 1996.

10. Lagnado, *Wall Street Journal*.

11. Adapted and reprinted with the permission of The Free Press, a Division of Simon & Schuster from *COMPETITIVE STRATEGY: Techniques for Analyzing Industries and Competitors* by Michael E. Porter. Copyright © 1980 by The Free Press. p. 35.

OUTCOMES

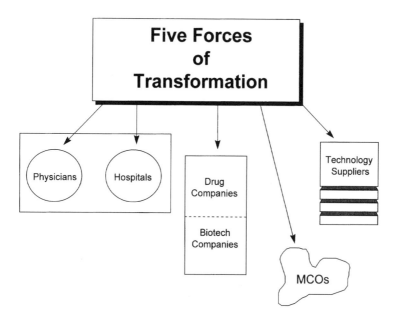

Part IV on "outcomes" focuses on how the inevitable if belated rationalization of the U.S. health care system through the five forces of transformation will affect various players. Each chapter of this part attempts to apply the lessons gleaned from the analyses of the previous chapters to an individual component of the health care system. Separate chapters are dedicated to the impact of the system's prognosis on hospitals, physicians, pharmaceutical companies, medical/surgical suppliers, and MCOs. In business generally and the health care business in particular (as in all things in life), there are neither threats nor opportunities; there is only change. How an institution or organization (or person) reacts to each change casts it, ultimately, as a threat or opportunity.

6

THE UN-HOSPITAL

Last year, we paid $1.6 billion in taxes and provided $1.2 billion in uncompensated care.

From the reverse side of former
Columbia/HCA business cards

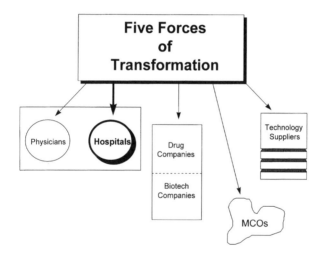

It was conventional wisdom by the mid-1980s that hospitals were the dinosaurs of the U.S. economy. They were barely profitable and tottering on the brink of extinction due to growing overcapacity and the sudden appearance of managed care. The end was only a few short years away: the introduction of less invasive versions of traditional surgeries would drive the bulk of patients to outpatient settings; major changes in the way the federal government reimbursed hospitals for Medicare patients would force hospitals to operate at a loss on a third of the patients remaining;[1] managed care would wipe out their profits on the other two-thirds. A decade later, hospitals are enjoying record profitability, they derive 37 percent of their revenues from outpatient services,[2] and they are aggressively building the EHOs that will spell the end of their managed care tormentors. However, it is still conventional wisdom that hospitals are dinosaurs on the brink of extinction.

No doubt many continue to jump to this wrongheaded conclusion if only because they have watched somebody try to manage a hospital today. Because of the constant change that swirls about them, the institutions as a class are slow to act, organizationally inert, and hopelessly bureaucratic. They are hobbled by a two-headed organizational structure—one administrative, the other clinical—that requires a constant, delicate balancing of physician and executive egos. The result is a continual struggle between those who champion better patient care at all costs and those who champion greater business efficiency—as if they were mutually exclusive goals. This bifurcated organizational design, unlike that of any other industry (except perhaps the MCOs, interestingly enough), guarantees turf battles at all levels over every aspect of hospital management. The resulting gridlock is typical of organizations with zero-sum-game budgeting.

But there have been a number of factors keeping hospitals afloat and prosperous, seemingly despite themselves and if only by default.

1. The rapid consolidation of capacity has held inpatient occupancy steady for the past decade, despite drastic reduction in lengths of stay and the migration to outpatient settings.
2. The noisy, aggressive rise of the for-profit systems has introduced the more hardheaded traits of a true business culture to hospital administration—among the for-profits and mirrored among the competing not-for-profits.

3. Reimbursement reforms adopted by Medicare and managed care have imposed cost disciplines on hospitals for the first time in their modern history.

Hospitals have also been helped mightily by their enormous power of incumbency. Inpatient services continue to be the single greatest health care expense, accounting for 40 to 50 percent of the typical MCO's medical costs and more than 50 percent of total federal spending on health care.[3] With this formidable economic pull on the system, hospitals have always had a knack for perpetuating their own existence. Historically, it was their ability to mold clinical practice to serve their own objective of maximizing inpatient resource consumption. As Starr notes, "the standard for hospitals was impervious to changes in medical practice, such as the growing belief in early ambulation instead of extended bed rest after surgery."[4] Today, it is the knack of hospitals—through a long-standing community presence—for controlling the flow of patients, even those thousands of patients who never cross the thresholds of their inpatient facilities. The persistent incumbency of hospitals flows in large part from a capital incumbency. Hospitals are central repositories for diagnostic and surgical technology, physician education and training facilities, community outreach resources, and research dollars. As a result, hospitals have invaluable contacts across a local market; they generate good will with the professional community, and they masterfully exploit the local media.

Hospitals have also responded well to the revolution in outpatient care. In 1991, for the first time in the history of modern American medicine, more surgeries were performed in outpatient settings than inpatient.[5] But hospitals were prepared for this statistical watershed well in advance: as usual, they took their cues from Medicare reimbursement rules which, starting in 1982, paid 100 percent of a physician's fee for ambulatory surgery, but just 80 percent for inpatient surgery for a large group of procedures, thus motivating patients to select outpatient facilities.[6] Employers have also been driving the migration to outpatient settings for obvious reasons. As the marketplace has evolved in general, hospitals have been forced to evolve in parallel; their responsiveness to the outpatient exodus serves as a model for the hospital industry's ability to adapt in the new century's health care system.

THE ACUTE CARE HOSPITAL AS ICU

The first step in exploring strategic options for hospitals in the new century's health care system is to take a hard look at the traditional hospital and ask, "what is left?" As the exodus to outpatient settings continues, acute care begins more and more to resemble intensive care. Patients still undergoing types of surgery major enough to require inpatient stays are stabilized after the procedure in the hospital, but are quickly transferred to lower-cost, subacute facilities for the longer recovery period and rehabilitation work that for generations occurred only in the hospital. Integrated Health Services and others have masterfully rushed to fill the void between the acute care setting and the patient's home; using fallow nursing home capacity, one day of "subacute" care costs a fraction of one more day in the hospital.

As a result, those patients left behind in the hospital are far sicker than in previous years, a fact that has been well documented using severity-of-illness measures.[7] This trend will continue as

- demographics make the average hospital patient older and sicker;
- new drugs are developed and marketed that extend the survival rates of patients who would have died a generation ago; and
- more aggressive treatments like chemotherapy and organ transplants create greater numbers of more physically compromised, chronically and terminally ill patients.

Thus, the pressure toward greater severity and higher per patient cost that may seem unique to the 1990s, a one-time event for the hospital industry, will actually prove to be a continuous process.

The only possible end to this upward spiraling of hospital patient acuity would be a collective, conscious turnabout in the way the majority of Americans confront the inevitability of the end of life. For now, as a culture steeped in optimism, fitness worship, and age denial—not to mention a limitless faith in the powers of technology—we view death as much a personal defeat as a personal loss. Because of our cultural refusal to accept death without every last ounce of fight, the acuity of hospital patients will surely rise for the foreseeable future.

Absent the transformation described in this book, the typical hospital's intensive care unit (ICU) would be its fastest growing revenue center. *Because* of the transformation described in this book, the typical hospital in the new century will have no revenue centers to grow at all, only cost centers. And as changes in the industry cannot change underlying cultural attitudes toward dying and death, the hospital's ICU is certain to be the fastest growing among these. In the new century's health care system, this growing disproportion of sicker and sicker inpatients will be accelerated not by patients' families, or managed care, or technology, but by the hospital itself. When hospitals cease to exist as hospitals *per se* but rather as key building blocks of EHOs, the most successful "hospital" will be the emptiest. The most prosperous hospital within a market will be the one with the fewest beds per dollar of revenue. Indeed, this very measure—beds per dollar—is a reversal of the traditional measure used to judge the financial performance of a hospital which, under the old fee-for-service system was rewarded amply for driving up its dollars per bed. The fully realized EHO will seek to drive *down* the same measure expressed in reverse—its beds per dollar. This ultimately will translate into fewer beds and fewer admissions under the fixed portion of the capitation payment allocated to the hospital. Successful reductions in the beds-per-dollar measure will thereby increase the hospital's and EHO's return on total assets.

The fully realized EHO increases the return on its assets by rewarding physicians with financial incentives for keeping patients *out* of inpatient facilities. (How deliciously ironic, after the millions of man-hours the government has invested in the promulgation, interpretation, and enforcement of laws barring hospitals from inducing physician referrals!) The results of such incentives are well documented across the literature. In one very typical study, physician practices with close ties to integrated health care systems reduced hospital days for MCO enrollees by 44 percent, from 269 to 151 per 1,000 members.[8] Other studies throughout the clinical and management literature have found precisely the same results, with reductions as dramatic.

Consistent with these economics and the notion of vertical integration in general, hospitals should seek to provide as little traditional "hospital care" as possible, and in its place provide as much nontraditional hospital care. They have all the leverage they need prebuilt into their market and capital incumbency: legacy relationships with purchasers, access to financing, research infrastructure, relationships with physicians, and information systems. Much of the typical hospital's clinical infrastructure is highly portable across the EHO's continuum of care. As an industry, hospitals need simply to respond as creatively and aggressively to the advent of risk-based care as they did to the outpatient exodus, but by another order of magnitude. A hospital, in short, should seek to become an "un-hospital," a community institution that seeks to keep people healthy, not just treat them when they fall ill.

"CONTINUUM CONUNDRUM," SAID THE CAT IN THE HAT

The vertical integration of what remains of inpatient hospital care with outpatient services, subacute care, ambulatory rehab, and home health care is not so much a bold reform of the health care system, as it is a belated correction of a historic accident. Paul Starr finds the origins of this fundamental problem manifesting itself early on in the U.S. health care system's development: "while corporations at the end of the nineteenth century became multi-unit operations, hospitals remained at an earlier stage of industrial development."[9] It has taken a full century to counsel the hospital industry out of this state of arrested development. As argued earlier in this book, the vertical integration of care is not so much a bold new move for the industry, but a bold fix for its traditional "dis-integration."

For patients and covered populations, ownership and successful integration of nonhospital clinical services represent a major reform of the system because they enable a long-needed coordination of the delivery of care. For hospitals, they are a classic business survival strategy. Why? Because outpatient surgery, subacute care, ambulatory diagnostic imaging and testing, and home health care services all represent substitute goods. Each is a service that was once either delivered on an inpatient basis, or was conducted only as an ancillary business for the hospital. But the economics of these substitute goods, delivered stand-alone, make a compelling case for hospital ownership of them: they are far cheaper than the inpatient services they displace.

This is consistent with Michael Porter's analysis of substitute goods: those that are the most critical strategically, he argues, are those that are "subject to trends improving their price-performance tradeoff with the industry's product, or are produced by industries earning high profits. In the latter case, substitutes often come rapidly into play if some development increases competition in their industries and causes price reduction or performance improvement."[10] This describes precisely what occurred following the seemingly overnight appearance and proliferation of both subacute providers and home health agencies: both offered significant price-performance improvement over inpatient care and thus generated initially high profits. These profits in turn attracted new entrants and drove down market prices for both types of new providers, thus making both even more of a competitive threat to inpatient services.

The rapid introduction and maturation of various types of outpatient providers—subacute and home health in particular—has spurred consolidations that have paralleled the consolidation of hospitals over the past decade. As discussed earlier in this book, Integrated Health Services (IHS) successfully "rolled up" a fragmented subacute care industry, emerging as the industry's largest provider of rehabilitation and other services for patients following their early discharge from full-blown acute settings. Because of consolidating MCOs and other purchasers who demanded "one-stop shopping"— not to mention flattening growth and profitability curves—IHS moved vertically in 1996 by purchasing Coram, which had rolled up an even more fragmented home health market. IHS is now one of the country's largest home care providers, serving patients from more than 1,000 sites in 47 states.[11] IHS's aggressive moves to own pieces of the continuum are paralleled by HealthSouth's 1997 acquisition of Horizon/CMS for $1.6 billion.[12] The deal combines the largest provider of outpatient surgery with the third-largest provider of re-habilitation services, providing a one-two punch of surgery and post-surgical rehab along the continuum.

The obvious strategy for a large, well-financed chain like Tenet or the Daughters of Charity would be to buy or align with a nonhospital chain like IHS or HealthSouth to solidify its grasp of the continuum in markets across the country. A combined Tenet and HealthSouth and/or IHS would create, overnight, the facility infrastructures for EHOs in markets across the country. But like the physician practice management companies—with their aggressive growth plans and associated high market valuations—IHS, HealthSouth, and the other nonhospital chains have grown too large and expensive for outright purchase by any of the national hospital chains. There is another problem: Columbia/HCA embarked on precisely this strategy, for all the right reasons. Unfortunately, with Medicare predominantly reimbursed on a fee-for-service basis for home health services, the chain has been accused of shifting costs from the inpatient business over to the home health business, to improve profitability on the former while pumping up the cost-plus reimbursement for the latter.

With the temptation to commit the same sins in the short-term neutralized by the misfortune that befell Columbia, the other hospi-tal systems should still pursue the same level of integration, for the same soundness of strategic reasoning. In so doing, they have three alternatives:

1. compete directly with the nonhospital chains through local acquisition/creation of nonhospital facilities in every market;
2. cooperate across the country through blanket deals with the nonhospital chains, an alternative increasingly described as "virtual" integration and one that is easy to set up, but complex to administer (and should be of particular appeal to the smaller chains still focused on inpatient care); or
3. match strategies to local markets, competing where their owned hospitals have developed the continuum and cooperating with the nonhospital chains where their hospitals are still inpatient focused.

Two of these strategic alternatives translate directly into options available to the locally owned EHOs that compete in individual markets with the chains. Given the parallel consolidations of hospital and nonhospital chains, local hospitals and their EHOs can:

1. compete against the national continuum consolidators with their own local version of the continuum, attempting to trump the trickle-down effects of the chains' national marketing clout in the EHO's local market; or
2. cut deals with the nonhospital chains for selected services in the EHO's market area, a local version of virtual vertical integration.

The utter magnitude of the strategic, operational, financial, and marketing uncertainties associated with these choices certainly underscores why hospitals have consolidated to their current degree and why they will continue at the same pace for the foreseeable future. In fact it is precisely the inevitability of this "continuum conundrum"—as health care moves at breakneck speed to integrate vertically—that drives a key observation of Lutz and Gee: "the question will not be whether to align with a larger network, but rather which network to choose…the issue is not whether a facility should select a for-profit system or remain independent, but whether it should select a for-profit system over another system in the market."[13] Indeed, how a hospital chooses to align itself with the continuum is not an optional next step for a network or EHO: it is a strategic imperative for perpetuating its existence in the new century's health care system.

IS THERE A DOCTOR IN THE CORPORATION?

The complications associated with a hospital's choices regarding integration with nonhospital facilities are mere trifles compared to the financial and legal complexities—not to mention egos, emotions, politics, and power struggles—surrounding that same hospital's options for integrating with physicians. Nothing less than a long, complex, uneasy history, characterized by stormy coexistence, stands between hospitals and physicians. Starr points out that both have always depended on each other, with the balance of power generally tilting toward the physicians. "The hospitals needed the doctors to keep their beds occupied," he writes. "In this context, as in group practice, the physicians' authority with patients and their strategic position in the system represented a resource that gave them power over institutions."[14] Much has changed in health care since the decades when this imbalance first arose, but not the imbalance itself. Patient primary relationships are still with the physicians. Under fee-for-service, this translated into referrals for the hospital; under risk-assumption, it translates into customers for the EHO.

The chronic uneasiness inherent in the physician/hospital relationship has suffered a number of acute flare-ups as consolidations of the two groups work their way through individual markets. The radical nature and coincidence of these parallel consolidations—combined with the blunt trauma rendered to both groups by the MCOs—are forcing hospitals and physicians to contemplate the once unthinkable after a century of standoffishness: integration. Integration has become "thinkable" now, if only because physicians and hospitals finally recognize that they will sink or swim together, thrown as they have been into the same turbulent, unforgiving waters of a self-correcting marketplace. As a reaction to the cost crises of the 1980s and early 1990s, government and private purchasers—directly and through their MCOs—have blamed both hospitals' and physicians' self-serving clinical behaviors, inefficient practices, and excess capacity as the main driver of their own health care spending woes. This is precisely why the purchasers turned the MCOs on them in the first place. This is why MCOs have been positioned as the enemy of both types of providers. And the enemy of my enemy is my friend, or so the thinking goes.

There is an ongoing and ferocious debate over the nature of hospital and physician integration. Should the EHO own, manage on an exclusive basis, or simply contract at arm's length with the physicians? This debate is complicated further by the prevalence of ridiculously antiquated but still intractable laws in numerous states against the "corporate practice of medicine," a legal device designed in the 1920s to prevent financial considerations from affecting clinical decision making. (The long view of history frequently provides us with a good laugh at the innocence and idealism of earlier generations, embodied in so many attempts to legislate away normal human behavior.) As a result of these archaic laws and the infectious uncertainty and anxiety of an industry as it crosses unfamiliar terrain, there is today a plethora of models of hospital/physician integration (staff, foundation, PHO, IPA, MSO, MOUSE, etc.), ranging from pure salaried and owned physicians at one extreme to open-ended contracting at the other. Because each model has been analyzed in depth in the industry literature, a repetition here would shed no new light on the subject, nor inform our selection of broader strategic choices and actions. Rather, it is better to ignore the specifics of legal form and instead develop a few abiding principles that will transcend all of them and thus surely outlast their continued mutation—still on a fee-for-service basis, of course—in the capable hands of the nation's attorneys.

Put simply, the economics and organizational challenges associated with developing and managing an EHO are too complicated for any arm's length arrangement with physicians. Between the EHO's hospitals and physicians, a marriage of some variety is essential. This may take the form of salary, salary plus quality and efficiency performance incentives, equity participation or, preferably, some combination of all three. But at rock bottom *the physicians must be captive if they are to be effective partners in the economics of risk-assumption.* Stoline and Weiner make the point rather bluntly: under full risk-assumption the physician who is "financially rewarded for performing a procedure on an inpatient basis in the end penalizes the hospital, which must pay for the institutional costs associated with the procedure out of its fixed payment."[15] Nonetheless, numerous forms of integration have failed to execute successfully, due to their inability or unwillingness to resolve this fundamental economic disconnect. This is the single most critical challenge facing those charged with developing and running an EHO.

Why? Because there is tremendous financial leverage associated with the proper alignment of physician and hospital incentives. This concept has been borne out in numerous studies of physician practice patterns under capitation, framed by two landmark studies in the *New England Journal of Medicine.* The first, published in 1989, found conclusively that the use of capitation as opposed to fee-for-service payments resulted in decreased hospitalization rates.[16] The second, published in 1995 and widely publicized, found that, for every 1,000 non-Medicare MCO enrollees in California, those whose physicians were paid under capitation spent 120 to 149 days in the hospital, compared to 232 for non-Medicare MCO enrollees across the state of California generally and 297 across the United States in 1993.[17] While the one-year difference between the study and comparison groups may account for some small fraction of the difference, it hardly explains this enormous gulf in inpatient utilization patterns.

Such a gulf in clinical behavior represents a gulf of money for a plan, its physicians, and its members. Hospitalization is and always will be the most expensive component of any risk-bearing entity's medical costs. The savings associated with modification of physician hospitalization patterns, via the proper alignment of their financial incentives, are consequently enormous. For the median California hospital in 1995, an inpatient day carried an operating expense of $1,359 after adjusting for higher wage levels in the state;[18] the reduction of 83 days per 1,000 members (a conservative calculation, based on the high end of the range for the capitated study group compared to the California norm) multiplied by this expense means that a provider-based plan covering 50,000 non-Medicare lives can save $5.6 million in inpatient costs—a whopping $9.40 per member per month. In today's brutal price competition for covered lives—with consumers ultimately feeling more and more of that pricing pain as their employers pass along plan costs—this translates into $23.51 per month in potential premium savings for the average insured family.[19] With the typical employee picking up half the premium through payroll deductions, this difference will—sooner rather than later—make or break a plan in a fully mature, competitive managed care market.

Those are just the obvious dollars. Physician "ownership" of the EHO's success also translates into other important cost savings for the sponsoring hospital. Hospitals for years have been struggling to standardize purchasing and use of medical devices and supplies. The more successful they are at reducing the variety of items within a class of supplies—brand of balloon catheters for angioplasty, for example—the lower the hospital's per unit purchasing and total inventory costs for those supplies. Financially "captive" physicians can be much more readily brought into purchasing decisions, and are much more likely to comply with them in the clinic. Such compliance translates into product standardization and better utilization, which in turn translates into significantly reduced supply costs. Driven by this logic, Tenet Healthcare embarked on precisely such a program in late 1997.[20]

There is also a positive relationship between physician ownership and quality—and quality of the variety that generally translates into cost savings because it involves standardization of *process*, not just product selection. The forces of industrialization described earlier are much more likely to take root in the clinic if physicians participate in their development and implementation, two factors much more likely with those who are financially "captive." An essay in *JAMA* notes that "guidelines are most likely to be translated into better care in settings in which physicians and their organizations have assumed responsibility for medical management from the payers. Such delegation of medical management almost invariably requires that physicians assume some measure of financial risk."[21]

The EHO can indeed be structured between hospitals and physicians not only to avoid the disasters of excessive medical utilization, but to create mutual benefit. If physicians do in fact engage in clinical behavior that seeks to earn them the controversial "target income" described earlier in this book, then so be it: acknowledge the economic reality and weave it directly into the EHO's financial and operating structure. The mechanisms used to exploit this ultimate driver of physician behavior will be far more effective than any other system of utilization or cost controls, regardless of how enlightened in design or implementation.

This view is fully confirmed by researchers who have studied the effectiveness of various hospital/physician models closely. One of the more forceful advocates of close integration, Douglas Cave, argues in *Integrated Health Care Delivery* that the equity model— whereby physicians are actual shareholders in the EHO—provides the best alignment of physician interests, and thus is key to successful integration. "Physician bonds are strongest when health systems maximize income, control revenues, and are owned and operated by physician peers," Cave writes. "Health systems founded on the equity model meet all three objectives. The for-profit and legal structures of the equity model allow physicians to maximize income through highly competitive salaries, bonuses, and equity positions."[22]

Designing and actually building a model of this sophistication requires a major leapfrogging of the current state of the art. Hospitals contemplating EHO formation tend to take half-steps in this direction, goaded forward by their consultants but held back by the horror stories of failures of EHO-like experiments in the trade press. Such half-steps result in all of the administrative complexity of—but little of the clinical and cost reform promised by—the fully realized EHO. Half-steps generally mean an additional layer of policies and procedures, not the wholesale reinvention of the outdated, counterproductive ones. They also mean that incentives probably have not changed, or at least have not changed sufficiently to modify clinical and financial behavior in general across the physician population and hospital staff. Lutz and Gee refer to these half-baked "physician joint ventures [as] little more than window dressing. Physicians received a financial stake but not a true say in the business."[23] The result of these half-steps in so many cases is failure—one that makes for a good horror story in the trade press.

By contrast to these half-steps, full-scale EHO formation usually occurs not because of bold risk taking of a visionary leadership, but in response to the threat of a sudden and significant loss of business to a competing EHO. These threats often come compliments of one or another of the national chains. Regardless, the shock to the market—like the shock of managed care to the health care system in general—is the impetus for real institutional reform.

TAMING A TWO-HEADED MONSTER

A principle struggle in hospital management has always been the constant complicating factor of a certain veto power by a hospital's nonemployees over nearly every aspect of day-to-day operations. Physicians drive the bulk of a hospital's costs and have *de facto* control over nearly all of its line employees, while traditionally having little vested interest in the hospital's success. Legal and financial disunion from physicians has always made hospitals vulnerable to the vagaries of physician behavior and performance, leaving them vulnerable, in the worst case scenario, to economic recklessness and substandard clinical practices. Traditionally, however, it did not matter: in the fee-for-service world, sloppy physician practices made more money for the hospital. Substandard medical care or surgical technique—when it does not kill patients or entice malpractice attorneys—will almost always result in longer stays, more drugs, longer detours through the ICU, and bigger bills.

But as reimbursement has undergone methodical reform since the middle 1980s, sloppy physician practices have begun to hurt hospitals. The use of *per diem* payment (a set fee for each day of a patient's stay) or per case reimbursement puts the physician's substandard clinical behavior at odds with the hospital's financial health. As reimbursement reform proceeds toward the logical conclusion of global capitation, and as physicians and hospitals assume financial risk for entire populations of patients, hospitals can no longer afford to ignore the central reality of physicians: they control nearly all clinical resource consumption, including the decision when to admit and when to discharge. This puts hospitals in the most financially and operationally tenuous of all positions. As a consequence, making physicians "captive" within the hospital's EHO is essential. Given the impact of physician independence from hospital management over the years, such an alignment is not so much a radical step forward as it is a badly needed reform to a flawed organizational design.

When contemplating the specific options for aligning with physician groups, hospitals and hospital chains face the exact same set of strategic alternatives as detailed with regard to their alignment with the nonhospital chains. As with the decision to acquire local nonhospital facilities versus cutting "virtual integration" deals with the national chains like HealthSouth, locally owned EHOs seeking integration with physician groups have two choices:

1. purchase or align with local group practices; or
2. align with local group practices that have been purchased by the national physician practice management (PPM) companies, which—like the non-hospital facility chains—have also emerged as publicly traded behemoths after rolling up physician group practices across the country.

The national hospital chains have the same option on a market-by-market basis, plus the option of a national alignment with a PPM for virtual integrations across all markets where both partners have a presence. A good example of precisely such an alliance is the one struck in the spring of 1997 between the second largest hospital chain, Tenet Healthcare, and MedPartners, the largest PPM. The agreement ties together 33 hospitals and more than 4,000 physicians in the Southern California market, and is worth $80 million in the first year of the deal for Tenet, as it serves as the hospital system of choice for the 100,000 members of a local MCO affiliated with MedPartners.[24]

The decision to align with physicians is not a question of why, but rather a question of when and how. As will be discussed at length in the next chapter, the physician has traditionally been and once again will be—after the industry's transformation is complete—in control of the health care system, the temporary incursions of managed care notwithstanding. This fact is central to the social and institutional history and future development of the U.S. health care system. As Starr points out, "patients develop a personal relation with their physicians even when medical care takes place in a hospital or clinic…The doctor's cultural authority and strategic position in the production of medical care create a distinctive base of power."[25] Hospitals that do not align themselves completely and properly with this base of power will find themselves baseless and powerless in the new century's health care system.

THE COMPETITIVE ADVANTAGE OF A LEGACY "INFOSTRUCTURE"

If physicians ultimately have control of their patients, and the most financially successful inpatient facility ultimately will be the emptiest, beyond operating surgical suites and an ICU for the sickest patients, does a hospital have any real birthright to ensure its relevance in the future health care system? Certainly: it possesses all the power that can be derived from that old cliché about information. If only through an infrastructure incumbency and inherent capital intensity, hospitals have a critical lock on the one thing that defines a truly integrated delivery system: clinical and financial information.

In their preemergent phase (the "beta stage" market outlined in Part III), an EHO is still a purely contractual rather than corporate phenomenon. As such, it is defined by three things: at-risk contracts with MCOs, employers, and consumers; intra-EHO operating agreements that govern clinical protocols and cash flows; and *patient data*. In the end, this last element will prove to be the hospital's greatest source of power; they will be the only institutions able to support, in a sustained way, the integration of clinically rich data on patients across the continuum. As enterprise-wide information networks come to serve as the EHO's nervous system, the hospital's current information system at its center is destined to comprise its brain.

The disjointedness and resulting inefficiencies that continue to haunt traditional medical delivery in the United States (described in the "Integration" chapter of Part II) will not be resolved until the system deals with the disjointedness and inefficiencies of medical information. Why? Because the successful resolution of a patient's illness or injury is not a series of independent clinical encounters; it is a complex and interrelated narrative that occurs over time. One's current medical condition is the sum total of a lifetime of medical care; one's physical history and health care is a never-ending story, as contiguous and consequential as his or her daily intellectual and emotional development. In stark contrast to this reality, however, there is scant integration of real medical data gathered on a person over time. While the richness of a patient's medical history is captured in physicians' memories and scrawled across dozens of paper charts stored in as many medical facilities, to the digital world a patient exists only as a series of unrelated encounters, then ceases to exist until the next episode requires another series of unrelated encounters. The patient is a stream of claims, submitted *a la carte* by providers and paid by whichever insurer happens to cover them that year.

Today's hospital information systems have only begun to attempt to resolve this problem. But they do possess, far and away, the greatest capacity for resolving it eventually. In contrast to all other types of information systems in the health care industry, those built and operated over the years by hospitals

- have enormous storage, relational, and computational capacity;
- accommodate the richest levels of patient data in terms of diagnostic, clinical, treatment, and financial information;
- enjoy the most concentrated, dedicated, technical support internally and externally; and
- are supported by a consolidated, well-capitalized community of vendors, led by HBO & Company, Shared Medical Systems, Cerner Corporation, Phamis, and IDX.

In contrast to the hospital industry's capital-intensive and well-supported "infostructures," physician office systems have been built to perform little more than patient billing, scheduling, and business management functions. As a result, these systems are small; functionally and developmentally limited to make them cheaper and more user-friendly; and not well supported internally due to the size of the typical group practice. Also, because physician groups have had neither the working capital nor the complex operational control needs of hospitals, their information system needs have not been technologically compelling. As a consequence, the associated market opportunity has not been very profitable, resulting in a highly fragmented industry of systems vendors.

Despite their much greater operational control needs and capital resources, most MCOs also suffer from weak infostructures, if only because of their collective organizational laziness and/or shortsightedness. Most MCOs have failed to invest in information systems of any clinical depth, with rare and notable exceptions—like HSI's Fourth Generation system, the automated patient records systems built by Kaiser, Cigna's aggressive computerized proliferation of care guidelines across all of its plans nationwide, and attempts by United Healthcare to develop a health care informatics business. MCOs generally equip themselves with mission-critical applications like claims processing, utilization management, and financial reporting systems, based on off-the-shelf systems installed and customized by systems integration companies. But few MCOs move beyond these infostructures, despite all their marketing talk about tracking and managing the medical risks and quality of care provided to their members. The failure to do so is understandable: with 20 percent of the covered population turning over every year, why invest in such systems? With no competing MCO investing in such a system this year, why put yourself at a cost disadvantage for a system that will not pay off for three to five?

By contrast to the fragmented vendors that sell physician practice management software and the systems integrators that build systems to support day-to-day MCO operations, the concentration of vendors to the hospital industry, by contrast, have invested billions of dollars building, marketing, and supporting complex financial and clinical management systems. All are moving aggressively to develop enterprise-wide systems that radiate outward from their installed hospital bases to capture and integrate information from across the continuum of care. At the prodding of these growth-hungry vendors—and based on the legacy infostructures already provided and serviced by them—hospitals hold this mostly unplayed trump card in the formation and control of EHOs. (How ironic, given that the large information systems of hospitals are often erroneously viewed as albatrosses for their cost and portability problems!)

How critical is a hospital's infostructure advantage relative to those of physician groups and health plans? It can be the basis for their entire fate. A good example is the decision in 1996 by HSI to acquire Graduate Health Systems, a network of seven hospitals in Philadelphia. In covering the now highly unusual example of backward integration by a health plan into the provider business, a Wall Street research report touted as one of the benefits of the deal the high level of information integration among the hospitals via a Wide Area Network (WAN). According to the report, the purchase will allow HSI to deploy and test its leading-edge Fourth Generation system of telephonic patient routing, described in the "Industrialization" chapter, within an integrated care network.[26] The resulting system, which marries sophisticated clinical decision support capabilities with emerging WAN technologies adopted by hospitals to map and track the care process, represents a critical competitive advantage for any integrated provider network.

That HSI would rush out only months after implementing Fourth Generation and purchase an entire hospital system so as to test this radical new approach to managing patient care underscores the leverage inherent in the infostructure of today's hospitals. Such moves also call attention to a key but often overlooked strategic weapon for hospitals: if exploited intelligently, the hospital's infostructure will prove to be their single most important source of strength in their death struggle with the MCOs. In the end, *as health care integrates across the continuum and moves inexorably toward industrialization, clinical control will equate to information control.* Incidentally, trade press reports cite the power of Fourth Generation as a major inspiration for Foundation's eventual purchase of HSI.[27]

As EHOs come to represent the integration of previously unrelatable clinical information across the continuum, they will be further positioned to compete successfully with MCOs. Their complex, expensive infostructures—brimming with rich clinical and financial information—will emerge as what Porter calls a "dimension of strategy in which competitors are ill-prepared, least enthusiastic, or most uncomfortable about competing."[28] Such infostructures will flow not from any independent initiative of the EHO, but from a key legacy technology currently in place in today's acute care hospital.

THE GROVES OF ACADEMIC HOSPITALS

Do the market challenges and solutions described in this chapter apply to academic medical centers (AMCs)? The answer is yes—by an order of magnitude. The typical AMC endures all the problems of confronting hospitals in general, but with far greater acuity. They are burdened by their larger cost structures, especially complex organizational designs, and a teaching and research mission that serves the entire health care system while penalizing the institution in the marketplace for the high costs associated with that mission. This is particularly problematic as local markets mature.

- Only 5 percent of the services provided by major teaching hospitals are unique to those institutions.
- Only another 15 to 20 percent are complex cases that such facilities can handle better than other hospitals.
- The remaining 75 to 80 percent of what these hospitals do can be done elsewhere, as effectively and for less money.[29]

If the problems facing hospitals are magnified for AMCs, so is the potential impact of their resolution. AMCs can benefit even more than the typical community hospital from a well-managed alignment with physicians: the physicians likely to join the academic EHO (those on its faculty) represent a prestige-based drawing card for the facility that, if managed and marketed properly, is collectively stronger than the prestige of the facility itself. AMCs also collect and store vast amounts of clinical information—much of it often cutting-edge—that can be used as a potent strategic weapon. The medical and surgical techniques developed at the AMCs and eventually proliferated to the medical community at large can represent a significant competitive advantage in a local market—a true "first-mover advantage"—if properly captured and communicated through the academic EHO's (A-EHO's) infostructure to all affiliated physicians.

Beyond the obvious need to pursue with even more vigor the same strategies available to all hospitals, major teaching hospitals must overcome a plethora of institutional issues, not the least of which are the awesome twin burdens of their own history and their own egos. The development of the health care system in this century set up the AMC as an anomaly, one that was protected in the world of fee-for-service medicine, but one grossly mismatched to the brutalities of today's market-driven system. According to Starr, "universities became the umbrella organizations for America's regional medical centers, which instead of being organized around the immediate needs of patients, were oriented primarily toward research and training…What was remarkable about this arrangement is how little remarked it was."[30] The arrangement is remarked upon frequently now: by lower-cost hospitals competing for patients; contemptuous managed care executives reviewing aggregate claims expense; and respectful but unsympathetic self-insured employers looking to balance choice and quality with cost.

This section will offer three survival strategies unique to academic medical centers. All three presuppose what many at academic medical centers still refuse to accept, judging by the ever-widening river of *mea culpae* from academic physicians and researchers in the medical journals. Fact: the health care system in America is undergoing an inexorable transformation from a cottage industry that once cherished and protected the academic medical center, to an unsentimental, market-driven business that is essentially philistine, a brave new commercial world that has no regard for medical research for research's sake, and will not subsidize it. Given this reality, there are a wealth of opportunities for academic medical centers to adapt to the new environment, differentiate themselves to survive its harshness, and perhaps even flourish. The following survival strategies are multifaceted and need to occur simultaneously.

Imitate and conquer. The academic medical center will survive and thrive only if it follows the market evolution described in the "Prognosis" part of this book and evolves into an A-EHO. The A-EHOs need to aggressively develop their own continuum of care, integrate with their own physicians, and assume medical risk for populations. The A-EHO must focus on variable costs with regard to pricing for EHO-type business, i.e., isolate and ignore the cost structure of its research and teaching mission within its budget, meeting the marketplace's conditions on the marketplace's terms. In many cases, to offer market pricing, the formation and operation of the A-EHO will require the blending of its academic facilities and physicians with other providers in the community. Such a combination provides the AMC with the marketing muscle and geographic coverage it has lacked over the years, and also helps attenuate the cost disadvantages of the A-EHO going it alone. In such instances, the AMC needs to accept its diminished role within the EHO. As the highest cost facility in the EHO, when it cannot handle cases as economically as its siblings, it needs to back off.

An excellent example of this strategy is the consolidation of 554-bed University of Minnesota Hospital with 693-bed Fairview Riverside Medical Center. Together, the two-facility system is a financial and marketing powerhouse positioned to serve the entire metropolitan Minneapolis-St. Paul market. Through the merger, the two hospitals consolidated their capacity and rationalized their specialization and divisions of labor: the University Hospital focuses on complex, high-technology care and still remains viable within the market; the non-University hospital enjoys the benefits of positioning at the high-end of the market and can exit the technology arms race without suffering any market damage. Culturally, the merger has resulted in some pleasant surprises for both hospitals: after graduating from the University, many of the Fairview doctors "swore they would never direct patients to the haughty university physicians," according to an administrator. Yet, inevitably, half their referrals now go to the University Hospital. "Now one-half of our out-of-network problem goes away," the administrator said.[31] As the Twin Cities area was an early stronghold of managed care and is now dominated almost completely by MCOs and direct employer contracting, this merger in a bellwether market represents a preview of coming attractions for academic medical centers.

Another example of marketplace alignment (or capitulation, as some might argue) was the quick response of famed cancer center, Sloan-Kettering Memorial, to an incursion into its Greater New York market by a low-cost managed care interloper. Sloan had long been protected from the realities of the marketplace by sheer prestige, its ability to provide radical treatments for late-stage cancer that had evaded most managed care controls up to that point, and by an endowment of $1.4 billion—a clear benefit of operating as a not-for-profit institution in a city full of millionaires, many of whom will die of cancer. Despite these legacy advantages, between 1993 and 1996

Sloan closed three patient floors with 148 beds, almost 25 percent of its inpatient capacity.[32] As a result, when cancer "carve-out" company Salick Health Care invaded its turf with cut-rate pricing for guaranteed volume to competitor St. Vincent's, Sloan-Kettering had little choice: it quickly countered by cutting a deal with Empire Blue Cross and Blue Shield, New York's largest insurer, accepting a reduction in rates of up to 30 percent, in exchange for guaranteed patient flow.[33]

Differentiate the brand. In order to survive and prosper as a full-blown EHO, the A-EHO needs to position itself as *the* quality provider in a consumer-driven market, matching its prestige to the "differentiator" segment of the market described earlier. The A-EHO needs to market the fact that, in clinical terms, it is the provider of best and last resort, trumpeting and expanding upon findings showing that, for the toughest medical cases, the most complex facilities always do the best job. They need to exploit the central fact of health care purchasing: when faced with a medical crisis, the specter of permanent disability, or the loss of a loved one, *price is irrelevant.*

For example, an A-EHO with a level III neonatal intensive care unit (NICU) should market itself by publicizing findings that survival rates are far higher for high-risk babies in level III NICUs than in less intensive ICUs. If it wants to throw off the gloves, it will also point out that mortality is 29 percent greater for high-risk infants covered by MCOs.[34] This latter point underscores the core clinical findings of the former: MCOs are less likely to include in their networks the large tertiary care facilities with a level III NICU. ("When you're picking the cheapest managed care network in town, you get what you pay for.") What does this mean for consumers? It means that unless one can absolutely guarantee a perfect pregnancy and delivery, consumers might want to think twice about the few dollars they are saving with their coverage from the MCOs or directly with the lower-end EHOs. These findings are typical, serious quality-of-care issues, and reveal what is really at stake in the selection of health insurance.

As these discoveries circulate, patients will demand access for high-risk situations; but as markets divide up, the only avenues for such access will be through the EHOs. A report on the NICU study in *Medicine & Health* points out that "market forces rather than regulation may be the most likely mechanism for implementing the study's findings."[35] Thus, the uncompetitive cost structure associated with maintaining high-costs facilities like level III NICUs inverts a competitive problem: what hobbles the A-EHO with a price disadvantage can actually help position it as a market differentiator. This is a clear competitive advantage that academic medical centers can and must exploit. They can do so in a pretransformed market by pressuring plans to include coverage, marketing their differentiation directly to consumers with a patient "pull-through" strategy. As the market then evolves and the full A-EHO emerges, they can market this positioning directly to the higher-tiered consumer: in a segmented market. Indeed, the "name-brand" academic medical center is the Mercedes.

Leverage the brand. Once the "name-brand" has been developed and marketed as such, the A-EHO needs to leverage it, aggressively and creatively. The cutting-edge research and clinical work that serves so often as a drain on teaching hospitals under reimbursement in the United States, represents a significant marketing opportunity overseas. Because of the superiority of American medicine generally and the reputations of the academic medical centers in particular, numerous AMCs have embarked on marketing programs that bring wealthy, cash-wielding patients to the United States for bypasses, major orthopaedic surgeries, and the like. An even more ambitious and intriguing step in this direction was taken by the University of Pittsburgh Medical Center in 1996. The pioneering organization in liver transplants in the early 1980s, by the 1990s Pitt was losing money on the procedure, which cost $140,000 to perform versus the predominant Medicare reimbursement of $120,000.[36] In need of new sources of business to subsidize its current program and continued research, Pitt decided to build up its liver transplant business overseas. But unlike other AMC initiatives, Pitt did not seek to bring foreign patients to the United States for the procedure; rather, it is bringing the procedure to foreign patients. Because of the general shortage of organs—and a 5 percent cap on the total U.S. supply available to foreigners—Pitt is taking its brand overseas. It has established a joint venture in Sicily, which has been seeking creative ways to rebuild its own economy.

Pitt's exportation of what is essentially an intellectual property mirrors similar moves by the University of Virginia Health Sciences Center in its move to open a facility in Saudi Arabia, and a like move by the Johns Hopkins Hospital into South Korea.[37] The Sicilian government, eager to keep health care dollars in the local economy and create high-skill–level jobs associated with health care, is investing $80 million in the transplant facility. Fixed costs are covered by the local government and Pitt is paid for performing the surgery. Translation from the Italian: it's all margin. Pitt expects to replicate its U.S. business, which amounts to $150 million annually. The numbers work, given that Sicilians spent $170 million for health care abroad.[38]

These all represent "export" business strategies: they help amortize further the huge fixed costs of research, staffing, and teaching for AMCs like Pitt, Virginia, and Hopkins.

ACUTE FLARE-UPS OF CHRONIC "BUREAUSCLEROSIS"

Yes, the opportunities to survive and thrive within an ultimately consumer-driven marketplace may well be, paradoxically, the greatest for the academic medical centers—with their enviable market presence, reputations for quality, and full gamut of the best clinical resources. But the playing field quickly relevels when we poke inside the typical AMC and look at how well they operate. Why? Because AMCs tend to suffer from the most advanced stages of the disease that threatens hospitals of all stripes across the United States: "bureausclerosis." Traditionally, the AMCs are institutions of applied science first and business second; this means they are hobbled by the worst version of this dreaded disorder.

But bureausclerosis affects, to varying degrees, all hospitals. Why? Because the hospital culture has always had an academic flavor: they tend to be run by consensus, and hobbled by a legacy of collegialism, inclusiveness, and intellectual purity, all death to a business enterprise navigating treacherous, ever-changing waters. Hospitals are also burdened with a complex, often self-defeating decision-making apparatus: each incremental step toward progress made by a hospital's administration is forever jeopardized by the veto power—either explicitly through declaration or tacitly in foiled implementation—of the shadow power structure of the facility, its physicians, and other clinicians.

The typical hospital's cultural problems are reinforced by its extensive dealings with government as regulator, financier, and single largest customer. Hospitals have been coping with government rules, oversight, second-guesses, audits, intrusions, and paperwork for so long that their managerial personalities have come to represent much that is onerous about government itself. They can be resistant to change, beholden to protocol over common sense, and stifling of innovation. This general organizational dysfunctionality does much to explain several things about hospitals: why they have been so slow to respond to their various afflictions, such as overcapacity; why their initial response to the emergence of managed care in the 1980s consisted of little more than institutional self-pity, passive-aggressiveness, and strategic paralysis; and why most have not successfully leveraged things like their infostructures to take on managed care more aggressively.

Collective bureausclerosis of hospitals across the United States helps explain why the industry, in general, appears so incapable of honest self-analysis. Back in 1987, the Joint Commission for the Accreditation of Healthcare Organizations (Joint Commission), a self-regulating organization set up to police hospitals for quality and safety practices in support of hospital marketing to payers, attempted to incorporate a meaningful performance-based analysis into its hospital accreditation process. The result was a monstrous political backlash; the Joint Commission backed off, watering the initiative down to a paperwork exercise that assessed a hospital's *capacity* for providing quality care, not any actual measure of it. Ten years later, the Joint Commission was trying again.[39] The new initiative to measure actual quality performance was introduced, but with the following conditions: no requirement to make the data public; no comparison of hospitals against any norms or benchmarks; and a hospital's poor performance cannot affect accreditation. With self-assessments this toothless, the hospital industry continues to beg for the harsh scrutiny of payers. It persists in its reluctance, internally and as a group, to standardize what it does, while abdicating any accountability for it.

Recalling Starr's analysis of the history of the hospital as institution, this reluctance may stem from the fact that the hospital embodies the "familiar American paradox of a system of very great uniformity and very little coordination. The absence of integrated management made it incumbent upon individual hospitals to develop a more elaborate administration than hospitals in other countries where administrative functions are more centralized."[40] Such elaborate, difficult-to-integrate, and ultimately inefficient approaches to administration do much to explain why the national chains—with their organizational templates and industrialization models—would eventually come to dominate the markets they entered. The chains simply supplanted many of the overly individuated, outdated, and suddenly uncompetitive institutional behaviors—with the clearer lines of authority and unsentimental taskmastering of a modern corporate culture. That goes for the Catholic systems as well as the investor-owned ones.

In contrast to the cultural revolution sweeping through half the hospital industry in the wake of the chains, the other half continues to bog down in its own politics. The industry abounds with a repetition of a few sad stories. The power struggles that plague much of the hospital industry tend to be most acute within teaching hospitals; while no component of the health care system stands to benefit more from the consolidation and integration dictated by the new order in health care than teaching hospitals, their cultures make them the least likely to implement these changes effectively. As of this writing, several years after the historic merger of the Massachusetts General Hospital and Brigham and Women's Hospital in Boston there have been no reductions in the combined facilities' scope or size. "Charges remain high, and there is little progress toward the elimination of overlapping clinical services," reports the *New England Journal of Medicine.* "Indeed Mass General opened an obstetrical service after the merger was announced."[41]

This inability to do the hard work and make the hard choices associated with consolidation and integration can kill a merger before it is even consummated. The most spectacular example of this occurred in 1997, as the highly publicized marriage of New York University Medical Center and Mount Sinai Medical Center fell apart at the altar. All accounts of the dissolution of the deal—conceived to help the prestigious facilities survive the coming onslaught of managed care in a grossly overbedded market about to experience pricing deregulation—attribute the failure to warring senior clinical and administrative egos.[42]

Like alcoholics and drug addicts who refuse to seek treatment that everyone around them knows they desperately need, some hospitals will remain incorrigibly trapped in their self-destructive behaviors until they have hit bottom. In too many markets, still numb from decades of fee-for-service medicine and insulated with the fat of endowments, many hospitals have not felt enough pain, yet.

REFERENCES

1. Medicare discharges as a percentage of total discharges for the median U.S. hospital in 1991, calculated in *The Comparative Performance of U.S. Hospitals: The Sourcebook,* 1996 ed. (Baltimore: HCIA Inc.).

2. Outpatient revenue as a percentage of total gross patient revenues for the median U.S. hospital in 1995, calculated in *The Comparative Performance of U.S. Hospitals: The Sourcebook,* 1996 ed. (Baltimore: HCIA Inc.).

3. A.M. Stoline and J.P. Weiner, *The New Medical Marketplace: A Physician's Guide to the Health Care System in the 1990s* (Baltimore: The Johns Hopkins University Press, 1993), 104. © 1993. The Johns Hopkins University Press.

4. P. Starr, *The Social Transformation of American Medicine* (New York: Basic Books/HarperCollins, 1982), 350.

5. 1991 survey data from the American Hospital Association.

6. Stoline and Weiner, *The New Medical Marketplace: A Physician's Guide to the Health Care System in the 1990s*, 73. © 1993. The Johns Hopkins University Press.

7. Stoline and Weiner, *The New Medical Marketplace: A Physician's Guide to the Health Care System in the 1990s*, 122. © 1993. The Johns Hopkins University Press.

8. From the Medical Group Practice Digest 1995, sponsored by Hoechst Marion Roussel, Kansas City, MO, in "Large Medical Groups Make Integrated Systems Competitive," *Health Care Strategic Management*, January 1996, 18.

9. Starr, *The Social Transformation of American Medicine,* 177.

10. Adapted and reprinted with permission of The Free Press, a Division of Simon & Schuster from *COMPETITIVE STRATEGY: Techniques for Analyzing Industries and Competitors* by Michael E. Porter. Copyright © 1980 by The Free Press. p. 24.

11. C. Snow, "One-Stop Shopping," *Modern Healthcare*, 25 November, 1996.

12. C. Snow, "HealthSouth's New Horizons," *Modern Healthcare*, 24 February, 1997, 20.

13. S. Lutz and E.P. Gee, *The For-Profit Healthcare Revolution* (Chicago: Irwin Professional Publishing, 1995), 152.

14. Starr, *The Social Transformation of American Medicine,* 218.

15. Stoline and Weiner, *The New Medical Marketplace: A Physician's Guide to the Health Care System in the 1990s*, 175. © 1993. The Johns Hopkins University Press.

16. A. Hillman et al., "How Do Financial Incentives Affect Physicians' Clinical Decisions and the Financial Performance of Health Maintenance Organizations?" *New England Journal of Medicine*, 13 July, 1989, 86.

17. J. Robinson and L. Casalino, "The Growth of Medical Groups Paid through Capitation in California," *New England Journal of Medicine*, 21 December, 1995, 1684.

18. Operating expense per adjusted discharge for the median U.S. hospital ($4,580), divided by average length of stay for non-Medicare discharges (3.22). Figures for 1995, calculated in *The Comparative Performance of U.S. Hospitals: The Sourcebook*, 1997 ed. (Baltimore: HCIA Inc.).

19. Assumes a total covered lives ratio of 2.5 per insured employee, a standard actuarial assumption for insured families.

20. S. Hensley, "The Deciding Vote," *Modern Healthcare*, 24 November, 1997, 42.

21. T. Lee, "Translating Good Advice into Better Practice," *Journal of the American Medical Association* 278 no. 23, 17 December, 1997, 2109.

22. D. Cave, "Vertical Integration Models To Prepare Health Systems for Capitation," in *Integrated Health Care Delivery: Theory, Practice, Evaluation, and Prognosis*, ed. M. Brown (Gaithersburg, MD: Aspen Publishers, 1996), 167.

23. Lutz and Gee, *The For-Profit Healthcare Revolution,* 81.

24. R. Rundle, "Tenet and MedPartners Agree To Form Health Network in Southern California," *Wall Street Journal*, 10 April, 1997.

25. Starr, *The Social Transformation of American Medicine,* 217.

26. From a research report, "Health Systems International," by Volpe, Welty & Company, 22 July, 1996, 16.

27. "Information System Sweetens Foundation-HSI Deal," *Modern Healthcare.*

28. Adapted and reprinted with permission of The Free Press, a Division of Simon & Schuster from *COMPETITIVE STRATEGY: Techniques for Analyzing Industries and Competitors* by Michael E. Porter. Copyright © 1980 by The Free Press. p. 70.

29. S. Andreopoulos, "The Folly of Teaching-Hospital Mergers," *New England Journal of Medicine*, 2 January, 1997, 62.

30. Starr, *The Social Transformation of American Medicine*, 361.

31. L. Scott, "Can Marriage of Academic, Community Hospitals Work?" *Modern Healthcare*, 17 March, 1997, 26.

32. L. Lagnado, "Famed Cancer Center Gives In to Managed Care," *Wall Street Journal*, 25 October, 1996.

33. Lagnado, *Wall Street Journal.*

34. "Tertiary Care Saves Lives, Money in Treating At-Risk Newborns," *Medicine & Health*, 7 October, 1996, 2.

35. "Tertiary Care Saves Lives, Money in Treating At-Risk Newborns," *Medicine & Health.*

36. S. Baker, "Transplanting the Transplant Biz," *Business Week*, 25 November, 1996, 130.

37. Baker, *Business Week*, 130.

38. Baker, *Business Week*, 128.

39. D. Moore, "JCAHO Tries Again," *Modern Healthcare*, 24 February, 1997, 2.

40. Starr, *The Social Transformation of American Medicine*, 177.

41. Andreopoulos, *New England Journal of Medicine*, 62.

42. L. Lagnado, "Elite Medical Centers Seemed Perfect Mates, Except to the Doctors," *Wall Street Journal*, 21 March, 1997.

7

MD, MBA

Yea, though we walk through the valley of managed care and our business (if not our soul) is traded on the floor of the New York Stock Exchange, we are lucky to be here, doing what we do, still students of medicine, tending to the afflictions and infirmities of those who call us doctor.

David Loxterkamp, MD
New England Journal of Medicine[1]

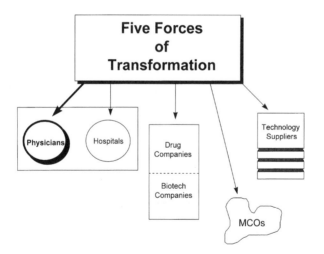

The multiple and sustained shocks to the U.S. health care system described in *Bleeding Edge* often seem like so much bitter medicine for the nation's physicians. Most distressing to doctors confronted by this and other frank discussions about what has gone awry with the medical system—and about the wrenching fixes that a rationalizing marketplace has imposed upon it—is the profession's collective perception of a sudden helplessness: *we are health care*, they collectively decry, *and everyone is now in control of it except us!*

Indeed, the debate over how best to reform the U.S. health care system rages on; national MCOs penetrate and dominate still more and more markets; remote control systems have come to dictate ever harsher new rules and conditions on patient mobility and physician clinical behavior. At the end of the year, physician incomes—especially those for specialists—are either flat or lower than the year before.[2] Physicians react to changes against their will and threats against their material well-being the way most normal human beings do—through variations of denial, rage, and resignation:

"Managed care is a bad dream that will go away."

"Managed care is evil!"

"Managed care has destroyed my profession. I should go work for a consulting firm."

Underlying these clearly counterproductive reflexes is an outdated presupposition, one that physicians need to confront and exorcise before they can cope successfully with the brave new world of health care: they must cease clinging to an outdated identity, to what Stoline and Weiner call the "romanticized image of the seemingly selfless and inexhaustive practitioner...the very attachment to such an idealized image makes it difficult for physicians and others to be objective about changes in the delivery of medical care."[3] Letting go of this archaic collective self-image is the first step to coping with the inevitable convulsions of the present and seizing control of a radically realigned future.

This is no small task, as the present is perhaps the worst time in the history of medicine to be practicing as a physician. Physicians spend their working days on the whipsaw end of the massive transformation of the system, a still nascent historic process that has generated few benefits at the close of the 1990s, aside from the flattening of health care costs. And while the reduction of health costs is of benefit to almost everyone else, it is a direct hit to physicians. Period.

Because the transformation is only gathering momentum, all the old systems are still in place. They operate in parallel to—and often in direct conflict with—the specific transitional systems arising to deal with those old systems. Consider the continuing practice of utilization management, which still exists to the degree that fee-for-service medicine still predominates. Utilization management—whereby a 50-year-old, Board-certified, widely published physician waits on hold for five minutes to finish explaining her clinical judgment to a 25-year-old MCO clerk with a two-year nursing degree—is the perfect example of a system in the throes of a messy transition. Such cumbersome practices, and the managed care "revolution" that gave rise to them, represent a kind of Dark Ages of medicine. This is a truly medieval process that the civilized medical community must endure between the days of its fallen, fee-for-service empire and the restraint of an enlightened, more responsible era—one under which physicians are paid to manage patients' health rather than treat their illnesses. As Richard Shinto, MD, and Harriet Press write in *Health Care Strategic Management*, this transitional era has "produced a new generation of physicians who have joined managed care networks as a strategy to compete and survive, but who aren't quite sure where they fit in the picture."[4]

On one hand, given the size, scope, and complexity of the $1 trillion industry in transition, it is little wonder how long the transition is taking. On the other hand, given the self-accelerating power of both marketplace economics and information technology to effect industrial and cultural revolutions, it is of greater wonder why this transition is taking so long. This paradox doubtless flows from the two-faced nature of any wholesale change: one constituency's threat is another's opportunity. Thus, it can readily be argued that much of the health care system's specific progress through this transitional period is the sum total of the collective will of the medical profession to hasten or retard that progress. In this regard, 1996 may be viewed as a critical breakthrough year: for the first time since such data were tracked, physicians led the total number of merger and acquisitions executed in the health care industry. In 1996, physician group practices were involved in 218 transactions, up a whopping 73 percent from the 126 posted the previous year.[5] Most tellingly, these deals outpaced the still expanding merger and acquisition activity of the nation's hospitals, MCOs, and home health companies.

The sudden uptick in physician group practice transactions illustrates how the profession is finally positioning to deal with the five forces of health care transformation to align itself with the new era, beginning with the first critical step of consolidation. Such alignment is the only hope for physicians in the long run: play by the new rules or be subject to them. All the old managed care tools, systems, and gamesmanship are headed for the scrap heap where they belong. The next wave of tools—the five forces of health care transformation described in this book—are the real curatives for what ails the system, and thus are here to stay. The faster physicians embrace these tools, the faster the transformation of the system will be complete.

Surviving this transformation will require a massive reorientation by the medical profession. As Stoline and Weiner aptly put it, "it is not only pointless but also counterproductive for physicians to resist the new era, because the interest of all parties is served best by their full participation."[6] This chapter should help elicit full participation by physicians, if only because its analysis provides a good antidote to much of the faulty conventional wisdom propounded by the managed care industry and public policy makers alike.

HOW MANY DOCTORS IN THE HOUSE?

Wrongheaded predictions about the future of the medical profession come in such number and at such volume that they seem almost a conspiracy to disarm physicians. Exhibit A: if you want to threaten someone into submission, tell them they are in oversupply. This strategy seems to have worked wonders in managed care negotiations with providers.

The health care business literature abounds with observations and predictions (as opposed to empirical facts) that, as with hospital beds, the United States has too many physicians—and that this over-capacity inevitably will undercut their bargaining power and ultimately their prices. Much of this belief stems from a historic parallelism between the rapid build-up in hospitals and medical school capacity, due exclusively to a concerted effort to expand the supply of physicians by the federal government in the 1960s and 1970s. As a result of this build-up, the number of practicing physicians increased by nearly 35 percent between 1960 and 1975, while the general population grew only 15 percent.[7] Growth of this magnitude, the thinking went, *had* to generate oversupply. Right?

This suspicion was confirmed in a large-scale study by the federally funded Graduate Medical Education National Advisory Committee in 1980. The study's conclusion that the United States had more physicians than it needed was widely publicized and circulated throughout the health care industry as the definitive conclusion on the subject. A decade later, as the keepers of the conventional wisdom came to understand how MCOs worked—with their core "care management" strategy of restricting access to physicians—this belief was galvanized. No doubt, the thinking went, the oversupply of physicians will get only worse as the nation converts to managed care and the demand for services is systematically reduced by its methods. Others backed into the same conclusion, pointing to the larger dysfunctional market dynamics that would sustain an oversupply of physicians, just as they had sustained too much hospital capacity: the system subsidized excess resources through artificially higher prices because there was no efficient, rational market mechanism in place until the advent of managed care.

Those so readily convinced that the system was littered with too many physicians and too few patients might have considered supplementing their "research" with a visit to the waiting rooms of a few physician offices.

Or tried to schedule a first visit with a pediatrician in any suburban market this month.

Or tried to find a new obstetrician in a major metropolitan market. Or tried to find a gynecologist taking new patients, anywhere.

While conventional wisdom leads one to the conclusion that the U.S. health care system is burdened with too many physicians—and conventional experience of trying to find one to deliver your baby or treat your child's ear infection leads to the belief that there are too few—a landmark study published in 1997 found that the actual number may be just about right. With the goal of anticipating physician needs under a fully mature managed care system, authors in the leading public policy journal *Health Affairs* analyzed physician-to-member ratios in Group Health Cooperative of Puget Sound and HealthPartners in Minneapolis, two large, well-established MCOs in what are considered leading-edge health care markets in the United States. The study found that the two MCOs maintained the equivalent of 180 physicians per 100,000 enrollees, which is "near the national average and far above figures that are typically reported in the literature."[8]

After rigorous analysis of the data and painstaking adjustments to account for everything from part-time physicians to the contributions of those out-of-network, the authors find "a remarkable similarity between the supply of physicians at the two MCOs and the supply of physicians within the United States as a whole for the same time period."[9] The study's authors speculate that contrary to expectations and traditional managed care practices, these more progressive MCOs may actually *promote* labor-intensity of physicians—which is actually more cost-effective than knee-jerk use of expensive medical technologies and other resources. "If promising access to both generalist and specialist physicians is a substitute for the use of expensive technologies and hospitals, or if physicians are effective in their health promotion and disease prevention activities, investment in health professionals may actually reduce some downstream costs," the study's authors conclude.[10]

Those who prefer theory to empiricism and are thus still convinced that the future system will be hobbled by too many physicians and too few patients should study more closely the theory of supply and demand as it pertains to risk-assumption. As prices decrease, so does supply. In the case of risk-assumption, prices not only decrease with an increased supplying of medical services, they actually invert. When paid on a fixed-fee basis per covered life, the more time a physician supplies per patient, then the lower his or her price drops per hour. In this sense, with prices set by capitation rates, physicians will adjust their supply of hours per patient downward; with this adjustment they are reducing their total number of work hours, all for the same market rate. The result will be fewer total physician hours available in the aggregate supply, and the need for as many or more physicians in that market.

Writing in *Integrated Health Care Delivery*, Richard Johnson points out this phenomenon in practice: "unless a patient is truly an emergency, the primary care physician probably is going to develop 9-to-5 practice hours. Under capitation, the physician enjoys no economic reward for working 12 or 14 hours per day, or 6 or 7 days per week."[11] Johnson extrapolates this reduction to its inevitable conclusion: the system actually needs *more* physicians. Because a family practitioner works on average 58.5 hours per week, and the general practitioner 62.2 hours per week, the decision by these physicians under capitation to reduce their work weeks to 40 hours "would require an additional one-third to the supply of primary care physicians."[12]

This phenomenon is already showing up in the data. By the end of 1996, the median workweek for office-based physicians in private practice had dropped to 57 hours, after averaging 60 hours per week "for longer than many can remember," according to a report on the numbers in *Health Care Strategic Management*.[13] The same study also found that the median number of weekly patient encounters fell to 95 in 1996, compared to 108 per week in 1988, constituting a sizable 12 percent decline since the five forces transforming the health care system began to work their charms. Most revealing, the geographic patterning of this drop-off corresponds perfectly with the regional penetration of managed care: the study found the shortest work week and greatest reduction in the number of weekly patient encounters occurred in the West, where managed care influence is the most fully entrenched.[14]

IS THERE AN ADVANCED NURSE PRACTITIONER IN THE HOUSE?

If a strong consistency between physician-to-population ratios in mature managed care markets and the United States as a whole flies in the face of conventional wisdom, then MCOs are doing much to restore at least a portion of this conventional wisdom with regard to how they organize and allocate clinical labor. If there is a preference for labor-intensive resource use among MCOs (though the creation of systems like telephonic triage are inconsistent with that position), then the managed care industry is developing and implementing numerous ways to channel their use of labor away from full-fledged physicians, toward "physician extenders." MCOs have recognized that physicians are a high-cost component of the system; as a consequence they have been aggressively seeking to manage these costs by promoting the use of these clinical alternatives to physician labor.

"Physician extenders" include the nation's 35,000 physician assistants (PAs), who perform first-line diagnoses and procedures in physician offices and emergency rooms. The number of graduates from PA programs has been increasing 13 percent annually for the last five years, and shows no signs of abating.[15] Physician extenders also include a variety of advanced nurse practitioners, such as certified registered nurse anesthetists, who administer anesthesia and monitor patients during surgeries under the supervision of anesthesiologists; certified nurse-midwives, who provide prenatal care and deliver babies; and other types of nurses with advanced clinical experience and training.

While this "de-doctoring" of clinical care may frighten the average patient, the analysis of data of alternative providers ought actually to provide them some comfort. In a study of the effectiveness of certified nurse-midwives, birthing procedures attended by these nonphysicians resulted in C-section deliveries only 11.6 percent of the time, half the normal rate. Even more disproportionate was the occurrence of normal vaginal births for mothers who had previously delivered via a C-section, a "VBAC" rate 68.9 percent higher than normal. While many would suspect these findings to be skewed by lower-risk patients, this was not borne out in the data: 87 percent of the midwives involved in the study comanage moderate- and high-risk births with physicians.[16] Such findings, when extrapolated to entire populations, equate to significant dollar savings on high-volume procedures like childbirth. With training that emphasizes natural approaches and surgical interventions only as a last resort, the use of nurse-midwives is—to put it in the crass calculus of managed care—a much better "buy" for the insurer, the patient, and the system.

Such findings drive the closely watched efforts of MCOs like Oxford Health Plans, one of the most aggressive innovators in the managed care industry, to push the envelope as far as its markets will bear with regard to using physician extenders. In 1997, Oxford began developing a corps of advanced practice nurses to diagnose and route patients to specialists, a practice that reportedly saves patients time, frees up doctors, and reduces paperwork.[17] This initiative, which positions nurses as *de facto* gatekeepers to the treatment system, is being pursued to its logical conclusion under a deal—entered into on an exploratory basis in 1997—between Oxford and Columbia Presbyterian Medical Center. Under the deal, Columbia's most highly trained and well-paid nurses will have actual primary care responsibility for Oxford members.[18] This is tantamount to an outright revolt against the traditional practice of medicine by licensed physicians.

So what do these changes mean for the profession? They mean that the fundamental role of physicians is changing radically, from one of practitioner to one of practitioner-manager. The use of "physician extenders" represents the leveraging of physician talent, time, and resources; it signifies that the primary role of physician shifts from one of caregiver to manager of a host of caregivers; it also means that physicians will be less involved in the easiest cases, and will devote a greater proportion of their direct clinical time working on the more complex cases that the physician extenders by necessity pass along. After this process is complete, in the new century's health care system

- the most successful primary care physician will be the manager of the largest number of physician extenders;
- the most successful obstetrician will be the best manager of pre-natal care, diagnostician, and manager of high-risk pregnancies, and deployer of nurse-midwives; and
- the most successful anesthesiologist will be the manager of the best stable of certified registered nurse anesthetists.

Though this describes a role dramatically different from the one normally associated with physicians, it is already beginning to emerge in their collective self-image. A 1997 survey of doctors found watershed changes in this regard: in 1992, 13 percent of all physicians viewed themselves as "leaders" first and 80 percent as "clinicians" first; by 1997, those numbers had flip-flopped, with 47 percent viewing themselves as leaders first and 42 percent as clini-cians first.[19]

This change has enormous implications for the future of medical training in the United States. If indeed the role of today's physician is mutating toward one that encompasses leadership and manage-ment responsibilities, then physician education will need to mutate accordingly. Medical residency, whereby physicians learn to master the subtleties and complexities of disease, should also expand to in-clude training on managing people and resources—a challenge sig-nificantly different from doctoring and often every bit as subtle and complex.

THE 50/50 RULE

Of the many bogus homilies about the U.S. health care system propounded by the Clintons in their campaign for federal control of that system, few have persisted at face value longer than the following: there is an oversupply in the number of specialists relative to primary care physicians (PCPs). This interesting bit of folklore, also a staple of the less enlightened MCOs, flows from the impeccable reasoning that specialists make more money than PCPs, health care in the United States is too expensive, and therefore the United States has too many specialists. Granted, specialists predominate in the United States: in 1945, approximately half of all U.S. physicians were general practitioners;[20] today, the share has dropped to 36 percent.[21] This percentage has held since the Graduate Medical Education National Advisory Committee calculated its physician-to-population ratios in the fee-for-service world of 1980—ratios that have served as a baseline for staff planning for health care organizations ever since.

The theory underlying the idealized MCO—specifically, the proactive maintenance of a population's health, rather than reactive treatment of only its sick—would logically support a call for more PCPs. Closer examination, on the other hand, of the many forces driving today's real world of managed care would argue for a little caution. Such caution is particularly important given the enormous expense—in both economic and human terms—of tinkering with public funding for medical education *and* given the many years required to measure and recorrect the effects of such tinkering.

Caution is even more warranted if we pause for a moment to unravel the serious contradictions in the entire PCP thesis: *as managed care and the EHOs eventually growing out of the managed care movement attempt to push patients from specialists back to PCPs, the advent of care automation tools and physician extenders is simultaneously reducing the need for PCPs.* Telephonic triage nurses, the use of patient routing systems like HSI's Fourth Generation, and the aggressive deployment of advanced practice nurses to function as nonphysician primary care providers, all presage the evolution of a system where patients may not have direct, immediate access to specialists on demand; but what will be standing between them and those specialists will *not* be PCPs. All of this restructuring and automation of the care delivery process is poised specifically to eliminate vast numbers of what would have been PCP patient encounters.

Reductions in the total number of PCPs through the automation of care and use of lower-level clinicians is the first of a one-two punch. The second is the sudden proliferation of findings on the relative clinical ineffectiveness of PCPs on the sickest patients. One such study of adult asthma patients, released in 1997 by the Managed Health Care Association Outcomes Management Consortium, found that patients treated by asthma specialists had better health status over time than those treated by generalists.[22] Another study, released in 1997 by the American College of Cardiology, showed that, after adjusting for relative clinical risk, patients hospitalized with heart attacks are 26 percent more likely to die if managed by an internist and 29 percent more likely to die if managed by a family practitioner.[23] And numerous studies of those with chronic disease have found that clinical ineffectiveness is more costly over the long run (meaning employers and consumers care) *and* short run (meaning MCOs care).

Nonetheless, in the early 1990s, when the use of PCPs as gatekeepers for the entire system was a *fait accompli* under the "managed care revolution," it was the rare contrarian view (not counting the protestations of specialists themselves, of course) that gatekeeping via PCPs for a covered population may reduce the use of specialists—but ultimately costs more for the entire covered group. Why? Because whatever savings flow from that fraction of patients that PCPs *can* filter out and treat more cost-effectively than specialists—will always be outweighed by the costs of using PCPs as gatekeepers for all those other patients they *cannot* filter out and treat. Using a PCP to sort through all presenting patients in a population adds one more encounter per patient illness for all those patients who end up requiring a specialist anyway—and thus one more blanket layer of cost.

This is the obvious thinking behind the decision by Oxford Health Plans in early 1997—once again incorporating leading-edge findings into its business practices—to use specialists rather than PCPs to manage the total medical needs of its chronically ill members. Such a break from the traditional MCO's model of patient control is based on Oxford's recognition of clinical findings like those cited above, and its corollary understanding that PCPs are not effective at managing all the treatments, expenses, and options for the chronically ill, a group that represents $1.7 billion of the company's $2.2 billion medical loss ratio in 1996.[24] Oxford also recognizes that consumerism plays a major role in this drama: the publicization of data on the superior clinical effectiveness of specialists versus PCPs serves only to heighten demands by consumers for direct access to specialists. Without such access, they will vote for other plans with their feet.

As explored earlier, the rise of consumerism merely exacerbates the marketing problems of MCOs, increases demands for greater flexibility within existing plans, and helps accelerate the ultimate demise of the managed care industry. In order to preserve market share and grow their overall populations, MCOs cannot help but participate in their own destruction. A telling example is the publicization by United Healthcare—within a few weeks of Oxford's announcement about specialist management of its chronically ill members—that it provides members with direct access to specialists without PCP authorization in United plans in 18 states.

"Such plans are the fastest-growing part of United Healthcare's non-Medicare business," James Carlson, executive vice-president for the MCO's health care operations told the *Wall Street Journal*.[25] Direct specialist access is, like the choice of individual physicians, highly cherished by the American health care consumer. This preference is destined to increase as health care consumers grow older and sicker, and as they become more educated about their own health care thanks, paradoxically, to the wellness and prevention efforts of the MCOs themselves.

Unfettered access to specialists is particularly important among women, given the unique nature of specific women's health issues and the enormous variations in care inflicted upon female patients (e.g., hysterectomy rates) by the health care system over the years. In fact, because "women's health" is central, rather than peripheral, to many female patients' views of their own medical care, the OB/ GYN specialist often serves as the *de facto* PCP for women. An illustration of this pattern is the fact that 23 percent of all antidepressants and 12 percent of all cholesterol-lowering drugs prescribed for women are done so by OB/GYNs. The first class of drugs is only obliquely related to the OB/GYN's sphere of clinical concern (e.g., depression after hysterectomy or childbirth), the last almost not at all. And as the introduction of care automation tools and physician extenders successfully inserts a battery of nonphysicians into the medical equation, then the "managing PCP" for most women may one day consist exclusively of OB/GYNs (and, later in life, gerontologists)—with general and family practitioners removed entirely from the process.

All of these market forces toward specialization notwithstanding, there must be some force more fundamental at work driving the supposed imbalance in specialists to PCPs in the current health care system—given the inroads of managed care over the past decade, with its initial emphasis on PCPs. The old fee-for-service system, supportive as it always was of supply-side medicine, simply does not explain the persistence of this "imbalance" into the late 1990s; nor does the additional income and prestige associated with specialization, especially given the rapid and well-publicized descent of the former. The real driving force behind the historic, current, and consistent "disproportion" of specialists is the simple fact that medicine is too complex, and the compounding fact that it is becoming only more so with each new wave of medical technology. The clinical community does not have a fixed number of drugs to use; when a new one is launched, another does not go away. The proliferation of new technologies like MRIs, which are extremely complex to interpret, does not mean that physicians no longer need to know how to read X-rays. Rather, they need to know how to utilize yet one more generation of technology. Each new medical breakthrough is additive: there are that many more choices, that many more benefits and side effects to consider, that much more data to digest.

The compulsion to specialize is not unique to medicine; it affects all fields with complex and continually evolving technologies. What *is* unique to medicine is the sudden confluence of the five forces of its transformation, as described in this book; *rigorous analysis of these forces indicates that what the health care system needs is more specialization, not less.* The very concept of health care industrialization compels specialization: the information tools and real-time clinical process analyses at its heart represent yet another new wave of technology for all physician specialties to absorb.

An excellent example of how the process of health care industrialization drives physician specialization is the introduction of the "hospitalist" specialty. Hospitalists specialize in inpatient care, long a fixture in the Canadian and British systems with their state-owned facilities. As of this writing, hospitalists are being introduced into those U.S. markets with the longest histories of managed care penetration, notably San Francisco.[26] The goal of the hospitalist is focus and efficiency. Because they are stationary in the hospital, hospitalists can manage patients in ways that are consistent with the spirit of health care industrialization: they practice via protocols and best demonstrated practices, mindful of the new era of cost-economics and the imperative to optimize resource consumption.[27] The advent of the hospitalist echoes that of intensivists, another specialty focused not on a specific physiologic system, but instead on coordinating the treatment of the entire patient within a specific medical setting. Both hospitalists and intensivists are generalists from a clinical standpoint; their specialization is a specific *process* of care.

Taken together, the rise of hospitalists and intensivists for acute care—and the radical restructuring of all other care through automated systems and nonphysician clinicians—point to one highly paradoxical conclusion: in the new century's health care system, the United States will probably need *more* specialists, not fewer. Taken to its logical extreme, one could easily argue that—contrary to the views of policy makers and the keepers of the conventional wisdom across the health care industry—the future of American medicine will not witness a greater emphasis on primary care physicians, but a near elimination of them.

HOLY (AND SECULAR) ALLIANCES WITH HOSPITAL SYSTEMS

If, as described earlier, the typical health care market inevitably segments into two to four local EHOs based on price, then each EHO's affiliated physicians obviously segment as well. Under such a market sorting, the physicians perceived as the most highly skilled will be part of the most highly differentiated system. How individual physicians end up in the higher-end EHO will be a natural extension of the ongoing filtering process that occurs all along the gauntlet of formal medical education, beginning with the rigors of premed competition for admission to the best medical schools and ending with the quest for a "match" with the best residency programs. This process creates a pecking order based on grades, honors, fellowships, research work, and faculty recommendations; and the subdivision of markets into differentiated EHOs will create a logical extension—one with far greater permanence and financial implications—of this preprofessional sorting.

The rudiments of a pecking order of physicians based on hospital affiliation exist within today's looser, but still ultimately differentiating, system of hospital privileges. As Starr notes, "because the hospital was essential to successful practice, its various grades could be used as delicately calibrated rewards to signal the progress of a career."[28] The stratification of physicians by vertically integrated, hospital-based EHOs—rather than by horizontal, stand-alone hospitals—represents the impact of consumerism on what was once a homogeneous, quasi-public enterprise.

No doubt those who believe that medicine is a public service and should be available equally to all as part of an expanded welfare state—and by extension that physicians are interchangeable public servants within that welfare state—will find the segmentation of physicians within a market somewhat offensive. Indeed, it represents a further polarization of the U.S. health care system. The sorting of physician by market segment is one more example of how the health care system is coming, more and more, to resemble any other product market served by corporate America. The goal here is not to pass judgment on this end, merely to anticipate and explore its ramifications for physicians and others with a real stake in the outcome.

Underlying this process of segmentation is one foregone conclusion about the new century's health care system: all physicians will be aligned with a system of hospitals through a financial/legal structure that is still only emerging. While the whole notion of such an alignment would have seemed absurd only a generation ago, the competitive pressures that drive the business behaviors of both parties will make it critical for the next. Such is the power of the system in flux: it has the potential of clarifying and focusing the long, complex, ambivalent relationship between physicians and hospitals, a relationship that historically has operated along a continuum of outright hostility, tangential competition, and guarded co-existence. With the emergence of the indemnity insurance system, the power pendulum eventually swung in favor of the physicians, as they made treatment decisions, directed admissions, and ultimately controlled the blank checks offered up by the sick and well-insured patient. "The private practitioners, who had first seen hospitals as a threat to their position, had succeeded in converting them into an instrument of professional power," Paul Starr observes.[29]

The pendulum is in the process of swinging back as EHOs engaged in consumer marketing—not the traditional insurers and MCOs—ultimately emerge as the source of business for physicians. The hospitals at the heart of an EHO have the marketing clout, capital, and information and control systems necessary to assume and manage medical/financial risk. This inherent power of the hospitals will be counterbalanced by the American consumers' prerogative to choose, whenever possible, their personal physician, following him or her into their affiliated EHO with their premium dollars. The end result will be an unprecedented symbiosis between physicians and hospitals, one necessary to deliver truly integrated patient care across the continuum of medical sites. The mutual interdependence of this arrangement cannot help but galvanize physician self-determination, as the EHOs come to rely on them for leadership more than their member hospitals ever did. This increasing level of participation is evident in the governance structure of today's physician-hospital organization (PHO), the antecedent structure of the fully realized EHO. Whereas physicians make up at best 20 percent the typical hospital's board, in PHOs they typically comprise up to 50 percent.[30]

Getting to this promised land of shared risk, responsibility, and rewards will require massive reorientation in the way hospitals and physicians have worked together historically. Board participation is a good start, but it hardly translates into smooth management of the EHO's clinical and business operations. What is required is a sea change in the way physicians approach the hospital, inserting themselves more forcefully and proactively into day-to-day management rather than remaining at the periphery, providing only reactive feedback to the initiatives of the traditional administrators. Physicians should also be incorporated into the business development process of the EHO, particularly given the newness of the terrain that all EHOs will be charting in the next decade. Consummation of all the clinical and financial improvement promises that EHOs make to employers and other purchasers during contract negotiations is contingent upon the medical staff's ability to deliver—to implement the changes that will improve quality and/or reduce costs. Thus, physician participation is the critical success factor for the entire enterprise. As with the advent of physician extenders, physicians will be expected to assume increasingly managerial roles within the operation of the EHO.

Fulfillment of these expanded roles by physicians underscores the economic dynamic driving their relationship with hospitals in an EHO. Given their discretionary power over medical costs, these dynamics cannot help but work in favor of the physicians. This power will allow them, according to Montague Brown, writing in *Integrated Health Care Delivery*, to "move their prices up a notch and shift the hospital's down a notch or two...The physicians determine nearly all of the hospital's costs through their individual utilization patterns."[31] This is the physician trump card in the endgame with hospitals. Enlightened hospitals know this; enlightened physicians know how to play it.

EQUITY, EQUITY, THAT'S OUR CRY

At the heart of Karl Marx's theories is the belief that the root cause of all human unhappiness is the alienation of labor from capital. Though mostly unbeknownst to their champions in today's organizations, a variety of corporate phenomena—ranging from employee stock ownership programs to the marketing of employee-owned airlines—represent an application of Marx's core belief. And though they too would be remiss to admit it, when it comes to Marx's principle of economic self-determination, most physicians are not all that different from car rental company employees, only more so: a real ownership stake in the enterprise diminishes the sense that one is not in control of one's own economic destiny.

Such ownership is important given the large proportion of the medical enterprise defined by the cost of clinical labor; the significant dollar value of total resources controlled by physicians; the profound impact that physician behavior has on consumer satisfaction; and how notoriously difficult physicians are to manage as traditional employees. An essay in *Health Care Strategic Management* sums it up best:

> As a group, physicians are noncompliant and they do not readily accept change. They are self-directed, autonomous individuals whose personal standards are paramount and who tend to practice defensively. It is not surprising that organizations value a wholly different set of characterizations and seek out individuals who are: collaborative and adaptable; knowledgeable about the practical demands of operating a business; supportive of managed care principles and practices.[32]

That physicians should give a whit about their attractiveness to "organizations" would have seemed preposterous a generation ago. Yet, in a few short years it has become tantamount to their survival in the new century's health care system. A landmark study published in the *Journal of the American Medical Association* in 1996 found that between 1983 and 1994, the percentage of physicians working as employees nearly doubled, from 24.2 to 42.3 percent; the proportion of physicians self-employed in solo practices dropped from 40.5 to 29.3 percent.[33] This is nothing short of an earthquake beneath the feet of the profession; more than anything else, this shanghaiing of physicians into employees embodies the very transformation of health care from cottage industry to corporate business.

With the tough-minded, independent physician set in potential conflict against the compulsion of an organization to control and direct its employees, a radical new approach to organizing physician "labor" is in order. Such an approach is embodied in the fully realized EHO. Although physicians are recruited and managed as employees of the EHO, they are employees with large financial stakes in the success of the enterprise, not unlike partners in law firms or senior executives in the best managed corporations. They are paid a base salary, but a substantial portion of their final compensation is tied to the EHO's overall profits. Such an alignment transcends all the micromanagement of resources, utilization, and admissions of current managed care networks and all the partially realized structures like independent practice associations (IPAs) and PHOs operating as predecessors to EHOs. Physicians with a direct and meaningful bottom-line stake in the enterprise are motivated to participate actively in EHO management, hospital administration, clinical cost reduction initiatives, and business development. In practice, they have every interest in keeping the EHO's covered population healthy and out of the hospital.

An EHO built and run partially on physician equity stakes exploits the entrepreneurial instincts that are wholly consistent with the self-reliance and autonomy of the physician personality. It preserves the notion of physician self-determination, aligns physician's interests with that of the hospitals, and gives them a chance to reap the capital gains associated with building a viable business. As Brown points out, equity participation allows physicians to build up value in the enterprise and then cash out of it. "Equity markets provide liquidity," he writes in *Integrated Health Care Delivery*. "Physician investors ultimately need liquidity. Many locally owned not-for-profit firms have too little interest in providing physicians with the kinds of return their assets might command in a public market."[34]

The best argument for the equity model is how grossly mismatched it is to the dysfunctional economics of the legacy health care system, and the strongest proof of all that this model will provide a long overdue correction to those economics. Columbia/HCA jumped on it too quickly, in markets that were still predominantly fee-for-service, and was burned badly by the government for trying to "buy referrals." But as risk-assumption emerges as the only product sold by EHOs—i.e., as the health care system transforms into a more functional, rational industry—the equity model will emerge as the best way to align the economic interests of all parties: purchasers, hospitals, physicians, and patients. The last thing physicians with a financial stake in a system at-risk for a population wants to do is admit a patient to "their" (the physicians') hospital.

GOING NATIONAL: GOING FOR BROKE?

The soundness of strategies that exploit the advantages of physician equity is proven in the inverse—in the cumbersome financial structuring between the national physician practice management (PPM) companies and their physician affiliates. The growth of PPMs echoes many of the themes discussed in this book.

The PPM represents the consolidation of physicians, with the explicit goal of increasing the bargaining power of both these sellers of medical services and these buyers of medical supplies, insurance, information systems, and other products. According to *Health Care Strategic Management*, affiliation with a PPM "gives doctors more leverage at the negotiating table with MCOs. Rather than having to negotiate and contract with multiple MCOs, physicians have access to all of the local players."[35] The PPM also allows previously fragmented groups of physicians to engage in a collective process of industrialization: the PPM represents a *potential* repository of clinical and financial data that can be used to generate and proliferate outcomes analyses, best practice standards, physician versus group versus PPM-wide benchmark clinical performance, and the like. Above all else, the national PPM embodies the triumph of organized business culture over the go-it-alone attempts of the cottage industry physician practice.

PPMs are publicly traded vehicles that, based on their superior economics and other business advantages, enjoy market multiples two to three times those associated with the valuations of private physician group practices.[36] As such, PPMs represent—if nothing else—a pure-play form of physician group arbitrage. This multiple constitutes a liquidity premium; the practice is supposedly worth this much more because there is an active market for it; there are buyers ready every day, around the world, to buy shares; and there is a valuation with nothing less than the collective energy and market wisdom of Wall Street behind it. Of course, such valuations suffer from a certain arbitrariness, namely accounting. PPMs have been pumping up their stock prices by pumping up their earnings in a variety of ways that have not escaped the notice of federal regulators.

The first of these financial engineering strategies is the way they amortize (or deduct from earnings) the intangible assets of their acquired practices over 40 years. Such assets represent the usually enormous difference between what the PPM paid for the practice and what its hard assets (computers, office equipment, etc.) are actually worth. Those intangibles—namely the "goodwill" of the practice, its contracts with MCOs, its presence in the community, and the commitment of its physicians to continue practicing—are expected to contribute to the earning power of the practice, and so they represent assets with value. But how long will they contribute? The way the typical PPM accounts for it, they are expected to contribute for

40 years from the date the practice was purchased.[37] That means no early retirement for any of the practice's physicians, no reductions in fees on current services, no adverse change in payer mix, no changes in the local market that would pull patients away. Yes—it's a stretch. Which is why the federal Securities and Exchange Commission (SEC), after investigating the PPM's accounting, is pushing to shorten the period of which the intangible assets can be amortized to 10 years.[38]

The second financial engineering strategy used by PPMs is to give physicians restricted equity shares in the PPM instead of salary, so as to reduce operating costs and improve the bottom line—temporarily. This pumps up the PPM's numbers for Wall Street. Unfortunately, while the physicians are waiting to cash out those restricted shares, they're working for less salary and still have personal bills to pay, so the PPM lends them cash, using the private shares as collateral.

Now do you feel like taking a hot shower?

Perhaps all the financing shenanigans that have come to define the PPM industry are inevitable, given the weakness of all strategic arguments for their existence. As has been demonstrated throughout general academic business literature and was discussed at length in Part II, horizontal consolidation ultimately requires vertical integration. The added bureaucratic costs associated with managing horizontal consolidation can be carried by the enterprise only through its attainment of the economies of vertical integration. As of this writing, there appears to be no coherent strategy for vertical integration of the PPMs at the national level. Specifically, there have been no mergers between one of the national hospital systems or MCOs with any of the PPMs. The only deals that come close, as of this writing, are alliances between Tenet and MedPartners to serve Southern California, and between Aetna/US Healthcare, supposedly to serve everybody.

But why no major national move by Tenet, or Daughters, or Columbia (before the scandal), or any other national hospital system? Because merging a national hospital group with a national group of physicians would contradict the hospital chains' core strategies of tailoring local market structure to local market conditions. As discussed at length in Part III ("Prognosis"), local EHOs all need to hedge on physician integration, aligning with a local group, or exclusively with one of the PPMs, or through a mixture of both. This makes a one-size-fits-all national PPM model difficult to impose on heterogeneous markets.

Perhaps recognizing this problem, MedPartners has tried to integrate on the national level in the other direction. Through a corporate-wide deal with Aetna/US Healthcare, MedPartners physicians will serve the MCO's covered populations in markets across the country. If ever fully consummated, a consumer who chooses Aetna/US Healthcare's plan in a local market would then be forced to choose a MedPartners doctor. This is exactly backwards. While this arrangement will work fine for those consumers whose current or preferred physician is already part of MedPartners, it shuts Aetna/US Healthcare out of the rest of the market. Eventually, it will also come to represent Aetna/US Healthcare's preselection of entire EHOs for its members, i.e., those EHOs affiliated with MedPartners' physicians. Existing members will chafe against this restrictiveness; prospects will refuse to join the plan; and Aetna/US Healthcare will eventually have to contract outside its own deal, thus defeating its original purpose.

In contrast to developing a national template and imposing it onto every local health care market, PPMs need to approach each market with the nimbleness of a franchisee. But it remains to be seen if PPMs can give up sufficient control to accomplish this, while retaining enough of the consolidation rationale to justify their continued existence. This is a bit of a squeeze play, and the PPMs are probably not equipped to pull it off. For hospitals, the capital intensity, large supply budgets, complex information systems, and big-ticket pricing negotiations of the stand-alone facility more than justify national consolidations. Does the same hold true for physician practices, which are far more labor-intensive, local service-oriented businesses?

Many PPMs also violate the principle of equity discussed earlier. The widely publicized struggles of one pioneering PPM, Coastal Physician Group, is a case in point. Coastal traditionally imposed pure employee status on its physicians after purchasing their practices. The result was a sea change in physician behavior. According to a report in the *Wall Street Journal*, "once the company paid a fat sum for their practices, many of the physician-owners-turned-salaried-employees weren't as eager to pull in business as they had been."[39] Coastal's near market collapse in 1996—which turned its founder against the Board in a nasty, public fight for control of the company—has served as an object lesson for the other PPMs to build equity into their models.

Apprised of Coastal's management difficulties, most of the other national PPMs have converted their acquired physicians into equity participants. Unfortunately, this equity tends to take the form of the PPM's publicly traded shares. In sharp contrast to EHO equity participation, whereby individual physician clinical behavior has a meaningful financial impact on the EHO's bottom line, the impact of more cost-effective decision making by a physician working in a 10,000-physician national practice is greatly diluted. (An even half-conscious physician would also recognize how little impact his or her clinical effectiveness would have on the PPM's share price relative to the often bizarre "Street" logic and daily histrionics of the stock market.) As a result, physicians have no greater ownership stake—or individual profitability leverage—in their PPM than the typical employees in a stock ownership program have in their corporation. Granted, this arrangement is better than the full alienation of labor from capital in a pure employee-employer relationship. But how much better?

This begs the most troubling question of all about PPMs: how does a business manage so many different physicians from afar, when they are barely manageable locally? Is equity—even a substantial stake in the local franchise of the national PPM, as practiced by a few PPMs—sufficient alignment and motivation? PPMs are, at bottom, growing through the acquisition of existing businesses, practices that had been run independently by the most independent-minded of all professionals. Their imposition of management control systems on those former entrepreneurs leads to nothing short of a cultural revolution.

At least so far, it does not appear to be an issue, as MedPartners proves itself incapable of running local practices effectively. For the fourth quarter of 1997, it took an unexpected charge of $145 million against earnings, to account for "overutilization" within clinics in Southern California, and to build up reserves for further losses on at-risk contracts.[40] Here, the company has proven itself supremely incapable of running its clinical operations under risk-based contracts—*the single most critical success factor for physician practice managers in the new century's health care system.*

So what happened in Southern California, an important market for both MedPartners and everyone else seeking to build a national health care company? The smart money would attribute this chaos to the well-publicized tussle between MedPartners and the leaders of Friendly Hills Healthcare Network. One of the largest, most progressive, physician-based managed care systems in the country, Friendly Hills was acquired by Caremark, which in turn was acquired by MedPartners in the deal that catapulted MedPartners into the leadership position in the PPM industry. Typical of many acquisitions, MedPartners inherited a number of management challenges that it neutralized with a number of management promises, including that of continued autonomy for the founders of Friendly Hills. The founders chafed against the new regime and, according to *Modern Healthcare*, "had a major clash with their new employer on various management and cultural issues."[41] The result was a raft of lawsuits and countersuits, a disruption to operations, and enormous uncertainty for a key part of the nation's largest PPM.

This is the first episode of its kind to spill out into the daylight, if only because Friendly Hills is a high-profile, bellwether group practice in one of the nation's most competitive health care markets. Indeed, the episode may turn out to be a fluke of outsized egos, bad corporate chemistry, and gross miscommunications. On the other hand, given that MedPartners has grown only bigger and more complex since the problem arose—and given that each subsequent practice left for MedPartners to acquire will consist of physicians who held out that much longer for whatever reason—this may be a preview of coming attractions.

THE UNBEARABLE LIGHTNESS OF RISK BEARING

One final word about the relationship between MCOs and physicians: though they have been whipsawed by the managed care regime, in the end physicians will prevail over that regime, if only by default. MCOs will slowly but surely fade away because of their inherent contradiction: they are in the first and final analysis, health insurers; they are *not* care providers. Their almost exclusively financial agenda has created an irreconcilable distortion in the way any rational producer would "manage care"—distortions they have imposed upon physicians.

Separate health plans devise and propound their own "guidelines," forcing physicians to practice one way for one patient, a different way for another patient, and still a third way for another. While this perverts the clinical decision-making process, physicians' collective rage at this perversion has fallen on deaf ears. Try with relish as they might, legislators simply cannot make the MCOs abandon the practice in general; consumers can, however, by abandoning the MCOs. As consumers are only now beginning to discover how violently managed care operators have interjected themselves into the physician-patient relationship, they will vote with their premiums. And where better to take those premium dollars than directly to "your" physician?

One of the more celebrated and egregious examples of the clinical schizophrenia imposed on providers by MCOs is the arbitrary use of autologous bone marrow transplants as a last-ditch effort to save late-stage breast cancer patients. Perpetuating the most extreme version of this abuse was Health Net, later a part of HSI, and now a part of Foundation Health Systems. In an episode reported by George

Anders in *Health against Wealth*, Health Net denied a bone marrow transplant for a patient based on guidelines written for the MCO by the very same physician who had recommended the procedure for that very same woman.[42] Why did he recommend it? Because he was unaware that she was covered by Health Net when examining her, and was thus free to exercise his full clinical judgment. This is nonsense. Physicians should practice medicine one way and one way only: the way that works best. Period. The vagaries of who happens to insure a patient should not matter!

When the current transformation of the system is complete, such clinical schizophrenia will have evaporated along with the MCO layer that generated it. Thanks to the fluidity of a more rationalized health care marketplace, physicians will have reconciled the schizophrenia in their own practices, using the very same sticks that MCOs have been beating them with over the years: risk-assumption and performance measurement. Under the assumption of medical/financial risk, the calculation between cost and clinical effectiveness is no longer a struggle between doctor and insurer; rather, it becomes unified within the physician's own clinical decision-making process. Medical choices become subject not to the arbitrary intrusions of managed care, but rather to a physician's own professional judgment and conscience. What will inform this decision making is the source of another great irony: it exists in all the utilization management systems, physician performance analysis software, and other apparatus of MCO scrutiny into physician clinical and financial behavior. It is a treasure trove of data and tools for analyzing that data.

Such technologies embody the essential spirit of health care industrialization that the idealized version of the MCO meant to bring to the care delivery process. Lee Newcomer, MD, the national medical director of United Healthcare, describes the origins of this spirit in a *Health Affairs* essay:

> As a medical oncologist, I can still name all of the Hodgkin's disease patients I lost. Cure rates for this disease are 92 percent in its early stages, so an oncologist considers a death from this disease his personal failure. I constantly

reviewed and examined the decisions that I might have made differently in those cases. I am not unique; every physician is his or her own toughest critic. Regrettably, I cannot tell you whether I was a good or a mediocre oncologist. The practice did not track the actual percentage of patients cured; I was measured only by anecdote. Like most of my colleagues, I never received any objective measure of performance.[43]

This is a powerful expression of the rationale for the many tools that MCOs have attempted to use to analyze their network providers. A burgeoning industry of "medical informatics" vendors is emerging to develop and market these tools to the MCOs. They compile and analyze hard data on what works best—from a clinical, financial, and outcomes perspective—in the care of patients. Such tools are commercially available to physicians, hospitals, and, ultimately, the EHOs to conduct these very same empirical analyses on their own practices. When physicians are willing to embrace these tools as fearlessly as the MCOs do—and incorporate their findings into their medical practices to improve care while managing costs—they will have completed the revolution that the MCOs themselves began.

Armed with these tools, physicians will be fully equipped to make the fundamental fixes outlined in the previous sections of this book. After doing so successfully, physicians' fortunes will be a modified replay of their good fortune over most of this past century in which, as Starr puts it, "not only did physicians become a powerful, prestigious, and wealthy profession, but they succeeded in shaping the basic organization and financial structure of American medicine."[44] In the new century's health care system, this history is destined to repeat itself.

REFERENCES

1. D. Loxterkamp, "Hearing Voices," *New England Journal of Medicine*, 26 December, 1996, 1992–1993.

2. In 1994, the average physician income fell for the first time in decades, by 4 percent, according to a report on physician income survey released in 1996, as reported by R. Winslow, "Doctors' Average Pay Fell 4 Percent in 1994 with Drop Attributed to Managed Care," *Wall Street Journal*, 3 September, 1996.

3. A.M. Stoline and J.P. Weiner, *The New Medical Marketplace: A Physician's Guide to the Health Care System in the 1990s* (Baltimore: The Johns Hopkins University Press, 1993), 11. © 1993. The Johns Hopkins University Press.

4. H. Brown and R. Shinto, "Making Physicians Networks Work," *Health Care Strategic Management,* April 1996, 1.

5. Health Care Mergers and Acquisitions Report for 1996 (New Canaan, CT: Irving Levin and Associates) reported in *Modern Healthcare*, 19 March, 1997, 3.

6. Stoline and Weiner, *The New Medical Marketplace: A Physician's Guide to the Health Care System in the 1990s*, 140. © 1993. The Johns Hopkins University Press.

7. Stoline and Weiner, *The New Medical Marketplace: A Physician's Guide to the Health Care System in the 1990s*, 26. © 1993. The Johns Hopkins University Press.

8. G. Hart et al., "Physician Staffing Ratios in Staff-Model MCOs: A Cautionary Tale," *Health Affairs*, January/February 1997, 56.

9. Hart et al., *Health Affairs*, 61.

10. Hart et al., *Health Affairs*, 68.

11. R. Johnson, "HCMR Perspective: The Economic Era of Health Care," in *Integrated Health Care Delivery: Theory, Practice, Evaluation, and Prognosis,* ed. M. Brown (Gaithersburg, MD: Aspen Publishers, 1996), 46.

12. Johnson, *Integrated Health Care Delivery: Theory, Practice, Evaluation, and Prognosis,* 46.

13. "Physicians Working Smarter, Not Harder," *Health Care Strategic Management*, February 1997, 14.

14. "Physicians Working Smarter, Not Harder," *Health Care Strategic Management*, 14.

15. *Physician Assistants: Statistics and Trends, 1991–1996*, published by the American Academy of Physician Assistants.

16. "Encouraging the Use of Nurse-Midwives," *Public Citizen*, November 1995.

17. K. Hammonds, "Oxford's Education," *Business Week*, 8 April, 1996, 110.

18. R. Winslow, "Nurses To Take Doctor Duties, Oxford Says," *Wall Street Journal*, 7 February, 1997.

19. Survey data included in "The New Physician Executives: Leadership for the Future," *Health Care Strategic Management*, February 1997, 11.

20. Stoline and Weiner, *The New Medical Marketplace: A Physician's Guide to the Health Care System in the 1990s*, 23. © 1993. The Johns Hopkins University Press.

21. J. Merritt, "How Many Docs?" *Modern Healthcare*, 10 March, 1997, 110.

22. N. Jeffrey, "Doctors Battle over Who Treats Chronically Ill," *Wall Street Journal*, 11 December, 1996.

23. Study from *Journal of the American College of Cardiology*, as reported in *Modern Healthcare*, 17 March, 1997.

24. R. Winslow, "Oxford To Give More Control to Specialists," *Wall Street Journal*, 25 March, 1997.

25. Jeffrey, *Wall Street Journal*.

26. R. Wachter and L. Goldman, "The Emerging Role of Hospitalists in the American Health Care System," *New England Journal of Medicine*, 15 August, 1996, 514.

27. Wachter and Goldman, *New England Journal of Medicine*, 514.

28. P. Starr, *The Social Transformation of American Medicine*, 168, quoting Glaser, "American and Foreign Hospitals," from *Hospital in Modern Society*, ed. E. Freidson (New York: Free Press, 1963), 54.

29. Starr, *The Social Transformation of American Medicine*, 169.

30. M. Brown, "Commentary: The Economic Era: Now to the Real Change," in *Integrated Health Care Delivery: Theory, Practice, Evaluation, and Prognosis*, ed. M. Brown (Gaithersburg, MD: Aspen Publishers, 1996), 55.

31. Brown, *Integrated Health Care Delivery: Theory, Practice, Evaluation, and Prognosis*, 55.

32. Brown and Shinto, *Health Care Strategic Management*, 21.

33. P. Kletke et al., "Current Trends in Physicians' Practice Arrangements," *Journal of the American Medical Association*, 21 August, 1996, 555.

34. Brown, *Integrated Health Care Delivery: Theory, Practice, Evaluation, and Prognosis*, 55.

35. S. Campbell, "Physician Practice Management," *Health Care Strategic Management,* June 1996, 13.

36. A. Bianco, "Doctors Inc.," *Business Week*, 24 March, 1997, 204.

37. M. Jaklevic, "Reining in Docs," *Modern Healthcare*, 31 March, 1998, 41.

38. Jaklevic, *Modern Healthcare*, 41.

39. N. Deogun, "Network of Doctors Touted as Panacea, Develops Big Problem," *Wall Street Journal*, 26 September, 1996.

40. A. Sharpe, a report on MedPartners, *Wall Street Journal*, Interactive Version, 19 March, 1998.

41. R. Shinkman, "Two MedPartners Execs Out of Jobs, Facing Lawsuits," *Modern Healthcare*, 2 December, 1996, 8.
42. G. Anders, *Health against Wealth* (New York: Houghton Mifflin, 1996), 124–125.
43. L. Newcomer, "Measures of Trust in Health Care," *Health Affairs*, January/February 1997, 50.
44. Starr, *The Social Transformation of American Medicine,* 8.

8

PANACEAS R US

We're part of the cure.

Promotional slogan for Pfizer Inc.,
fourth largest pharmaceutical company in the world

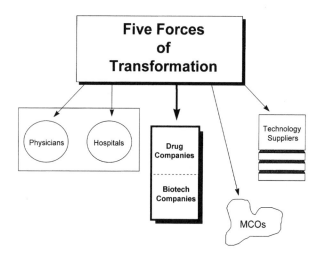

This will be a short chapter for good reason. The last three decades have witnessed lockstep cycles of diversification and divestiture by the major pharmaceutical companies. Since the 1970s these cash-rich companies have moved into and out of vaguely related businesses: nutrition, animal health, cosmetics, a brief flirtation with generics, continuing flirtations with medical informatics, and wrongheaded attempts at forward integration into pharmacy benefit management, all punctuated by quadrennial rounds of generally inspired consolidation. Having tried every other conceivable corporate development scheme, what will prove to be the best strategy for today's drugmakers seeking to compete in the new century's health care system? *Make more and better drugs.*

Unlike hospitals, doctors, MCOs, and most technology suppliers, drug companies have one distinct advantage: they sell expensive, highly proprietary products that pay for themselves in the medical equation many times over. The *net* value of each new generation of pharmaceuticals—and of most variants within each generation—is enormous. Compared to the cost of the diseases remediated, hospitalizations prevented, and surgeries forestalled, even the most expensive drugs are a bargain. The sheer economic leverage inherent in most pharmaceuticals explains why, protestations about price aside, expensive new drugs are eagerly and actively embraced almost universally—not only by consumers, but also by hospitals, physicians, and MCOs.

This economic leverage also explains why the body blow to the industry expected from the weighty trajectory of managed care never landed. In fact, just the opposite has occurred: the advent of managed care—the supposed bogeyman to the drug companies because it represents the consolidation of drug purchasing at steep discounts—has actually proven a boon to them. According to a report in the *Wall Street Journal* following a tide of positive earnings news from major drugmakers near the end of 1996, "growth in managed care is actually good for the growth of pharmaceuticals because managed care emphasizes less expensive, preventive types of treatment."[1] Such emphasis is embodied in the benefit plan structures for MCOs, which typically charge nominal amounts or nothing for drugs, versus the much larger copayments under traditional insurance. "Managed care insurers are paying for the prescriptions of more patients…and those patients are filling more of their prescriptions," the report continues.[2] Why? Because the end result of more prescriptions written, filled, and taken is a healthier, less costly population for the insurer.

This has been confirmed in numerous studies of drug utilization and total health care costs for covered populations. One study in par-

ticular, conducted by researchers for the managed care industry, provided the best vindication for drugmakers vis-à-vis the managed
care revolution: it found and quantified the unintended, negative
economic consequences associated with the maintenance of a restrictive "formulary" of prescription drugs.[3] These formularies—
lists of pre-approved products—have been held out by MCOs as an
effective way to reduce drug costs: by channeling all patients in a
therapeutic class toward one type of drug, the MCO can leverage
deep volume discounts from manufacturers and reduce excess utilization of more expensive brands. The resulting clinical inflexibility
backfired: the managed care study found that patients with the most
restricted access to prescription drugs had the highest total medical
costs; those with the least restricted access, the lowest total medical
costs. The drug companies' core value proposition is thus vindi-
cated; the threat to the industry posed by the imposition of a formulary turns out to be a bigger menace to those who wield it.

In this sense, pharmaceutical products fulfill one of Porter's observations about price premiums: "If the product or service…can
improve the performance of the buyer's product, then the buyer will
tend to be insensitive to price."[4] Indeed, drugs reduce hospital stays,
eliminate emergency department visits, delay or preclude surgery,
and slow the inevitable progression of chronic conditions. They are
the health care system's best deal, which explains why MCOs and
employers have been far less likely to pick on the drugmakers than
they have on other "suppliers" of health care services. It is as if managed care has recognized, on some collective unconscious level, that
expensive drugs mean more and faster breakthroughs, better drugs,
and still lower health care costs in the long run.

In *The Death of Competition*, James Moore refers to this as a "social compact…In exchange for investing heavily in product and process innovation, drug companies have enjoyed comparatively high
margins."[5] Interestingly, Moore fears that this "social compact" is
now in jeopardy, as the government addresses the cost problems afflicting Medicare and Medicaid without recognizing what the MCOs
clearly have: that higher prices continue to drive product innovation,
the embodiment of the social compact in the private sector. This is

one more argument for privatization of the government's health care programs.

ON THE WINNING SIDE OF THE REVOLUTION

Just as the forces of managed care work in favor of the drug companies, so do all five forces of the transformation of health care in general. All bearers of medical risk recognize the inherent cost benefit of early and aggressive intervention of drugs in comparison to surgery, hospitalization, or more aggressive preventive therapies. This awareness only increases as risk-bearing moves closer to the actual delivery system. An MCO executive may be able to recite the favorable cost benefit analysis associated with expensive cholesterol-lowering medicines for people at risk of a second heart attack; the physicians who run an EHO can tell you exactly *why* this occurs clinically, precisely where those costs will be taken out, and how best to make sure the people at risk appreciate their good luck and express that appreciation through strict compliance with their prescription orders.

So too, the forces of integration and health care industrialization greatly favor the drug companies. The improved coordination of care embodied in the vertical integration of the medical delivery system places a particular emphasis on the timing and utilization of best therapies; a system of truly coordinated care also seeks to improve patient compliance with physician orders. Remember the map of the continuum of care in Part II? "Pharmaceutical care" stretched the length of the treatment system, because it pervades all aspects of medical care and needs to be coordinated as such. As EHOs seek to integrate and orchestrate medical care for the best possible outcomes and lowest possible costs, they place a particular emphasis on integrating information about patient drug compliance. Why? Because a missed drug treatment by a home health care provider can well mean a readmission to the hospital for a complication that the drug treatment was meant to preclude. Because drugs handed out in an emergency department for a routine ear infection can interact with drugs prescribed for routine allergies, resulting in a serious cardiac event in an otherwise healthy patient. Because the failure to refill a prescription for an antidepressant could well mean admission to a psychiatric hospital for an acute depressive attack or worse.

As the forces of integration tie together medical care across the continuum, the forces of industrialization provide the empirical knowledge that ties together the clinical decision making at each point along that continuum. Both place a special emphasis on protocols that seek to maximize outcomes and cost-effectiveness. Under both movements, drugs always prove to be just what the doctor ordered.

And of the five forces of health care transformation, none plays better to the industry's strength and positioning than consumerism. Well-versed in mass marketing and consumer brand management from their over-the-counter businesses, the pharmaceutical companies—aided by a relaxation of federal rules on adverse risk disclosure—have attacked the consumer market with a frenzy of advertising. In 1997, drugmakers spent $800 million on direct-to-consumer advertising, a ten-fold increase over 1992.[6] The principle behind this advertising is the same consumer "pull-through" strategy practiced by smarter health systems seeking to force their way onto MCO networks: if patients know about and demand specific drugs, then physicians—the traditional targets of drug promotion—will be compelled to prescribe them.

Consumer marketing also taps into our strong cultural belief in the power of technology—the latest version of which is always perceived (correctly or not) as the most advanced. Backlash against managed care has served only to galvanize this sentiment: numerous doctors report that patients have begun to demand the latest, branded drug within a class of near-equivalents—because they "know/heard that the HMO will skimp if it can," switching them to a substitute. They automatically expect this of their MCO, and automatically recoil against it, convinced by their experience in most other product markets that more expensive is more effective. If this were not the case, then SmithKline Beecham would not be allowed to charge twice the price of generic coated aspirin for its Ecotrin brand, precisely the same chemical, which consumers pay for out of pocket.[7]

THE EMERGENCE OF "BIG PHARMA"

So too, the force of health care consolidation works in favor of the drugmakers. Granted, the bargaining power of buyers has increased greatly with the consolidation of hospitals and physician groups—the drugmakers' industrial consumers—and the consolidation of MCOs, insurers, employers, and employer coalitions (all proxies for the drugmakers' retail consumers). But such power is easily held in check by drugmakers who

- are already consolidated to a large degree, relative to the fragmentation of providers;
- enjoy well-entrenched national marketing organizations; and
- have undergone their own consolidation in parallel with the rest of the health care industry.

The economies of scale that accrue to a major drug company help explain the general health and productivity of Big Pharma as a whole. James Moore in *The Death of Competition* cites Eli Lilly & Company as an example of a drug company with only one cash cow drug—Prozac—to reinvest in its business. This company has an ability to "plow these profits into further core innovation" resulting in "information and insight used to lead change. The drug companies are ideally positioned to fund and benefit from such efforts…they wield more power in setting standards than most of the managed care leaders."[8]

This leadership is not the result of incumbency or any other transitory advantage prone to erosion as the health care system transforms itself over the coming decades. This leadership, the profitability that continually stokes it, and all the competitive advantages that flow from it, are the result of the sustained and superior risk/reward profile associated with new drug development. This profile is built into the outsized research and development (R&D) spending of the drug industry—14.2 percent of net drug company sales, versus 3.2 percent for all U.S. industrial firms[9]—and to the high valuations of drug industry stocks, which consistently trade at a significant premium to the rest of the stock market. At the time of this writing, the price-earnings ratio for the top 10 drugmakers is 24.6 versus 18.1 for the S&P 500; this spread between the two is typical.[10]

The enormous amount of money spent on for-profit drug research in the United States has a long history. According to Starr, in 1945 the drug industry spent $40 million on basic research, compared to $25 million among not-for-profit organizations, including foundations, universities, and research institutes.[11] By 1996, the private sector number had grown to $15 billion for R&D.[12] (This figure represents only 1.5 percent of the nation's total spending on health care, inarguably a pittance of the total crop to dedicate to seed corn.) Given the magnitude of these costs, what is a bigger surprise: that a handful of pharmaceutical companies control the worldwide drug market—or how large that handful still is? Even after two waves of consolidation, the drug industry is still fragmented to a degree, at least in comparison to other capital- and R&D-intensive industries like autos, aluminum, glass, and semiconductors. As of this writing, no single drug company has more than four truly blockbuster products, and none controls more than 5 percent of the total worldwide market for pharmaceuticals.[13]

Nonetheless, the industry is still engaged in a consolidation-in-progress, a notion confirmed by the accelerating costs of drug development. In the aggregate, expansion of these costs serve to increase the industry's total fixed costs relative to revenue. Thus, Michael Porter's observation that "industry concentration and mobility barriers move together…if mobility barriers are high or especially if they increase, concentration almost always increases"[14] would indicate further consolidation in the future. Mobility barriers are higher for pharmaceutical companies than for almost any industry, save perhaps autos, utilities, chemicals, and steel—and they become increasingly so as the cost of R&D increases every year in real terms.[15] This concentration raises the stakes, decreases the mobility of Big

Pharma, and places ever greater pressures on the individual drug-makers to launch and market their brands successfully.

This helps explain why Big Pharma is renewing its focus on core research, after various forays into businesses vaguely (and sometimes genuinely) related to drug manufacturing and marketing. Such focus has paid off handsomely for Pfizer: steadfastly resisting the temptation to follow other drug companies into the pharmacy benefit management (PBM) industry via acquisition in the early 1990s, Pfizer overtook both Merck and Johnson & Johnson (J&J) as the fastest growing pharmaceutical company in the world, introducing a slew of new drugs for major diseases.[16] Merck, by contrast, sunk $6 billion in potential R&D spending into its acquisition of Medco Containment Services, the nation's largest PBM, and several hundred million into the creation of generic manufacturer, West Point Pharma.[17] When Ray Gilmartin took the helm of the company in 1994, the world's largest drug manufacturer was choking on Medco, struggling with West Point Pharma, and hemorrhaging key executives. Gilmartin assembled a broad, multidisciplinary executive team, the first act of which was to "affirm that Merck would remain a research-driven pharmaceutical company, eschewing diversification," according to a report in *Business Week.* "Backing up the words, Gilmartin quickly shut down the generic drug operation and has since sold off more than $1 billion in assets."[18]

This renewal of focus is nowhere more evident than the merger of Ciba-Geigy and Sandoz Pharmaceuticals into Novartis. While overall economies of scale have been held out as the most immediately tangible benefits of the merger, the real impetus is the streamlining of the two companies' research operations: according to a report in the *Wall Street Journal,* the combined company is engaged in a "battle that neither of its partners felt able to wage successfully on their own: how to spend and save wisely in the hotly competitive, cash-intensive business of pharmaceutical research and development."[19] While both companies have excellent products on the market, their pipelines are characterized by less than promising compounds. Also, both have been notoriously slow—with 11.4 years from lab to FDA licensing application for Ciba and 11.5 years for Sandoz,[20] versus an industry standard 9.8 years.[21] (How important is speed in this process? For the typical drug, every additional day of delay between patent application and product launch equals $1 million in lost patient-protected sales.[22]) Prior to the merger, both companies had undergone major restructuring of their R&D units in the same direction, including heavy pruning and an uncoupling of basic research from development—with the express purpose of speeding up the throughput of their most promising compounds.

Given the increasingly renewed focus of Big Pharma on breakthrough drug development, such consolidation will continue. R&D costs are increasing relative to sales, pushing the risk-reward curve of drug discovery still higher, as products move to market faster and their margins erode faster following patent expiration. As the drug companies continue to improve their performance in a transforming health care system, more investment capital will inevitably flow toward such discovery. Such inflows are the inevitable results of the market's recognition of the unique leverage of drugs in the overall economics of health care financing and delivery. After the next few cycles of such consolidation are complete, the pharmaceutical industry will eventually come to resemble a more profitable version of the worldwide automobile industry, which has many of the same characteristics in terms of decreasing product life cycles, mobility barriers, high fixed costs, and risky R&D.

Big Pharma's Virtual R&D

Macromanagement of the drug discovery process itself is the source of another paradox in health care today: as the drugmakers continue to consolidate into a smaller number of larger companies, more and more of their core product research is occurring outside their own walls. After Big Pharma has developed an infrastructure with the scale necessary to move a wide array of drugs from compound to marketed product, the size of this very infrastructure turns anathema to the cultural nimbleness, technological volatility, and creative serendipity that characterize breakthrough biochemical research. The move by Novartis to uncouple basic research from its product development is a defensive strategy that acknowledges this problem organizationally; it also symbolizes Big Pharma's need to diversify its basic research risk.

Such diversification is accelerated by Big Pharma's move to function less as a basic research house, and more as a shepherd for the basic research of others. Through licensing, equity stakes, comarketing agreements, and other alliances with start-up biotechnology companies, Big Pharma is "renting with an option to buy"—rather than building in-house—the riskiest part of the research pipeline. This hedge strategy supplies start-up research companies with the enormous amounts of cash they need to finance their hungry research missions. This funding of Big Pharma's "virtual R&D" through hundreds of deals in the 1990s fits a variety of models, ranging from straight licensing deals for future marketing rights to outright ownership of the biotech company, which then continues to operate independently to preserve its scientific culture. In an *Industry Week* interview, William Steere, chairman and CEO of Pfizer, describes his company's alliances with 30 to 35 different biotech companies. "Some are license deals, a whole variety, so we have a portfolio of the best and brightest leading-edge companies."[23]

Virtual R&D allows Big Pharma to fill, overnight, an empty pipeline. A good example is American Home Products' decision to purchase the balance of Genetics Institute, in December of 1996, for $1.25 billion. According to the *Wall Street Journal*, "the drug maker's decision to take full control of Genetics Institute signals the company's intent to bolster its own research capabilities by wrapping in Genetics' enviable research pipeline."[24] It also signals the company's intent to buy into a much more entrepreneurial culture. Pfizer's Steere reveals this desire for all of Big Pharma, when describing Pfizer's approach to licensing deals: "we buy just enough equity to keep people motivated, and it seems to work."[25]

Virtual R&D provides Big Pharma with research risk diversification with the stroke of a pen rather than the recruitment and equipping of hundreds of new scientists, researchers, and lab technicians.

The same principle works in reverse: it is much easier to kill failed basic research projects if they are investments on the balance sheet rather than a physical and psychological part of the organization. Delays in killing in-house projects are endemic to the industry; there is a good deal of emotion involved in the drug development process, often making it difficult for Big Pharma to expedite difficult decisions. As Roy Vagelos, MD, former chairman of Merck, told the *Harvard Business Review*, "most people work on ten projects at once and hope that one of them will succeed. And they are often not willing to put down one of the ten because that may be the successful one. That unwillingness is the fastest way to fail."[26]

There is also a technological rationale for outsourcing R&D through partnerships. In the 1990s, a number of competing schools of thought regarding drug design have emerged, resulting in quantum leap–type competition to find the best route to developing the best drugs. For decades, the process was simple and consisted only of "rational drug design," the methodical testing of molecules for biologic action. Core breakthroughs in both microbiology and information technology have ushered in two major competing approaches to basic drug discovery.

The first is combinatorial chemistry, a computer-generated matching of molecular agents and biologic targets that expedites the hit-or-miss labors of rational drug design. The technology was considered important enough for Glaxo Wellcome to plunk down $533 million in cash for five-year-old Affymax, the leading "pure technology" company in the arena of combinatorial chemistry.[27] The other is genome-based development, flowing from the concurrent mapping by scientists of the human genome, which consists of analyzing every possible genetic mutation at the root of human disease. This scientific revolution is, according to a report in the *Wall Street Journal*, "upping the ante by forcing industry leaders to shell out billions of dollars to buy fledgling firms that offer cutting-edge science."[28]

Some big ticket examples of this type of virtual R&D funding include: SmithKline Beecham's $125 million investment in Human Genome Sciences since 1993; Hoechst's $85 million investment in

Ariad in 1997; and Eli Lilly's $70 million investment in Millennium Pharmaceuticals.[29-30] All three licensers focus exclusively on translating the discoveries of the genome mappers into drugs that Big Pharma can develop and market. Combined with the emergence of bioinformatics, which meshes progress in the basic biologic sciences with parallel breakthroughs in information technology, these new approaches have greatly accelerated the process of core drug discovery. As importantly, they have revolutionized the *culture* of core drug discovery, and in ways that do not necessarily favor the traditional R&D scale of Big Pharma. This divergence is consistent with Michael Porter's observation that "technological change may penalize the large-scale firm if facilities designed to reap scale economies are more specialized and less flexible in adapting to new technologies."[31]

The decentralization inherent in the funding of virtual R&D both enables and accelerates the globalization of Big Pharma, already a factor as most major pharmaceutical companies are worldwide organizations. Licensing allows for greater geographic flexibility: countries can invest in new drug discovery technologies wherever they happen to emerge. Such investments are on the rise, as European drugmakers invested $2.6 billion in 52 different U.S.-based biotechnology companies in the 18-month period that ended June 30, 1996, compared to $1.6 billion in 32 biotech companies during the entire previous 24 months.[32]

Why all these investments from Big Pharma when the biotechs have been showered with tens of billions in venture capital and Wall Street cash? A small part of the answer involves some financial history, whereas the larger answer is steeped in strategy. Despite the enormous generosity and patience of the world's investors for most of biotech's history, there was a serious bear market in biotech stocks from 1993 to 1995. The bear was fed three kinds of red meat:

1. the threat of managed care, which—until consumers reasserted themselves—was initially hostile to the high prices of biotech compounds;

2. the specter of federal health care "reform," which had the Clintons specifically badmouthing the drug industry in general, and biotech segment in particular, for high prices and profits; and
3. a series of spectacular clinical trial failures for Centocor, Synergen, and others.

As a result, by mid-1995—when many of the biggest deals between Big Pharma and the biotech companies closed—the biotech industry was burning R&D money a lot faster than it could raise it through traditional channels.

But there is a more important rationale for these deals: taking a drug from lab bench to corner pharmacy requires one of the few things that cash cannot buy; it requires hard experience. Almost from the birth of the biotech industry, the most expeditious and obvious throughput of new products to the marketplace ran through Big Pharma. While the first generation of fledgling biotechs (Amgen, Genentech, Biogen, Chiron, and Genzyme) sought to develop into fully integrated pharmaceutical companies, they all still required licensing deals, equity funding, or a combination of both from Big Pharma. As of this writing, four of these five companies are still entangled to varying degrees:

1. Though fully mature and functional as a stand-alone drug company, Genentech continues to operate under the majority ownership of drug giant Roche.
2. Amgen continues, not to its pleasure, to market a version of its first product through a Johnson & Johnson subsidiary, as does Biogen through Schering-Plough.
3. After a number of marketing and product stumbles, generally successful Chiron was acquired in full by partial owner Ciba-Geigy (Novartis).
4. Only Genzyme managed to break free almost completely from Big Pharma for its marketed end products, if only because it owns and markets an extremely expensive niche drug, Ceredase, for the rare condition, Gaucher's disease.

Why this dependence on Big Pharma? Because the costs of turning a marketable biotech compound into a marketed drug has proven too expensive and organizationally complex a task for a start-up technology company. Big Pharma has the infrastructure and experience to ram drugs through the tortuous regulatory process; the product management machinery to package, launch, and promote the new brands; and the marketing muscle to move them.

Nonetheless, based on the persistence of the pioneers of the fully integrated model (Amgen, Biogen, and Genzyme)—and the relative operating independence of fully integrated Genentech and Chiron— the next generation of biotechs made an ambitious run at their own full integration. They tried to build companies that spanned core research, manufacturing and marketing, only to stumble as a class into the arms of Big Pharma partners. This acquiescence to the expediencies and economics of licensing versus full integration range from highly successful niche biotechs like Alza, which markets time-release versions of Big Pharma's drugs; to outright failed product companies like Synergen, the research remnants of which were acquired by Amgen; to scrappy contenders who overcame the failure of one product with the success of another, like Centocor, which licenses its products through Eli Lilly.[33]

Such acquiescence is now the rule in biotech. In its own anachronistic way, such acquiescence signifies biotech's participation in the health care industry's chain-reaction consolidation. Indeed, only when a biotech chooses to go it alone does the business press even take note. Start-up Agouron is one of those exceptions, and its odds are long: sales of its AIDS drug, the fourth in the class of protease inhibitors and finally approved by the FDA in early 1997, will have to reach the high end of Wall Street's estimates for the company to reach profitability by the middle of 1998. Such are the stakes for a company that consumed $500 million in investment capital over its 13-year R&D-stage life.[34]

Big Pharma's funding of virtual R&D via the biotech companies represents its attainment of an industrial maturity described by Porter in *Competitive Advantage.* "Basic product innovation is often less scale-sensitive than the subsequent rapid introduction of new product types and the incorporation of new features."[35] These more "scale-sensitive, subsequent" activities are the special provinces of the established drug companies, with their entrenched product lines, machinelike launch of line extensions, and sophisticated marketing organizations. By contrast, biotech focuses on basic product innovation, and its nimbleness offsets the disadvantages of smaller scale.

LIKE FATHER, LIKE SON

Even more interestingly, the once leading edge of the upstart biotech industry itself seems to have attained Big Pharma's "industry maturation" in less than a decade. The science of drug discovery is in such flux—and the economics in such overdrive—that the competitive advantages and working cultures of the first generation biotech companies themselves have hyperevolved to the point that they themselves now resemble Big Pharma in their appetite for virtual R&D. Many of the biggest promises in the pipelines of Amgen and Genentech—the pioneering biotech upstarts funded in large part by *out*-licensing their products to Big Pharma—are now *in*-licensed compounds from pure R&D-stage biotech companies. While Amgen and Genentech still have large and growing research operations, like Big Pharma, these labs are subject to all manner of scientific, clinical, and financial risks; also like Big Pharma, the companies have built major marketing forces, hungry for new drugs to sell. As a consequence, what were once the virtual R&D labs for Big Pharma have mutated into organizations dependent on the same strategies.

This mutation works in both directions. Access to the operations of its virtual R&D biotech partners provides Big Pharma with insights into how best to motivate and manage its own R&D. How? By replicating the freewheeling environments of small labs. Pfizer is attempting to do precisely this by sequestering its leading-edge researchers at a dedicated lab in Great Britain. A *Wall Street Journal* article points out that the facility's physical isolation from corporate headquarters in New York "may make it as important a source of novel ideas as fledgling biotechnology allies over the next few years."[36]

Taking this strategy full circle is the reverse–virtual R&D strategy of Sanofi. A major French drugmaker with $4.5 billion in 1995 sales,[37] the company is *out*-licensing its most promising drugs to other major drug companies, rather than *in*-licensing from the biotechs. This strategy allows Sanofi to subsidize its broader-based research efforts, the same way the biotechs subsidize their very existence with licensing from Big Pharma. Sanofi is engaged in this strategy, according to a report in the *Wall Street Journal*, because "even companies with productive labs such as Sanofi are under pressure to get bigger or get out of the costly research race."[38] Here is an example of Big Pharma reacting to the same economic pressures toward consolidation that all the major drug companies feel, not by consolidating, but by feeding down at the other end of the consolidation food chain.

A GREAT LEAP FORWARD? BIG PHARMA'S PBM FANTASIES

If risk-assumption emerges as the only transaction in the new century's health care system, how does Big Pharma position itself? For a time, the thinking in the industry was: move upstream in the health care system and capture premium dollars for patient drug coverage rather than revenue dollars for their drugs. Such thinking translated into strategic deal making in 1993 and 1994, when Merck, SmithKline, and Lilly spent, collectively, $13.1 billion purchasing three pharmacy benefit managers (PBMs).[39]

PBMs are risk-assuming entities, in essence "drug MCOs." They apply to pharmaceutical care the same purchasing economies and control systems that MCOs apply to doctors and hospitals. Like MCOs, the PBM—in theory—seeks to accomplish several (often contradictory) goals at the same time:

1. purchase drugs on the cheap, given the PBM's consolidation of buyer power;
2. offer drug companies guaranteed volumes for price discounts;
3. channel patients toward the most cost-effective drugs; and
4. reduce total drug costs for a population.

As an MCO or preferred provider organization (PPO) develops and manages a "panel" of discounted providers, a PBM develops and manages a network of contracted pharmacists and a "formulary" of discounted drugs. Like MCOs, the cheaper the total care delivered under this system, the greater the PBM's margins.

Big Pharma's purchases of the PBMs represent an expensive and risky attempt at forward integration. Such attempts are driven by three strategies:

1. The most obvious, if least articulated, strategy recognizes that, because PBMs exist to move market share via the imposition of drug prescription switches, they can make those switches over to products manufactured by the parent drug company; they can, in effect, load up their formularies with their parents' drugs. In this light, Big Pharma is simply neutralizing the consolidating buyer power represented by the PBM.
2. The most frequently articulated strategy argues that PBM ownership allows the purchasing drug company to leverage the drug utilization review apparatus at the core of the PBM's operations. Access to such an infrastructure is critical if the parent drug company enters into at-risk contracts with MCOs or self-insured employers to manage the pharmaceutical care needs and dollars for a certain disease within a covered population. Under such "pharma-capitation" deals the drug company has the financial incentive to provide fewer rather than more drugs for a fixed fee per member.
3. Finally, the most intellectually compelling, if most poorly thought-out, strategy argues that PBMs are really information companies. As a distributor of drugs for covered populations,

they maintain large repositories of data on patients and prescriptions. Such data will provide the parent drug company with an edge of strategic intelligence to drive its product-market research.

All three of these strategies are interesting and highly informative, as each encapsulates several of the themes that are either directly related to, or symptomatic of, the five forces of health care transformation. But at their core, all of these strategies are faulty.

Moving Market Share?

After sitting on the sidelines for the first two purchases of PBMs by Big Pharma, with the third deal, the Federal Trade Commission (FTC) sprang into action: it held up Lilly's acquisition of PCS Health Systems until the company agreed to institute organizational barriers and practices that would specifically preclude the implementation of this strategy. As a result, the FTC now guards the PBM henhouses owned by the Big Pharma foxes. It combs through marketplace data for any indication that the parent manufacturers are spiking the PBM's formularies with their own brands, muscling competitors' products out of their captive distribution channels.

The FTC can relax. Common marketplace discipline precludes any such distortions. MCOs and self-insured employers will not select a PBM owned by Big Pharma if it is not price competitive (1) within all classes of drugs in which the parent's drugs compete, and (2) across the board against the several other PBMs that are not owned by Big Pharma. A loss of such price competitiveness underscores how clearly the strategy of moving market share represents a conflict of interest: the PBM positions itself as an objective managed care company with the mission of providing the best drug for the best price to its MCO customers, not the parent company's drug at the next-best price.

The inevitability of such marketplace discipline underscores an even more troubling truism about PBMs, one that Big Pharma obviously overlooked when it purchased them at such rich multiples: *PBMs are glorified distributors*. And as distributors, they inevitably will be forced to turn ruthless over price, engaging in a battle royale that no distributor in any industry ever wins, except for the two pyrrhic victors that emerge as large companies with paper-thin margins. But until the inevitable occurs, they will pretend to emulate the MCOs. And just like the MCOs, the only value PBMs add is the concentration and control of medical resources on their formularies. (Unlike MCOs, such control governs only 7 percent of a covered population's total health care spending, greatly minimizing the potential impact of the PBM.) PBMs do not produce cures; they merely place the cures that somebody else developed and manufactured into little plastic containers.

One would be hard pressed to find a funnier punch line for this truism than the amusing irony of *declining* PBM market share of the parent companies' drugs in 1996. Three years after the deals were completed, two of the three Big Pharma acquirers actually *lost* market share in their captive channels. Lilly's share went from 2.0 to 1.7 percent of drugs at PCS; SmithKline's share went from 4.0 to 3.2 percent at DPS; and Merck's share went from 3.4 to 4.1 percent at Medco.[40] Randomness would produce the same or better results. In Lilly's case, it has: the company is actually performing better in the PBM marketplace generally than within its own corner of it; Lilly's product prescription volume grew 7.2 percent at all PBMs, versus a decline of 6.9 percent at PCS.[41] Bad execution of this strategy? Bad luck? Or is Lilly simply that hell-bent on pleasing the FTC?

These reversals of expected fortune notwithstanding, it may prove useful to assume that the experiences of Lilly and SmithKline are the anomalies and that of Merck the norm, achieved through better execution. This still begs an unpleasant question: are 0.7 points in share gains—earned through one outlet that competes within only one of several channels—worth the $6.6 billion Merck spent on Medco? Net present value analysis would certainly reveal not. Even assuming against common sense that the deal could pay for itself in shifted market share, does the magnitude of the requisite shift fall below the radar of the FTC? And the FTC is not the only regulatory bogeyman haunting the PBMs. Attempts to control drug choices more categorically, i.e., through the elimination of competitors' drugs from a PBM's formulary, are illegal. Lilly found this out in New York state, where a judge ordered that drugs manufactured by Pfizer, the plaintiff, be reinstated on the Lilly-PCS formulary.

Such has been the paralysis of the PBMs under the corporate umbrellas of Big Pharma parents. As the third and last major deal, Lilly's PCS unit has been particularly hobbled, garnering the harshest scrutiny and restrictions on its business practices by the FTC. With the $4.1 billion purchase not making an adequate contribution to Lilly's bottom line, analysts blamed it for Lilly's earnings shortfall in 1996.[42] It has since taken a sizable write-down on the deal, and for good reason: an analysis of Lilly's financial data indicates that the annual charges for interest and goodwill amortization for the PCS acquisition are greater than the net income thrown off by the unit, resulting in a dilution to Lilly's earnings per share.[43]

Bearing Risk for Drug Costs?

Defenders of the PBM deal argue that the real point of the PBM is not to move market share in a fee-for-service world, but to allow Big Pharma to enter the new century's health care system as a full risk-bearing provider. While on the surface this appears a rather seductive strategy, one consistent with the emerging role of risk in the health care purchasing equation, it is a classic example of the *au courant* thinking that tends to distract the pharmaceutical industry every few years. Because it completely ignores the unique cost-economics of pharmaceutical care, this is a structurally flawed strategy. As stated earlier, the competitive advantage of drug companies as a class is the tremendous economic leverage of drugs on total health care costs. Spending on drugs accounts for only 7 percent of a population's total medical costs, and yet it has a profound impact on the other 93 percent. Patients who do not take their "expensive" ACE inhibitors are far more likely to suffer heart attacks, enter the hospital, and require costly surgery.

The last thing a self-insured employer, MCO, EHO, or any other holder of global medical/financial risk wants to do is put a whole population's health and economics at risk to manage down 7 percent of total costs. Giving a drug company the financial incentive to reduce drug costs through its PBM would have monstrous economic displacement effects downstream in the medical economics of the covered population. Any MCO that, in effect, rewards Merck to use fewer and cheaper antibiotics is asking for a tidal wave of aggravated infections, physician visits, hospitalizations, and unhappy patients. *The entire premise of the PBM as a risk-bearing front for Big Pharma falls apart because the goal of the PBM is at odds with the fundamental risk management needs of its ultimate customers.* It also mutes the singular value of the entire pharmaceutical industry. Some have suggested that the way around this problem would be to put the drug company/PBM at risk for *all* medical costs associated with a covered population. While this is consistent with the economic leverage of drugs, it is hardly feasible from an operational perspective. Given how well drug companies seem to be running their PBMs, they may wish to think twice before trying to run entire managed care delivery systems.

Information Resources

When acquiring the PBMs, Big Pharma expected to find a wellspring of prescription data flowing into a raging river of detailed clinical data on medical resource consumption and outcomes. Such information would allow Big Pharma to study what drugs worked best—both clinically and financially—for which kinds of patients. This enormously valuable intellectual property would allow them to develop, test, redose, target-market, and promote their drugs with an unprecedented incisiveness and depth.

What they found instead was a wellspring of prescription data. The pharmacy claims data warehoused by the PBM rarely connects to all the medical and demographic information associated with a population. Pharmacy claims include the patient's ID, the drug prescribed, its dosing (in a very good database), and its cost. These claims are devoid of information on patient diagnoses, procedures, physician visits, hospitalizations, diagnostic tests, or outcomes. As the pharmacy information thus sits in a vacuum, it would require the MCOs, insurers, and self-insured employers to supply the PBMs with all the other patient data necessary to execute this strategy.

The hurdles to combining meaningful medical information with the PBMs' pharmacy data are probably insurmountable. They range from simple problems of incompatible information technology; to bureaucratic gridlock over data ownership, confidentiality, and commercial uses; to outright institutional mistrust between the PBMs and their MCO customers. Why this last problem? Because both the MCOs and PBMs recognize that the only truly proprietary business process associated with managing a population's care is how best to leverage the information about that population. Such information is a proprietary resource that all bearers of risk perceive as strategically critical, and treat it accordingly. The PBMs and MCOs thus remain frozen in a game of strategic chicken over who will use the integrated information more effectively to outbargain the other.

So much for the three strategies driving $13.1 billion in PBM acquisitions. The best confirmation of the foolishness of these purchases—aside from Lilly's write-off—is the experience of Pfizer in comparison to Merck, SmithKline, and Lilly. While steadfastly resisting the temptation to join the PBM purchasing mania in the early 1990s, Pfizer emerged as the fastest growing major pharmaceutical company in the world. Pfizer's Chairman William Steere attributes this success to the company's focus on its research mission. "We are not a distribution company," he told *Industry Week*. "We're not a generic drug producer. We're a research-intensive, value-added company, and that's where we're placing our bets, regardless of what the distribution system ultimately comes out to be."[44]

Steere's comment underscores the central, inescapable fact about PBMs: while they represent a smarter way to distribute drugs than dispensing them through the retail pharmacy, the PBMs are, in the end, still only distributors, and in any industry, margins for distributors stink. They stink because the value-add is negligible; the barriers to entry are small, at least relative to drug manufacturing; and the gaining and sustaining of competitive advantage is elusive, almost always the result of critical mass at the outset and sheer size in the end. Such is the essence of PBM industry structure. Consider, then, the dilutive effect of the distributor on the high-margin, research-intensive drug company's profitability. Medco represents an outsized one-third of Merck's revenue—about $6.5 billion—even though 1996 profits for Medco were estimated at $700 million. But Medco needs to earn $900 million per year for 15 years for Merck to show a return on the $6.6 billion consistent with Merck's long-run return on capital.[45]

The sustainability of sufficient profit margins for the Medco business—barely more than half of Merck's margin generally—are highly unlikely. As with any breakthrough approach to distribution, from just-in-time inventory to electronic data interchange (EDI) transaction processing, to Internet-based order entry, the one-time savings associated with PBM drug distribution are working their way through the system and becoming standard. When this process is complete, the PBMs will engage in the inevitable pricing wars typical of distributors in a mature market. The effects were already showing up by early 1997, when Columbia/HCA acquired Value Health at a 31.6 percent discount to sales ($1.3 billion versus $1.9 billion in 1996 sales), following a 7.7 percent drop in Value Health's net income.[46] (Columbia has since sold Value Health as part of its massive 1998 restructuring.) Only in 1997 did Medco's top line finally surpass what Merck paid for it in 1993.

Value Health's valuation is so much lower because the PBM business is stagnating. Despite its sexier product lines like information services and managed behavioral health care, nearly 80 percent of the company's revenues are generated by its PBM. And according to a report in *Modern Healthcare*, "this once lucrative business has lost much of its shine" as the PBM market has "little room for growth and a lot of competition, hence the shrinking margins."[47]

As PBMs are the drug version of the MCOs, they are destined to share the same fate. They are the middlemen between the supplier of the health care service—the drug company—and the consumer and purchaser of it. As with direct contracting with EHOs, self-insured employers and coalitions can contract directly with pharmaceutical companies for whatever configuration of risk-sharing program they believe would optimize the value of pharmaceutical care delivered to their covered members. Like those investing in for-profit MCOs when they neared their inevitable market top in early 1997, the drug companies will also learn this the hard way—the way Lilly already has—and sell off the businesses at a huge loss.

Such losses will be minimal relative to the size of Big Pharma's collective balance sheet. But what the final accounting will fail to capture is the most troubling aspect of this experiment in poorly reasoned forward integration: *what is the opportunity cost of the $13.1 billion spent on the PBMs?*

In the decade the pharmaceutical industry spent learning this hard lesson, what additional drugs could they have discovered with all that money? A gene-based approach to blocking the degenerative agony of arthritis? Cleaner chemotherapies for arresting juvenile leukemia? A drug delivery molecule that threads through the blood/brain barrier and slows the devastation of Alzheimer's?

Or maybe just a vaccine against AIDS.

READY-MADE FOR INDUSTRIALIZATION

The most interesting aspect of Big Pharma's PBM acquisition strategy was the theory that it would gain a wealth of insights into the financial and clinical impact of drugs on total health care costs and quality. Indeed, the coordination of pharmaceutical and other types of medical care, all for the purpose of optimizing the total value of a drug-based intervention, is central to the principles and practices of health care industrialization. But Big Pharma is already engaged in such efforts in the drug development, testing, and marketing processes, thus pre-positioning drugmakers for the loftier industrialization role carved out by Deming. "Deal with vendors that can furnish statistical evidence of control," he instructs manufacturers in *Out of the Crisis*. He indicates that the mobilization of such evidence may carry a pricing premium, coupling this with the dictate that companies "examine generic lowest-price buying."[48] (So much for the price-driven approaches of the PBMs.)

In addition to the intensive statistical exercises traditionally associated with clinical trials and cost benefit analyses for new drugs, pharmaceutical companies also contribute significantly to the industrialization of health care in three fundamental ways. They couple their products with value-added services such as patient education; "portfolio-ize" products with therapeutic complementarity through cross-licensing with other drug companies; and augment the clinical marketing of products with information about their use. All three activities have been mobilized as marketing and sales strategies—with generous funding because they work to increase sales.

Value-added services like patient education are packaged generically by the drugmakers as "disease management programs." Such programs increase the company's national account activity, i.e., their sales to the hospital chains and MCOs, because they do for the MCO precisely what the MCOs claim to be doing for their employer customers—improving wellness through patient education, illness prevention, and better disease-state management.

"Portfolio-izing" complementary products also often begins as pure marketing strategy—leveraging an existing field force, for example—but ultimately seeks to rationalize the vertical segment of care that the pharmaceutical company can directly affect. Such combinations may involve multiple lines of increasingly aggressive and expensive therapies, like multilines of antibiotics or ulcer medications (when the first line fails, the next line steps in); or they may involve the packaging of a chemotherapy and an antiemetic drug to prevent the nausea associated with chemotherapy.

Finally, the augmentation of drug products with information is the very *modus operandi* of a pharmaceutical sales force. In addition to the sheer promotional efforts for which they are known and generally derided, drug sales reps also provide clinical and financial outcomes information to doctors, hospitals, and pharmacists. This explains why Big Pharma continues to add to their field forces—long after the conventional wisdom predicted their extinction—despite the consolidation of purchasers into national accounts and the simultaneous rise of the PBM, MCO formulary, and other control mechanisms designed specifically to diminish the impact of direct-to-physician promotion.[49]

It is interesting to note that all three of these strategies are particularly critical to suppliers of medical and surgical devices and supplies. Because these products enjoy scant proprietary product advantages, at least in comparison to pharmaceuticals, their marketers focus much more intensively on all three strategies, as will be explored in the next chapter, "The Supply Chain Gang."

By using these three strategies, Big Pharma is no longer simply vending line-item products—it is helping rationalize the entire health care delivery system. This is a natural strategic response to the forces of industrialization; and it adds significantly to the value that MCOs, risk-bearing hospitals and physicians, and ultimately the EHOs derive from pharmaceutical products. This contribution is the embodiment of Porter's observation that "differentiation derives fundamentally from creating value for the buyer through a firm's impact on the buyer's value chain…The value created for the buyer must be perceived by the buyer if it is to be rewarded with a premium price, however, which means that firms must communicate their value to buyers through such means as advertising and the sales force."[50]

If anything, pharmaceutical companies have not communicated this value effectively enough. Instead, they tend to emphasize the purely clinical benefits of their products, rather than their aggregate economic benefits. This shyness at trumpeting the economic value of its products clearly hurts the industry when under siege by politicians who periodically demonize the drug industry—in a pandering to voters unaware that their $60 monthly prescriptions are not capsules of a simple chemical, but rather miracles of biochemical technology that preclude $30,000 surgeries. In the wake of the particularly damaging version of this demagoguery included in the Clinton health care reform circus, a rare and effective version of this communication found its voice in an ad campaign by Pfizer, which simply pointed out: "we're part of the cure."

THE BEST COMPETITIVE ADVANTAGE OF ALL: CLARITY OF PURPOSE

Pfizer's slogan underscores another clear competitive advantage of the drug companies: they have a resoluteness of mission rare for any industry. While there are numerous economic and structural factors that contribute to the tremendous productivity and sustained profitability of the drug companies, they also benefit significantly, if unquantifiably, from the solemn purposefulness associated with seeking to cure disease. In contrast to the hospitals, doctors, and others who deliver services to the sick using technologies invented by others—making progress for individual patients, but not for the public health as a whole—most of the drug companies are in the breakthrough business.

One can well imagine the motivational impact of this mission on an organization's culture when walking the halls of Genentech's corporate headquarters, past the unusual "decorations" that drape the length of 20-foot-high walls in every direction: pieces of the AIDS quilt. In stark contrast to all the corporate mission statement plaques in the world, these most human voicings of the devastation of uncured disease reminds Genentech employees with painful clarity the ultimate purpose of their work.

REFERENCES

1. E. Tanouye, "Managed Care Is Boosting Drug Sales," *Wall Street Journal*, 12 October, 1996.
2. Tanouye, *Wall Street Journal*, 12 October, 1996.
3. From S. Horn et al., "Intended and Unintended Consequences of HMO Cost Containment Strategies: The Results from the Managed Care Outcomes Project" in the *American Journal of Managed Care*, as reported in *Managed Care News*, April 1996.

4. Adapted and reprinted with permission of The Free Press, a Division of Simon & Schuster from *COMPETITIVE STRATEGY: Techniques for Analyzing Industries and Competitors* by Michael E. Porter. Copyright © 1980 by The Free Press. p. 115–116.

5. J. Moore, *The Death of Competition* (New York: HarperCollins Publishers, 1996), 249.

6. J. Kleinke, "Power to the Patient," *Modern Healthcare*, 23 February, 1997, 66.

7. No controlled study. An equivalent packaging of Ecotrin was twice the retail price at Hodel's Drugs on Colorado Boulevard, Denver, CO, 19 March, 1998. (Yes, I bought the generic.)

8. Moore, *The Death of Competition*, 251–252.

9. Aggregate pharmaceutical R&D spending figures included in "The Contribution of Pharmaceutical Companies," The Boston Consulting Group, September 1993, 84.

10. Calculations made using Dow Jones & Company Quotations and Summaries.

11. P. Starr, *The Social Transformation of American Medicine* (New York: Basic Books/HarperCollins, 1982), 339.

12. "Pharmaceutical Industry Survey," *The Economist*, 21 February, 1998, 5.

13. N. Nichols, "Medicine, Management and Mergers," *Harvard Business Review*, November/December 1994, 9.

14. Adapted and reprinted with permission of The Free Press, a Division of Simon & Schuster from *COMPETITIVE STRATEGY: Techniques for Analyzing Industries and Competitors* by Michael E. Porter. Copyright © 1980 by The Free Press. p. 185.

15. R&D inflation from "The Contribution of Pharmaceutical Companies," The Boston Consulting Group, September 1993, 74.

16. J. Weber, "Mr. Nice Guy with a Mission," *Business Week*, 25 November, 1996, 137.

17. Nichols, *Harvard Business Review*, 7.

18. Weber, *Business Week*, 132.

19. S. Moore, "Success of Ciba-Sandoz Merger Will Be Tested in the Lab," *Wall Street Journal*, 30 July, 1996.

20. Moore, *Wall Street Journal*, 30 July, 1996.

21. Years to FDA licensing for new drugs, from "The Contribution of Pharmaceutical Companies," The Boston Consulting Group, September 1993, 106.

22. "The Pharmaceutical Industry Survey," *The Economist*, 21 February, 1998, 5.

23. G. Smith, "Not That Easy: Even a Strong Hand Must Be Played Well," *Industry Week*, 3 June, 1996.

24. R. Langreth and J. Hirsch, "American Home Sets $1.25 Billion Price," *Wall Street Journal*, 18 December, 1996.

25. Smith, *Industry Week*.

26. Nichols, *Harvard Business Review*, 7.

27. M. Schrage, "Drugmakers Need To Find New Ways To Make Their Voyages of Discovery," *Washington Post*, 3 February, 1995.

28. S. Moore, "French Drug Maker Reaps Profits with Offbeat Strategy," *Wall Street Journal*, 14 November, 1996.

29. L. Johannes, "Hoechst Makes Large Investment in Deal with Ariad," *Wall Street Journal*, 7 March, 1997.

30. W. Bulkeley, "Eli Lilly To Invest up to $70 Million in Millenium Unit," *Wall Street Journal*, 25 May, 1997.

31. Adapted and reprinted with permission of The Free Press, a Division of Simon & Schuster from *COMPETITIVE STRATEGY: Techniques for Analyzing Industries and Competitors* by Michael E. Porter. Copyright © 1980 by The Free Press. p. 16.

32. M. Selz, "Enterprise: U.S. Biotechnology Firms Enjoy a Surge in European Alliances," *Wall Street Journal*, 6 August, 1996.

33. J. Bamford, "How a Near-Death Experience Forced Centocor into Strategic Alliances," *Financial World*, 11 April, 1995, 69.

34. R. Rundle, "Agouron Gets Go-Ahead To Join the AIDS-Drug Battle," *Wall Street Journal*, 17 March, 1997.

35. Adapted and reprinted with permission of The Free Press, a Division of Simon & Schuster from *COMPETITIVE ADVANTAGE: Creating and Sustaining Superior Performance* by Michael E. Porter. Copyright © 1985 by Michael E. Porter. p. 183–184.

36. S. Moore, "Pfizer's English Site Is Research Boon," *Wall Street Journal*, 6 September, 1996.

37. Moore, "Value of Some Drug Firms' Acquisitions Is Questioned," *Wall Street Journal*, 14 November, 1996.

38. Moore, *Wall Street Journal*, 14 November, 1996.

39. E. Tanouye, "Value of Some Drug Firms' Acquisitions Is Questioned," *Wall Street Journal*, 11 November, 1996.

40. Tanouye, "Value of Some Drug Firms' Acquisitions Is Questioned," *Wall Street Journal*, 19 November, 1996.

41. E. Browning and T. Burton, "Lilly's PCS Receives Rx: A Write Down," *Wall Street Journal*, 2 August, 1996.

42. Browning and Burton, *Wall Street Journal*.

43. From a research report on Eli Lilly & Company by *Rx Scrips*, 5 August, 1996.
44. Smith, *Industry Week*.
45. Analysis by Princeton health economist Uwe Reinhardt, as reported by J. Weber, "Mr. Nice Guy with a Mission," *Business Week*, 25 November, 1996, 139.
46. S. Hensley, "Valuing Value Health," *Modern Healthcare*, 3 March, 1997, 38.
47. Hensley, *Modern Healthcare*, 38–40.
48. W.E. Deming, *Out of the Crisis* (Cambridge, MA: MIT Center for Advanced Engineering Study, 1986), 201.
49. "Looking Ahead: Predictions for 1998," *CenterWatch*, 1 January, 1998, 3.
50. Adapted and reprinted with permission of The Free Press, a Division of Simon & Schuster from *COMPETITIVE ADVANTAGE: Creating and Sustaining Superior Performance* by Michael E. Porter. Copyright © 1985 by Michael E. Porter. p. 53.

9

THE SUPPLY CHAIN GANG

Speed is God and Time is the Devil.

Silicon Valley adage[1]

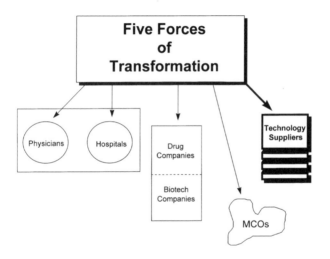

Manufacturers of medical and surgical devices and supplies face many of the same business challenges as those in the pharmaceutical industry while enjoying few of its strategic advantages. Like pharmaceuticals, almost all devices (and many types of supplies) are high cost, research and development (R&D) intensive, complicated to manufacture, and subject to costly regulatory approval and oversight. But unlike pharmaceuticals, which have active postlaunch life cycles of 4 to 12 years, the typical device or supply enjoys at best two to four years of supremacy.

Such is patent life. The chemical compounds that define branded drugs are qualitatively unambiguous, difficult to emulate, are thus legally well protected from imitation. By contrast, the mechanics and functionality that define most branded medical and surgical devices can be readily and cheaply cannibalized by look-alike products; the result is rapid commoditization across the device and supply industry.

Devices and supplies are also subject to frequent and wide-ranging substitution. Breakthroughs in surgical technique occur in waves; each wave moves quickly out from the epicenter of the surgical introduction (i.e., the academic medical centers), stimulating an industry-wide adoption at an ever accelerating pace. Such adoptions often begin as the "import" of a breakthrough technique into one surgical domain from an unrelated surgical domain. The result is still faster diffusion and chain-reaction product cycling across the entire industry. This rapid cycling generates exponential revenue growth for each new generation of technology, but those growth rates are mirrored by just as rapid a rate of revenue fall-off for the passing generation.

THE LEAST UNKINDEST CUT

Two movements in the recent history of surgery embody major variations on this theme. The introduction and widespread adoption of cardiac catheter-based procedures in the 1980s, and minimally invasive surgery in the 1990s, created enormous new product markets, quick profits, and just as rapid downdrafts. Intense competition from existing suppliers and aggressive new entrants sent the new technologies from both surgical domains into accelerated versions of classic technology product life cycles.

Two cardiac catheter-based procedures—angiography and angioplasty—involve threading a catheter, or wire-thin tube, up through a main artery in the body and into the delicate arteries that supply the heart with blood. (Blockages that build up in these coronary arteries cause chest pain and fatigue, a condition known as angina; if left untreated they lead to heart attacks.) The catheter performs a variety of functions, including

- the release of a special dye or "contrast agent" that allows physicians to see the extent of the blockages in the coronary arteries;
- the delivery of thrombolytic drugs (e.g., t-PA) that bust up and flush out the portion of those blockages due to blood clotting;
- the inflation of a tiny balloon (a "balloon angioplasty") to compress the blockages against the walls of the artery and restore the full flow of blood to the heart; and
- the use of a microscopic cutting device that grinds the blockage away (an "atherectomy").

Though their longitudinal effectiveness has recently come under fire in various studies, these procedures were originally sold as highly cost-effective alternatives to bypass surgery. As a result, their introduction created an enormous demand for the exquisitely engineered, high-priced cardiac catheters, balloons, and related products that, within 15 years, would grow into a $1.5 billion annual market.[2]

How quickly does this market move? Within three years of its introduction in 1993, the stent—a tiny wire cylinder delivered by the cardiac catheter into the newly opened coronary artery to keep it from reclosing—grew into an $800-million-dollar product market, dominated by Johnson & Johnson (J&J) and Cordis, which J&J quickly acquired.[3] While still in its infancy, the premium price charged for the now clinically standard stent is already starting its inevitable downdraft, as the device is replicated and improved upon by competitors.

In keeping with the principle of rapid diffusion to other surgical domains, all the technologies developed for cardiac catheter-based procedures have quickly been applied to surgery on the major blood vessels elsewhere in the body. In previous generations of technique, vascular surgeons were forced to open up the neck, thigh, or abdominal region to repair or replace clogged sections of the arteries and veins that transport blood between the heart and the extremities or brain, just as cardiac surgeons open patients' chests to perform bypass procedures. After the introduction of catheter-based technology for heart surgery, these "peripheral vascular" surgeons were able to apply the core breakthroughs designed originally for these less-invasive approaches to the heart—sparing patients the trauma of fully invasive surgery elsewhere. The new technology thus set off a chain reaction in the market for *all* cardiovascular devices and supplies: the catheter-based products ate quickly into the market share for all products used in bypass surgery. Then, almost as quickly, they ate into the market share for all those products used in peripheral vascular surgeries.

Precisely the same dynamic thundered through a number of surgical specialties in the early 1990s with the introduction of laparoscopic surgery. "Lap" surgery involves operating deep inside a patient's body without having to make a large incision for access. Instead, surgeons perform the procedure by following their movements with surgical instruments on a television image captured by a laparoscope placed inside the patient's body through a small incision. Like the laparoscope itself, the surgical instruments are delicate, high-tech devices placed down into the patient's body through small incisions. The result of this surgical approach is greatly reduced trauma to the patient, faster recovery, and drastically lower costs. As a consequence, within three years of the introduction of this new approach to gallbladder removal, the "lap choly"—for laparoscopic cholecystectomy—became the dominant procedure performed on more than half-a-million patients per year.[4]

While lap surgery did not revolutionize a host of other surgeries as quickly as the manufacturers of lap equipment told Wall Street it would, the technique eventually spread to include hernia repair, hysterectomy, and numerous other high-volume procedures. As importantly as this rapid uptake of lap surgery has proven within its primary surgical domains—mostly gastrointestinal and gynecological procedures—the technologies at its core (e.g., laparoscope visualization tools) are now driving breakthroughs in numerous other far-flung surgical domains. Most notable among these is the still experimental introduction of "closed" coronary bypass procedures. Like lap surgery and using tools built from the same types of technologies, a closed bypass allows a surgeon to operate directly on blocked coronary arteries without having to open the patient's chest. The new products for the procedure cost between $2,300 and $5,000 per surgery,[5] but their less invasive approach has the potential to knock five times that many dollars out of total hospital costs associated with the open heart version of the same surgery.

As this procedure is perfected and proliferated, the devices and supplies used in open bypass will experience further market erosion. And so we return to the very beginning of our story: even more rapid will be the market substitution of these new products—inspired by laparoscopic surgical technology—for the many devices used in the once-revolutionary cardiac catheter-based procedures. Such are the chain reactions of new medical technology around the human body and across the medical and surgical device and supply industry.

FROM CUTTING EDGE TO DULLED INSTRUMENT

As the surgical examples detailed above illustrate, the device and supply industry endures an unusually bowed version of what Porter describes as the "S-shaped substitution curve,"[6] illustrated in Figure IV–1.

In the normally early and flat part of Porter's curve, adoption of a substitute product is slow; the curve then steepens as the substitute gains momentum; it then flattens again when the substitute reaches a natural saturation point.

This curve applies perfectly to medical and surgical devices and supplies. Initial uptake is flat, due to the obvious risk factors associated with new surgical techniques. But once widespread adoption finally begins in earnest, it tends to do so in overdrive. It then tends to flatten just as quickly, due less to saturation than to the introduction of the next substitute technology. Applied to the example of "lap cholies," the product substitution process occurs as follows:

1. The earliest part of the curve is almost completely flat as the lap choly is experimental and performed only by research surgeons at academic medical centers.

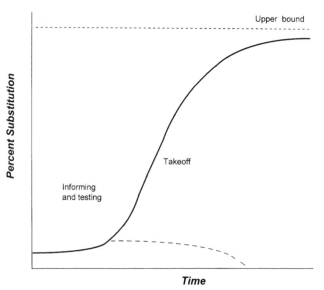

Figure IV–1 Product Substitution Curve. *Source:* Adapted and reprinted with the permission of The Free Press, a Division of Simon & Schuster from *COMPETI-TIVE ADVANTAGE: Creating and Sustaining Superior Performance* by Michael E. Porter. Copyright © 1985 by Michael E. Porter.

2. The curve starts to pick up as the lap choly is perfected, results are published, and surgeons at all teaching hospitals begin to adopt it on the clinically simplest cases.

3. The curve enters its steepest phase as vendors aggressively promote lap cholies to surgeons and payers across the United States and research surgeons test the procedure on increasingly difficult cases.

4. Finally, the curve flattens again as the procedure reaches clinical saturation, meaning the only cholies *not* performed using the laparoscopic technique are those that cannot be for clinical reasons (e.g., a ruptured gallbladder due to trauma).

A particularly steep substitution curve would be easier to cope with strategically and operationally but for the vagaries of regulatory oversight. The regulatory approval process has been particularly problematic to the medical and surgical device makers over the past decade. New devices and even simple product-line extensions—many of which are designed specifically to bring better cost-economies to their surgical domains—typically languish for years in the FDA's approval pipeline. Why? Because the FDA received political signals years ago that the rapid proliferation of new medical technologies has been responsible for escalating health care costs. While the advent of high-visibility technologies like CT and MRI machines *does* increase total costs (at least in the legacy fee-for-service world), the preponderance of medical and surgical devices and supplies represents major improvements in procedural technique, rather than the introduction of entirely new procedures. Most seek to minimize surgical invasiveness and accelerate patient recovery, not expand baseline surgical procedure volume—as the critics of the industry on Capitol Hill would have it.

In a health care system driven by cost containment, with return on investment serving as the driving force behind increasing share of new purchases by hospitals and other facilities, it should be too obvious to bother making the observation, but make it we must: this progress can only *lower* health care costs. If it did not, then hospitals placed at risk to perform surgeries for market-dictated fees would not adopt the new technology. It is also not too obvious, unfortunately, to make another observation: given the competitive pressures on medical and surgical technology manufacturers, the FDA's persistent general and arbitrary delays in the approval of new devices constitutes the cruelest sort of regulatory malpractice.

What is the cumulative result of accelerated product life cycles, a steep substitution curve, and chronic regulatory problems? The answer is relentless competitive pressure among nearly all the medical and surgical device and supply manufacturers. The situation is highly analogous to the vendors of information, software, and telecommunications technology, where today's hottest products are tomorrow's has-beens. Competitive pressure of this magnitude compels the industry toward one conclusion about strategy: the creation of value-added services to enhance the marketing of pharmaceutical products, described in the previous chapter, are not "enhancements" for the makers of devices and supplies—they are critical success factors. That these value-added services also help align the drug companies with the five forces of health care transformation redoubles the argument that the marketers of devices and supplies need to pursue their own versions of precisely these same strategies.

THE WHOLE SURGICAL KIT AND CABOODLE

As medical care is integrated across settings, the device and supply companies are confronted with integration challenges and opportunities of their own. Because of the leverage intrinsic in building a medical products portfolio, these firms have particularly strong motives to align their business strategies with the five forces of health care transformation, in particular consolidation and industrialization. Like the multiple therapeutic lines assembled by the drug companies but with even greater potential impact, the medical and surgical products companies are compelled by market forces and provider needs to develop and market turnkey sets of clinically related devices and supplies, rather than line-item products.

This is as often accomplished by acquisition as through product development. J&J's purchase of stent-pioneer Cordis allowed it to provide an end-to-end product line for balloon angioplasty. Now J&J can develop, market, and service the catheters, balloons, and stents, all in one package. This leverages everything from the company's research community, to its sales and service force, to its distribution channels. For its provider customers, this packaging creates an economic sum of the parts that is greater than the whole. The prepackaging and integrated training and service adds a value that supersedes the diminishing value of the component devices and supplies. Such product integration is consistent with much of Porter's analysis of product "complementarity." In *Competitive Advantage*, he observes that "a position in the complement [i.e., stents or balloons for a catheterization company] gives the firm a leverage point with which to influence the development of the complement's industry."[7] Precisely this rationale drove Urohealth's acquisition of 17 companies in two years, capping it off with the purchase of Imagyn Medical for $70 million in 1997: now the company markets a spectrum of surgical products that covers the full range of urology and gynecology.[8] The same strategy inspired US Surgical's decision to purchase Pfizer's Valleylab unit for $425 million, broadening its own surgical supply business to encompass a fuller suite of wound closure products.[9]

The speed of product development in the device industry makes the leverage of such "full spectrum" portfolios particularly critical. The integration of clinically related products also allows for piggyback marketing, creative packaging, and aggressive pricing, and it simplifies paperwork for the purchaser. Product integration also provides an important rationale for continued active participation in the physician-education process by the device or supply company's field representatives. This is important from a tactical perspective: the success of sales representatives from these manufacturers (and drug companies) is almost always a function of such participation. Finally, the packaging of integrated medical or surgical products is also implicitly a force of industrialization. The standardization of *products* into turnkey kits imposes an obvious standardization of *process* upon surgeons, anesthesiologists, nurses, surgical technicians, and, in some cases, the entire operating room.

The main obstacle to the strategic necessity of combining products into clinically coherent portfolios is usually cultural. Of all the entrepreneurs in health care, few as a class are more fiercely independent than the engineers turned CEOs in the medical and surgical device industry. As a result, even the most logical and successful deals are often consummated via hostile takeover. J&J's purchase of Cordis involved a protracted bidding war and nasty proxy fight. Another excellent case in point has been dragging on for more than a year and a half—and drags on still, as of this writing—as US Surgical struggles to acquire Circon.

US Surgical was the pioneering and once market-leading maker of lap-surgery instruments. But J&J moved quickly into the business through its Ethicon business unit, cut prices, and aggressively promoted the breadth of its product line. Now US Surgical is locked in a fierce competitive battle with its much larger rival; its future success hinges on its ability to match J&J's product breadth and enormous marketing machinery with even greater product breadth. Circon is a perfect strategic fit. The leading niche manufacturer of the video equipment used to visualize the surgery inside the patient through the laparoscope, Circon's products are key complements to US Surgical's portfolio of lap instruments.

The deal is designed specifically to counter J&J's product integration. Leon Hirsch, US Surgical's chairman and CEO, told the *Wall Street Journal* that "everyone who uses our products uses [Circon's] products."[10] It also helped that US Surgical's bid came at a difficult time for Circon, with sales down over the previous year. Nonetheless, despite this and the fact that the combination makes tremendous strategic sense, Circon is still resisting what it considers an insufficient offer, convinced it can work through its troubles on its own. But those troubles as a stand-alone vendor in a consolidating health care system underscore the entire case for a combination of the companies. Together the two can compete against the one-stop vendors like J&J; alone, they are both vulnerable. "We think the combination of their product lines and our product lines would make an attractive merger," Hirsch reiterated to the *Wall Street Journal* six months later as the deal dragged on.[11] The combination of product lines would finally allow both companies to move beyond the status of niche vendor, offering fully integrated product lines for their provider customers.

J&J's product breadth has inspired precisely the same countering strategy for another device company, Boston Scientific. Once a niche vendor of cardiac catheters, the company embarked on an aggressive strategy of both horizontal consolidation (acquiring smaller cardiac catheter makers) and vertical consolidation (acquiring niche makers of other types of catheters and microdevices). Like J&J and US Surgical, Boston Scientific is seeking critical mass by building a broad portfolio of related products: between 1995 and 1997 it spent

$2.5 billion buying or merging with nine companies involved in catheter technologies, allowing the company to apply its core R&D and manufacturing expertise to everything ranging from angioplasty to urinary incontinence to stroke.[12]

This strategy was capped off in 1997 with the company's acquisition of Target Therapeutics for $1.1 billion.[13] Target makes tiny catheters for stroke. Because Boston Scientific had only a nominal position in this clinical domain until the deal, the combination will leverage the company's wealth of technical, managerial, and marketing resources. As reported in the *Wall Street Journal*, the deal is the "latest and largest in a long string of deals" and is fully consistent with the Boston Scientific's stated desire for "'global leadership' in the less invasive surgery market."[14]

FROM ROCKET SCIENTISTS TO ROCKET SERVICERS

Global leadership and sheer size have particular advantages as an industry matures and the strategies of its participants evolve away from product innovation to encompass more value-added services. Just such a process is at work in one fairly well-consolidated corner of the medical products industry, the manufacturers of large diagnostic equipment. The makers of CT and MRI scanning machines, large laboratory analyzers, and the like have been on the whipsaw end of the transformation of health care, as consolidating providers seek to rationalize the purchase and utilization of these very expensive pieces of capital equipment. Indeed, one of the stated goals of hospital consolidation within a market is to eliminate excess technological capacity, based on the fee-for-service principle that the presence of expensive resources compels their utilization.

The result has been a major blow to all the makers of these high-dollar technologies—who are often compared, derisively, to medical "defense" contractors feeding a "medical arms race." Sales of new diagnostic imaging equipment, excluding ultrasound, crashed between 1992 and 1995, from nearly $3.5 billion to barely over $2 billion at the low point in 1994, as managed care's cost control bug worked its way down the food chain.[15] Now, as every local health care market struggles to "rightsize" the total technology capacity scattered across multiple care settings and sites, these manufacturers are scrambling to find new ways to add value and guarantee a continued presence in the facilities.

They are doing so by adding service to their value chains. Under multivendor service and asset management programs, these suppliers service not only the equipment they have sold and installed within the health care facilities, but also the equipment of their competitors. This seemingly counterintuitive strategy has a number of critical features, all of which are necessary to the long run viability of these companies, including

- redeploying and leveraging the company's excess technical expertise idled by the market slowdown;
- galvanizing relationships with a consolidating customer base;
- offsetting revenue losses associated with the slowdown in technology purchasing; and
- inserting the vendors into the care process.

According to a report in *Modern Healthcare*, revenues from this activity have grown to between 10 and 15 percent of the typical large vendor's total, "from almost nothing 18 months ago. Manufacturers predict the offerings could exceed 40 percent of their service revenues in five years, with large health systems the primary target."[16]

Aggressive pursuit of the service business, well beyond the servicing boundaries of their own products, is the medical product supplier's equivalent of the patient wellness and education programs provided by drug manufacturers. Of critical strategic importance, this new service business includes a risk-assumption component, in the form of underwriting the operating risk of the machinery: the companies receive a fixed fee to service all of a provider system's imaging equipment with its own technical staff and subcontractors.[17]

This is not a trivial opportunity—manufacturers already control 65 percent of the $2 billion spent on maintaining imaging equipment. (The rest of the market goes to independent service companies.) Full technical service represents a much larger market opportunity, estimated at $50 billion per year.[18]

HOW RISKY IS THIS SURGERY? ABOUT $18,546 WORTH

The integration of medical and surgical products into turnkey packages is a key steppingstone to another alignment by their manufacturers with the transformation of the health care system: it allows them to engage in medical/financial risk-assumption. As with the drug companies' approaches to the same opportunity, it does not make sense for these companies to assume medical/financial risk for an entire population. Like drugs, most of these products represent only a small fraction of total health care dollars, and reversing utilization incentives would have a perverse impact on total member health care costs. Product integration does, however, open the door to risk-assumption arrangements designed to support a manufacturer's claims of superior clinical effectiveness for specific types of clinical cases.

This is the leading-edge positioning and sales strategy for a new wave of medical and surgical technology. Under a risk-based marketing program, the manufacturers put their money where their sales reps' mouths are, a strategy that will have special appeal as more and more providers assume total financial risk for their patients. A good example of this strategy for a maker of turnkey angioplasty product kits would be to provide the EHO with free kits for all clinically necessary repeat angioplasties, above a baseline rate within a specified period of time. Such risk-based marketing obviously requires good integration downstream by at-risk providers, as traditional purchasing decisions are schizophrenic affairs that involve pure clinical promotion to surgeons, a process wholly unrelated to pure price promotion to the surgical facility's purchasing managers. Such marketing will also require the mobilization of reliable information: standardized, clinically detailed data on patient conditions and complications, measured against norms and contract-related targets.

Once these hurdles are cleared, by creating financial incentives for more rational, integrated purchasing by EHOs—and by developing and using better patient information—use of a risk-based marketing strategy represents a unique opportunity for the medical or surgical products company to contribute significantly toward the health care industry's progress.

REFERENCES

1. Common saying among Silicon Valley executives and investors, as repeated in *Net Gain*, J. Hagel & A. Armstrong (Boston: Harvard Business School Press, 1997), p. 7.

2. *Cardiovascular Device Update*, published by American Health Consultants, March 1998.

3. T. Burton, "Medtronic Profit Plunges on Big Charge for Restructuring Plants, Write Down," *Wall Street Journal*, 19 February, 1998.

4. Aggregate laparoscopic and traditional cholecystectomy (ICD-9-CM 51.22 and 51.23) procedure volume, compiled in the *National Inpatient Profile* (Baltimore: HCIA Inc., 1996).

5. R. Winslow, "Hope and Hype Follow Heart-Surgery Method That's Easy on Patients," *Wall Street Journal*, 22 April, 1997.

6. Adapted and reprinted with the permission of The Free Press, a Division of Simon & Schuster from *COMPETITIVE ADVANTAGE: Creating and Sustaining Superior Performance* by Michael E. Porter. Copyright © 1985 by Michael E. Porter. p. 298.

7. Adapted and reprinted with the permission of The Free Press, a Division of Simon & Schuster from *COMPETITIVE ADVANTAGE: Creating and Sustaining Superior Performance* by Michael E. Porter. Copyright © 1985 by Michael E. Porter. p. 420.

8. R. Rundle, "Urohealth Will Buy Imagyn Medical," *Wall Street Journal*, 21 April, 1997.

9. A. Latour, "U.S. Surgical To Buy Pfizer Division," *Wall Street Journal*, 10 December, 1997.

10. S. Lipin, "U.S. Surgical Launches Takeover Bid for Rival Circon, Valued at $230 Million," *Wall Street Journal*, 2 August, 1996.

11. S. Lipin, "U.S. Surgical To Reduce its Offer for Circon Due to Target's Results," *Wall Street Journal,* 16 December, 1996.

12. L. Johannes, "Boston Scientific Agrees To Acquire Target Therapeutics for $1.1 Billion," *Wall Street Journal,* 21 January, 1997.

13. Johannes, *Wall Street Journal.*

14. Johannes, *Wall Street Journal.*

15. L. Scott, "Like House Guests Who Never Leave," *Modern Healthcare,* 2 December, 1996, 51.

16. Scott, *Modern Healthcare,* 51.

17. Scott, *Modern Healthcare,* 52.

18. Scott, *Modern Healthcare,* 52.

10

WHAT WAS AN HMO?

HMO actions designed and intended to interfere with an existing doctor/patient relationship constitute extreme and outrageous behavior exceeding all bounds usually tolerated in a civilized society.

California arbitration panel, in 1995 review of breast cancer treatment denials of Health Net members[1]

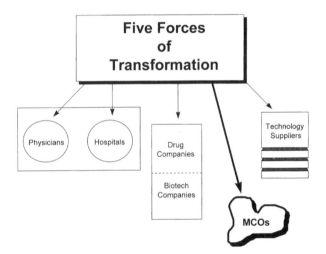

Until the revolution is complete and the fully transformed system described in *Bleeding Edge* characterizes more local health care markets than not, the bloodshed associated with this revolution will continue. The only phenomenon with the power to accelerate the inevitable passing of the traditional MCO is the panic associated with the passing of that phenomenon itself: as the last batch of Americans willing to convert to managed care does so, the MCOs will find growth opportunities increasingly scarce. Their margins will be squeezed by both the zero-sum game left in the wake of this market saturation and the emerging strength of the "substitute good" of EHO direct contracting. The result will be an increasingly embittered and adversarial relationship between the MCOs and providers, as both jockey ever more fiercely for leverage in price negotiations and the control of patient care. Such will be the final and fullest dose of medicine for a once sickly U.S. health care system nearing full recovery.

Managed care represents the last and most ruthlessly effective counterpunch to a century's worth of physician resistance to any external control or exploitation. As Starr observes, "doctors opposed corporate enterprise in medical practice not only because they wanted to preserve their autonomy, but also because they wanted to prevent the emergence of any intermediary or third party that might keep for itself the profits potentially available in the practice of medicine."[2] The emergence of those third parties was inevitable, with the MCOs their most strident form. Such stridency—this one-time shock to the system—will prove to have been a critical, transitory phenomenon in converting health care delivery from an unorganized and unpredictable enterprise into a rational system whereby providers act in the best interest not only of the patient, but also of the system's economic health.

The necessity of such a difficult, painful process is underscored by physicians' and hospitals' initial resistance to it. "Health care providers react with bewilderment, resentment, and—above all—anxiety to the numerous cost-control measures implemented by payers and policy makers in an attempt to bring health care costs under control," note Stoline and Weiner.[3] "Hospital administrators and physicians are like disturbed wasps," Lutz and Gee write, "angry and aggressive. If you want to stir up doctors in a hospital, cite the recent quarterly earnings of the local HMO."[4]

It is precisely this anger that emboldens providers to create previously unthinkable corporate entities and enter into business arrangements designed specifically to circumvent the "local MCO" and contract directly with employers and the government. In doing so, both the providers and ultimate purchaser recognize a mutual inter-dependence—one that transcends the shortsighted financial goals and petty antagonisms of classic managed care control strategies, and one that involves the long-run viability of each other's business, and the health and welfare of their common community. In doing so, they are acknowledging the essential irrelevance of the once-necessary intercession in their relationship by the MCOs. The U.S. economy is moving through a historic streamlining of distribution, a pandemic elimination of the middleman from countless purchasing equations—from catalog consumer retailing, to factory outlet stores, to direct sales of securities by companies, to Internet-based commerce. Given the comprehensiveness of this unique moment in our economic history, is it any wonder that the 20 percent of our health insurance premiums skimmed off by MCOs simply provides too easy a target for creative and ambitious people?

For the employers who are too small, unsophisticated, or un-nerved to move in this bold new direction, the purchasing coalitions in existence for more than a decade are ready and willing (if, in many cases, still not fully able) to provide the collectivization of purchasing, minus the margins, of the MCOs. As Alden Solovy, writing in *Health Care Strategic Management,* observes, "business coalitions that purchase for groups of employers will increasingly direct-contract with providers on behalf of employers, and the coalitions and providers will split the profits that have been going to HMOs."[5]

The object lesson in this process is taking place—like so much of note in the evolution of the health care system—in the leading-edge health care market of Minneapolis. In a shot heard around the health care world, in 1996 the Buyers Health Care Action Group, a coalition of Minneapolis–St. Paul employers, bypassed the local and national MCOs and contracted directly with local provider systems, through 14 agreements with hospitals, physicians, and outpatient facilities that organized into EHOs.[6] Such arrangements are the first few trickles in what will be a floodtide of direct purchasing in local markets.

The emergence of the phenomenon of direct contracting is of particular relevance to the thousands of large, self-insured employers who have avoided contracting through MCOs entirely, either because of provisions in union contracts or because of their own unwillingness to impose the rules and restrictions of managed care on their employees and dependents. Such companies are poised to leapfrog the MCO phenomenon entirely, moving from self-managed indemnity insurance to direct contracts with the EHOs. An excellent example of this process is the experience of General Motors (GM). Because of the richness of the benefit package won by union negotiators over the years, GM is obligated to provide its employees, dependents, and retirees with the richest flavor of health coverage—an open-ended, traditional indemnity plan. As a result, the company—which has bypassed the managed care system entirely—is working directly with providers to streamline, rationalize, and optimize the medical services delivered to its beneficiaries. Through such activity GM is acting precisely like MCOs claim to act, but with the longest of long-term financial self-interest in mind: preserving the lifelong health of their population of employees, dependents, and retirees.

A titan of the processes of industrialization in its core business for decades, GM is thus contributing significantly to the industrialization of health care described in this book. GM is also setting a key example for all other employers, either directly or via coalitions, to work in partnerships with providers rather than passively through managed care intermediaries. In the process, according to a *Wall Street Journal* report, through their direct work with providers such companies are "creating their own *de facto* managed care system, which ultimately could squeeze out insurers altogether."[7]

THE PARADOX OF PROFITABILITY

Of all the paradoxes in the brave new world of health care, none will prove greater than the ultimately self-defeating nature of its profitability. Indeed, there is little in the delivery of medicine at the local level that will drive down health care profits faster than the full emergence of for-profit medicine. In the typical health care market of today, there are too many competing entities; it is too easy to develop substitute financing goods; there is too much capacity; consumers have too much mobility; and there is too much information about costs, profits, and quality for highly profitable arrangements to persist for long.

Such is the end result of the introduction of competition into the delivery of health care via risk-assumption, consumerism, and industrialization: the health care system starts to look like any other industry, only in overdrive. As Porter points out, "competition in an industry continually works to drive down the rate of return on invested capital toward the competitive floor rate of return. This competitive floor, or 'free market' return, is approximated by the yield on long-term government securities adjusted upward by the risk of capital loss."[8] As such, the dominant model of health care delivery in the new century's health care system will regulate its own profits far more effectively than any government-controlled pricing strategy or regulatory apparatus.

The high level of MCO profits through 1996—followed by their sudden nosedive in 1997—describe perfectly this historic arc. In 1997, price competition continued to drive down premiums while medical costs continued to track with the rate of general inflation. As in most things in health care, California led the way. For the largest employers for the typical California MCO, 1996 premiums dropped 3 to 7 percent from 1995 levels.[9] As a demonstration of the fluidity of the marketplace, those MCOs that did not acquiesce on price paid for it with immediate limits on membership gains: according to a Wall Street analyst report, because of pricing discipline, HSI "suffered serious erosion in market share."[10] This was followed quickly by the larger national MCOs. As a result of their inevitable earnings' shortfalls, stocks in bellwether MCO plans United Healthcare, PacifiCare, and Oxford plummeted in mid-1997 due to unforeseen increases in medical costs amidst aggressive pricing strategies.[11] (The size of Oxford's hit outpaced the group because of special operations problems.) This is typical for the industry at large as premiums for the median MCO across the United States, adjusted for inflation, fell from 1994 through 1996.

This profitability arc underscores the generally transitional nature of the MCO phenomenon itself. National MCOs represent the creation of a new industry, formed specifically to rationalize one of the oldest nonindustries. The risk/reward profile generated by this moment in economic history attracted significant capital, worked to achieve the goals of the new industry, and accelerated its own erosion under the imminent maturation and passing of the process. The profitability soar-and-swoon of the 1980 to mid-1990s mirrors that of any other new and revolutionary industry: the oil companies and railroads in the 19th century, steelmakers in the first part of the 20th, computer manufacturers in 1970s and 1980s, and the networking equipment makers of today. Relative to these larger industrial cycles, the national for-profit MCO will prove to be the Betamax in the long, slow rationalization of the U.S. health care system—a good first stab at the technology, but not the eventual standard.

The temporary profitability of today's for-profit MCOs contrasts sharply with the social reform-oriented generation of nonprofit MCOs in the 1970s, which spent 94 percent of premiums of medical care. By the 1990s, this held steady around 90 percent for the nonprofits, but had fallen into the 70 to 80 percent range for the for-profits.[12] Why this tiering of the MCO world? Because the for-profits proved to be much more aggressive marketers and were flush with the capital—and the cultures to leverage that capital—to develop ever more strenuous systems for controlling costs and achieving economies of scale. Such "reforms" are a one-time event: even the not-for-profits can quickly and easily ape those "ever more strenuous systems," applying the very same tools developed through the higher risk/reward mechanism of the for-profit MCOs.

THE UNDERWRITING CYCLE: DEJA VU ALL OVER AGAIN

The MCO pricing problems described above represent history repeating itself. For decades, students of the health insurance industry have identified and tracked a phenomenon known as the "insurance underwriting cycle." The cycle involves the influx of new firms and underwriting capacity attracted by two to four years of profitability; this in turn creates two to four years of losses as the new competition holds premium increases below related increases in claims costs. These losses in turn shake out the weakest competitors and drive away many of the stronger ones, allowing for the next cycle of gains in subsequent years as insurers restructure, consolidate, and increase premiums against stabilizing claims costs.[13] This cycle affects *all* realms of underwriting, not just medical insurance.

In the 1990s, MCOs appear to have developed their own shortened version of this classic underwriting cycle. Indeed, the managed care industry's reaction to losses in 1996 was typical of the dynamics of the cycle: according to a report in *Medicine & Health*, "faced with shrinking margins and slumping stock prices, HMO executives are talking more these days about premium increases, benefit rollbacks, and exiting unprofitable markets as the way to deal with medical-loss ratios."[14] In the same report, *Medicine & Health* anticipates premium increases of 3 to 6 percent in 1997 in several markets.[15] This is consistent with the 2.5 percent uptick in premiums in the 1996 edition of the annual Foster Higgins survey.

While still lower than inflation, this is significant following an actual decline in premium costs, adjusted for inflation in 1995. In a report on the survey's findings in the *Wall Street Journal*, Joseph Sebastianelli, president of Aetna, noted that "after two years of flat or declining insurance premiums, 'there is a catch-up period' that must occur."[16] This "catch-up period" is the underwriting cycle incarnate. The fact that it is now turning on the short side of the normal two-to-four year period underscores the volatility of the MCO version of this phenomenon. It also indicates that the MCOs and other insurers may not have endured the full shake-out necessary for the market to sustain the uptick in premiums, especially in light of the emergence of the substitute good of direct contracting with lower profit needs and thus lower prices.

How long will the MCO version of the underwriting cycle play itself out? Perhaps not long at all, if the antidote—as with the

MCOs' historic displacement of indemnity insurance—turns out to be substitutes. If so, then the cycle is not a cycle at all, but a major realignment of market pricing. Were there no substitute good poised to siphon away market share, the 1994 to 1996 trough in premiums would represent the standard shift-to-upswing in the classic underwriting cycle. But the sudden presence of the direct-contracting EHOs inevitably will exert market pressure on the MCOs as they attempt to raise prices.

For the MCOs, the only alternative to raising prices—and thus losing market share to the EHOs—is no alternative at all: exert even greater cost-management pressure on patients and providers. This position represents a competitive impossibility, one aptly described by James Moore in *The Death of Competition*: "cutthroat competition between HMOs led companies to slash their prices to well below not only their current costs, but below any responsible cost projection...This sort of wildly unmanaged and ruthless competition among managed care ecosystems virtually assures the economic implosion of some of these networks, or else deplorable skimping on care."[17]

Over time, such price wars will drive all MCO net margins to zero. In the meanwhile, managed care will stave off the inevitable only through continued consolidation. Large national mergers and other tactics will become less strategic in the end; rather, they will be pursued exclusively and specifically to delay the shake-out at the end of the MCO's own foreshortened version of the classic health insurance underwriting cycle.

PROVIDERS' LAST LAUGH

In the past, the MCOs have been able to pass their underwriting pain along to providers. As Scott MacStravic observes in *Health Care Strategic Management*, "where MCOs themselves engage in price wars, they tend to pass on the price pressure to providers. Even after signing contracts...MCOs have come back with demands that providers lower their rates in the face of lower premium offers by the

MCOs' competitors."[18] Fortified by their consolidation into EHOs, providers will finally be able to push back.

The idea that providers will be more ably positioned to do so as EHOs—and thus stand to gain more sustainable market acceptance than MCOs—underscores a simple fact about managed care: it never truly realized its vision as an industry, nor was much strategic vision ever manifest with most of the individual MCOs. In their obsession with managing costs rather than truly managing care, the MCOs have fallen victim to a syndrome Porter recognizes as a broader affliction of numerous U.S. companies and whole industries during the past decade. In an incisive, contrarian 1996 *Harvard Business Review* article that borders on scolding, Porter argues that companies have confused operational effectiveness with vision: "almost imperceptibly, management tools have taken the place of strategy."[19] According to Porter, "driven by performance pressures but lacking strategic vision, company after company has had no better idea than to buy up its rivals…the result is zero-sum competition, static or declining prices, and pressures on costs that compromise companies' ability to invest in the business in the long term."[20]

While Porter is describing much of American business in general—or at least its low-growth, traditional sectors—this is an incisive description of precisely the cannibalism and lack of vision that has characterized most MCOs over the past few years. The only truly noteworthy exceptions to this rule—Oxford, Harvard Pilgrim Health Care, Kaiser, PacifiCare, and United—are characterized by the stark fact of their noteworthiness.[21] These organizations are exceptions in every sense of the word and, most tellingly, can be counted on one hand.

Much of the failure to realize the collective vision of managed care may prove to have been beyond the control of the plans themselves. Developing real business strategies, differentiating themselves, and creating sustainable competitive advantages—all the while making money quarter after quarter—is probably an impossible undertaking in the brief, tumultuous revolution that they themselves brought to health care. Under these conditions, as the typical

MCO's membership turns over 20 percent every year—and as new substitute goods (i.e., PPOs, EPOs, point-of-service HMOs, EHOs, etc.) are introduced as frequently—the typical MCO has had little choice but to obsess over operational effectiveness.

Such "effectiveness" however will prove to be the MCOs' own worst enemy: when all the window dressing is taken down, effectiveness for the MCO struggling to compete and grow means effectiveness at holding down costs and utilization, which translates to ever greater pressure on providers and members. This pressure will become increasingly important (and self-defeating) given the only populations still left for the MCOs to capture: the poor on Medicaid, the elderly and disabled on Medicare, and the "indemnity holdouts"—all those privately insured individuals who have been the most reluctant to join managed care until now.

Of course, imminent legislation that imposed legal accountability on MCOs for their meddling in the care process may make all of this moot. In 1997 numerous bills were introduced into state legislatures and Congress that would hold MCOs liable for medical malpractice, if their refusal to authorize care was tantamount to negligence.[22] So much for having your cake and eating it too. Absent such laws, MCOs have been able to direct physicians' clinical decision making, but at the same time be immune from lawsuits when those directions go awry.

HEALTH MAINTENANCE, NOT MENDING ORGANIZATION

While legal liability for its medical decisions may seem like the MCOs' worst nightmare, this will be nothing compared to their experiences with the "late adopters" of managed care—the poor, elderly, and the indemnity holdouts. Because of the preponderance of chronic medical conditions and sociomedical pathologies within their ranks, the unusual complexity of managing their health, or their simple collective spirit of self-determination in health care matters, these groups have either not had access to—or have outwardly resisted—managed care until the bloody end. These final waves of new members will be far more likely to be sick; they will be the most expensive members to serve in general; and they will be the most resistant to any and all attempts at management and control. These are the worst members for MCOs, not only from an economic standpoint, but from a medical management standpoint as well.

The sickest among these new waves of people will conjure up the MCOs' fundamental fatal flaw: managed care focuses on effective maintenance of health, rather than on effective treatment of the sick. The impact of this effectiveness eventually finds a point of diminishing returns among the healthy; among the sick—who constitute the bulk of the medical loss ratio—such effectiveness has only marginal value, if any. This is another paradox in the economics of MCOs, one that few recognized in their lemminglike rush to manage asthma, lower back pain, depression, and other broadly populated but relatively low-cost chronic conditions through high-profile "disease management" programs. In contrast to the members targeted by these programs, the truly sickest portion of an insured population offers an MCO the greatest leverage in terms of return on investment and medical management effectiveness. MCOs generally respond to this phenomenon not with sophisticated medical management, but rather with ham-fisted attempts to restrict rather than optimize their care.

The end result of managed care's market saturation problem is the inevitable onslaught of precisely these kinds of expensive cases. The medieval methods used for dealing with them will surely backfire with enormous lawsuits and the worst kind of public relations. Why? Because underwriting the costs associated with the rare but costly catastrophe is the whole point of group insurance, a principle that drives all the most basic law of insurance risk–pool economics. The MCOs never internalized this concept, instead focusing their efforts on incremental improvements in the health of most members while begrudgingly micromanaging the care delivered to high-cost members.

In his harsh critique of the managed care industry, *Health against Wealth*, George Anders refers to this phenomenon as the "strangely lopsided picture of medical care, filled with healthy patients getting check-ups but devoid of anyone fighting a serious illness."[23] Anders points out that this disconnect is built into the only major and sustained effort by the managed care industry to analyze its own performance, an exercise in data gathering and analysis called the "Healthplan Evaluation Data and Information Set (HEDIS)." "By the yardsticks of HEDIS," he writes, "a health plan could achieve a fine score without having the least ability to deliver good care in a crisis."[24] This is highly problematic for MCOs in general: a scant 1 percent of a covered population represents more than 30 percent of its total medical costs.[25]

This economic reality will prove highly lethal to the typical MCO as it starts insuring older, poorer, sicker members. With the elderly population, in particular, the tough economics of illness spread widely and rapidly, as a greater proportion of these populations fall victim to ever costlier diseases: 90 percent of Medicare beneficiaries incurred bills of just $1,430 each in 1993, while the other 10 percent had average bills of $28,000 each.[26] This skewing is the source of the enrollment bias seen for HMO patients in study after study. One such study, published in the *New England Journal of Medicine*, found that inpatient hospitalization rates for Medicare beneficiaries enrolling in HMOs was only 66 percent of rates for the traditional fee-for-service group; those who disenrolled from the HMOs had 180 percent higher hospitalizations while in the HMO than the fee-for-service group.[27] This means that HMOs have been particularly good at attracting healthier seniors—and driving out unhealthy ones.

The days of such enrollment bias, as the market saturates, are coming to a close. Managed care is ill-prepared for this challenge, as the traditional MCO has focused not on treating the very sick, but rather on keeping the healthy from becoming so. By contrast, the traditional provider has always focused on the very sick. Following the money under a hundred years of fee-for-service medicine, the medical and hospital communities have dedicated the bulk of their technical resources, basic research, process development, and training efforts on interventions for the sickest, most costly patients in society. Given these very different historical orientations and the intractable skewing of disease and dollars in the population, which group seems better positioned—the MCOs or the providers—to assume and manage the risks associated with disease and triumph in the end?

WHAT NEXT?

Change is the only constant in today's health care system. As demonstrated throughout this book, nothing changes faster than the economics of care delivery following corrections in the way providers are organized and paid. As the MCOs' cost advantages eventually crumble alongside the aggressive marketing of these corrections—as embodied in the mature-stage EHOs—the only thing sustaining MCOs will be their incumbency, their marketing presence, and their ownership of lives. MCOs' relationships with benefits consultants and corporate purchasers will make them difficult to dislodge—even though their competitiveness on price, in the end, will be sustainable only through increasingly brutal methods of cost-control. But despite the often torturous, bureaucratic decision making and market lags associated with annual benefits purchasing, such incumbency eventually wears out. Too many dollars and too many lives are at stake.

Given the inevitable unsustainability of the MCOs as currently marketed and managed, their only possible recourse is true innovation. As they provided a harsh, but necessary fix for much that was wrong with the health care system, the visionaries in the managed care industry may well be able to replicate this relevance through the development and distribution of tools that truly *manage care*. Such tools can range from care automation processes like telephonic triage, to useful chronic disease management programs with midterm, measurable benefits, to catastrophic or end-of-life case management systems. In this last regard, the MCOs culture of care denial actually helps patients: they have proven adept at restricting the use of heroic but ultimately futile interventions at the end of patients' lives. A study found that Medicare patients hospitalized in intensive care units (ICUs) were 25 percent less likely to undergo aggressive, expensive treatment destined not to work. And such restrictions did not have an impact on acute mortality rates for the two studied groups.[28]

Beyond these few clinical spheres that actually benefit from aggressive case management, what is left behind for the MCOs to manage may be nothing more than information: normative clinical and financial databases, analytical services, and informatics products they can market to the fully at-risk EHOs. To this end, the survival instinct of the MCO would compel a mutation from insurers and managers of care to vendors of care management systems and other tools that embody medical management intellectual property.

The rudiments of such future opportunities are embedded in the better MCOs' current organizations. The most progressive of them have developed clinically rich, useful tools for identifying and managing the medical risks of covered individuals. They have coupled these with empirically driven information systems that empower physicians with meaningful feedback, with the goal of practicing better medicine. As Anders reports on physician experiences with a certain MCO, it "did best when it could interest physicians themselves in analyzing their processes for handling common illnesses and making their own systems work better."[29] The aggressive development and marketing of such tools today—while designed to manage more effectively their own medical loss ratios, providers, and populations—will offer MCOs the opportunity to survive and thrive as transformed businesses over the long run. They will also allow the MCOs, in the short run, to provide more than lip service about the quality of care they currently manage.

This eventual role will dovetail perfectly with the other roles outlined previously regarding the Post-MCO (P-MCO). While the high costs associated with the sickest patients have helped doom the classic MCO model and will pose serious challenges to the EHOs, they also represent a significant business opportunity for the P-MCO: reinsurance coupled with catastrophic case management. This integrated product offering would provide an excellent value-add to the relationship between the EHO and the P-MCO. In effect, members are insured and cared for locally by EHOs who, as defined, have sufficient medical capacity as providers but restricted financial capacity as local insurers. Through this arrangement, the sickest members fall into large national reinsurance pools, and ultimately are insured by the national P-MCOs.

The quality of case management attached to their reinsurance business will ultimately drive the underwriting and financial success of the P-MCO. Those good at it will make more money, be able to price more aggressively, and—through a unique combination of two previously irreconcilable cost and care management competencies—garner market favor. The EHOs in this situation will thus be allowed to leverage the strengths inherent in their unique positioning as locally based insurer/provider and focus on what they are best equipped to do: deliver cost-effective medical care to their communities.

Driving this final divergence between what are today national payers and local providers is the assumption of day-to-day medical risk by those providers—a complete blurring of medical practice with the provision of medical insurance. This represents a historic correction to a decades-long disconnect in the U.S. health care system, created and compelled by physicians themselves. As Starr points out, in the early part of the 20th century health care reformers viewed health insurance as "an opportunity to subordinate medical practice to public health, to encourage the growth of group practice, and to change the method of payment from fee-for-service to salary or capitation...These changes the doctors would not accept."[30] Everything these reformers wanted—and that a subsequent generation of reformers wanted out of health insurance in the 1930s—they are now getting in a health care system almost a century later: providers rewarded financially for prevention, a kind of "privatized" public health; the consolidation of providers into ever-larger groups; and the conversion of payment from fee-for-service to capitation.

The difference between then and now? In the closing decades of the 20th century, we have witnessed a violent chain reaction across the health care system, one wrought by too many years of runaway medical inflation and the consequent task-mastering of the system under managed care. The impact of this chain reaction is less a power shift away from providers than an intensive exercise in behavior modification of those providers due to the temporary, partial shift of power to managed care. Providers will eventually succumb to this modification, if only because they recognize within managed care the seeds of an even more harshly disciplined system.

A fuller grasp of what is good and achievable in all of this is far more encouraging. Providers with that grasp will be fully prepared not only to accept and effect the critical changes the system needs over the long run, but will be *eager* to do so—if only because they will be the ones dictating the terms of those changes. In this, the self-determination of the physician class—the driving force behind much of the development of medical care over the past century—is emerging yet again as the driving force behind the system's transformation going into the new century.

REFERENCES

1. California Arbitration Panel, 1995, in review of treatment denial of Health Net breast cancer patients Nelene Fox, Christine DeMeurers, and Janice Bosworth, as reported in G. Anders, *Health against Wealth* (New York: Houghton Mifflin, 1996), 131.

2. P. Starr, *The Social Transformation of American Medicine* (New York: Basic Books/HarperCollins, 1982), 215–216.

3. A.M. Stoline and J.P. Weiner, *The New Medical Marketplace: A Physician's Guide to the Health Care System in the 1990s* (Baltimore: The Johns Hopkins University Press, 1993), ix. © 1993. The Johns Hopkins University Press.

4. S. Lutz and E.P. Gee, *The For-Profit Healthcare Revolution* (Chicago: Irwin Professional Publishing, 1995), 160.

5. A. Solovy, "Strategic Forecast 1996," paraphrased in "Consultant's Corner," *Health Care Strategic Management,* April 1996, 16.

6. K. Pallarito, "Babes in Managed Care Land," *Modern Healthcare*, 18 November, 1996.

7. R. Blumenstein, "Auto Makers Attack High Health-Care Bills with a New Approach," *Wall Street Journal*, 9 December, 1996.

8. Adapted and reprinted with the permission of The Free Press, a Division of Simon & Schuster from *COMPETITIVE STRATEGY: Techniques for Analyzing Industries and Competitors* by Michael E. Porter. Copyright © 1980 by The Free Press. p. 5.

9. A research report on Health Systems International, Volpe, Welty & Company, 22 July, 1996, 6.

10. A research report on Health Systems International, Volpe, Welty & Company, 22 July, 1996, 7.

11. A research report on Healthsource by Alex. Brown & Sons, Baltimore, 30 July, 1996, 1.

12. G. Anders, *Health against Wealth* (New York: Houghton Mifflin, 1996), 62.

13. "Do Blues Losses Signal Return of Insurance Underwriting Cycle?" *Medicine & Health*, 14 October, 1996, 2.

14. "Bargains on MCO Coverage—Get 'em While They Last," *Medicine & Health*, 16 December, 1996.

15. "Bargains on MCO Coverage—Get 'em While They Last," *Medicine & Health*, 16 December, 1996.

16. R. Winslow, "Health Care Costs May Be Heading Up Again," *Wall Street Journal*, 21 January, 1997.

17. J.F. Moore, *The Death of Competition* (New York: HarperCollins Publishers, 1996), 248.

18. S. MacStravic, "Price Wars Are No-Win Games for Health Care Systems," *Health Care Strategic Management,* May 1996, 19.

19. M. Porter, "What Is Strategy?" *Harvard Business Review*, November/December 1996, 61.

20. Porter, *Harvard Business Review,* 64.

21. These are based on personal observations of the level of medical management innovation demonstrated by these few MCOs, in comparison to their 500+ brethren, gathered in my work with MCOs while at HCIA Inc. Such innovations are embodied in the types of medical informatics systems HCIA and its competitors build for MCOs; these involve patient health status monitoring, risk screening, outcomes measurement, and clinical performance-based compensation for network providers. Only the handful listed were actively investing in these systems, though they were readily available to all MCOs.

22. L. McGinley, "Broad Battle To End HMOs' Limited Liability for Treatment-Coverage Denials Gains Steam," *Wall Street Journal*, 12 January, 1997.

23. Anders, *Health against Wealth*, 41.

24. Anders, *Health against Wealth*, 41.

25. Proprietary market research data developed by Franklin Health, Inc., a medical management company that provides catastrophic case management services to indemnity insurers, self-insured employers, and MCOs.

26. Anders, *Health against Wealth*, 176–177.

27. R. Morgan et al., "The Medicare-HMO Revolving Door——the Healthy Go In and the Sick Go Out," *New England Journal of Medicine* 337, no. 3 (1997): 169.

28. L. Lenert et al., *Journal of the American Medical Association*, 24 September, 1997.

29. Anders, *Health against Wealth*, 43.

30. Starr, *The Social Transformation of American Medicine,* 247.

SELECTED
BIBLIOGRAPHY

Anders, G. 1996. *Health against wealth*. Boston: Houghton Mifflin.

Brandenburger, A.M., and B. Nalebuff. 1996. *Co-opetition*. New York: Currency Doubleday.

Brown, M., ed. 1996. *Integrated health care delivery: Theory, practice, evaluation, and prognosis*. Gaithersburg, MD: Aspen Publishers.

Cassell, E. 1997. *Doctoring: The nature of primary care medicine*. New York: Oxford University Press.

Chandler, Jr., A.D. 1977. *The visible hand: The managerial revolution in American business*. Cambridge, MA: Harvard University Press.

Clayman, C.B., ed. 1989. *The American Medical Association encyclopedia of medicine*. New York: Random House.

Coddington, D.C. et al. 1996. *Making integrated health care work*. Englewood, CO: Center for Research in Ambulatory Health Care Administration.

Deming, W.E. 1986. *Out of the crisis*. Cambridge, MA: MIT Center for Advanced Engineering Study.

Flitter, M. 1997. *Judith's Pavilion: The haunting memories of a neurosurgeon*. South Royalton, VT: Steerforth Press.

Herzlinger, R. 1997. *Market-driven health care: Who wins, who loses in the transformation of America's largest service industry*. Reading, MA: Addison-Wesley Publishing Co.

Lutz, S., and E.P. Gee. 1995. *The for-profit healthcare revolution.* Chicago: Irwin Professional Publishing.

Millenson, M. 1997. *Demanding medical excellence: Doctors and accountability in the information age.* Chicago: The University of Chicago Press.

Moore, J.F. 1996. *The death of competition.* New York: HarperCollins Publishers.

Nuland, S.B. 1997. *The wisdom of the body.* New York: Alfred A. Knopf.

Porter, M.E. 1985. *Competitive advantage.* New York: Free Press.

Porter, M.E. 1980. *Competitive strategy.* New York: Free Press.

Rognehaugh, R. 1996. *The managed health care dictionary.* Gaithersburg, MD: Aspen Publishers.

Starr, P. 1982. *The social transformation of American medicine.* New York: Basic Books/HarperCollins.

Stoline, A.M., and J.P. Weiner. 1993. *The new medical marketplace: A physician's guide to the health care system in the 1990s.* Baltimore: The Johns Hopkins University Press.

Wennberg, J.E., and M. McAndrew Cooper, eds. 1996. *The Dartmouth atlas of health care in the United States.* Chicago: American Hospital Publishing.

ACKNOWLEDGMENTS

The observations, analysis, and begrudging optimism expressed in this book all flow from countless interactions with physicians, entrepreneurs, researchers, executives, allied health professionals, economists, attorneys—and the occasional iconoclast in the clinical and administrative trenches—during my first 10 years of work in the health care system. Without their insights, instruction, and commitment to making that system work better, I would have neither the understanding nor inspiration to rage at or lead cheers for the past, present, and future of our industry.

First, I wish to acknowledge the entrepreneur with the vision and courage to create and build a company that would afford me a rarefied vantage point for studying the health care system—above its political fray but neck-deep in its business problems. George Pillari of HCIA is a corporate Renaissance man in an era of technocratic CEOs: aggressive, literate, and passionate, at once a hardheaded number-cruncher, reflective man of letters, and consummate deal maker. Over many years and many hard miles, he has been a vigorous champion of my work, incisive editor, tough coach, and friend.

Next, I would like to express my profound appreciation and admiration for Kathleen Ford, my research assistant, editor, and graphic artist. As talented, resourceful, and thorough as she is patient, she has been crucial to the final assemblage of this book. Her skill with the language is my constant insurance against professional disaster, making her indispensable to the success of both *Bleeding Edge* and the more recent chapters of my career.

I would also like to acknowledge a few of the many talented people involved with HCIA over the years who have contributed to my understanding of the health care system and the realities of management: Jean Chenoweth; Taylor Dennen, PhD; James Dewey, PhD.; Henry Dove, PhD; David Foster, PhD; Donald Good; Ray Hanley; Tom Hutchinson; Phillip Lassiter; Tim Madden; Daniel Malloy, PhD; Catherine McCabe; Peg Molloy; John Morrow; Barry Offutt; Ralph Perfetto; Kurt Price; Steven Renn, JD; Sean Riley; John Robison; Mark Rogers, MD; David Rollo, MD; Carl Schramm, PhD; Leora Simantov, JD; Cherise Skeba; Theresa Whitmarsh; and Mark Williard.

At the risk of offending those I have worked with and cannot recall at the tail-end of my first 10 years in health care, I would like to acknowledge the contributions to my learning of those I *can* recall: Paul Epner of Abbott Laboratories; Michael Hoover of Actamed; Arthur Benvenuto and Jana Stoudemire of Advanced Tissue Sciences; Kelly Seither of ALZA Corporation; Robert Attila, Thomas Hardy, PhD, and Melanie Call of Amgen; Peter Lancer of Ancilla Health System; Robert Goldberg, PhD, of Brandeis University; Ann Gallo of BT Alex Brown; Timothy Cost and Richard McCloskey, MD, of Centocor; Neal Patterson and Tom Tinstman, MD, of Cerner Corporation; Kaylor Schemberger of Chandler Regional Hospital; Robert Riley of Chesapeake Medi-Tech; Allen Schaffer, MD, and Victor Villagra, MD, of Cigna Healthcare; Tracy LaBonte of Cigna Reinsurance; Alan Shusterman, MD, of CMG Health; Richard Scott, David Manning, and Herbert Wong, PhD, formerly of Columbia/HCA; Michael Hamilton of Ernst & Young; David Levy, MD, William Thar, MD, and Tom Hagan of Franklin Health; Henri Termeer and Dawn Renear of Genzyme Corporation; Hal Prink of the Healthcare Financial Management Association; Khahn Nguyen of HealthOne; Chris Umstadt of Johns Hopkins Healthcare; Gerald Anderson, PhD, and Earl Steinberg, MD, of the Johns Hopkins University; Simon Cohn, MD, and Allan Khoury, MD, of Kaiser; Michael Dalby and David Mahonney of McKesson; John Iglehart of the *New England Journal of Medicine* and *Health Affairs*; John Ware, PhD, of the New England Medical Center; Connie Perla of Novartis; Justin Edge of the *Opinion Research Corporation International*; James Richter of Oxford Health Plans; Sam Ho, MD, of PacifiCare; Jennifer Doebler, Paul Jeffrey, Mauri Rosenthal, and George Tsugranes of Pfizer; Gerry Oster, PhD, of Policy Analysis, Inc.; Tom Heimsoth and Steve Clements of RIMS; Sister Maria Verkhooven of Saint Joseph's Memorial Hospital; Bernard Salick, MD, and Michael Fiore of Salick Health Care; James Kean of Sapient Health Network; Phillip DeLoache, Susan Hahn, Jack Kent, Suzanne Reynolds, and Steven Sharfstein, MD, of Sheppard Pratt Health System; Spyros Stavrakos, PhD, and Vijay Aggarwal, PhD, of SmithKline Beecham; Susan Alt and Donald Johnson of The Business Word; Patricia Flannery of United Healthcare; Sherry Perkins, PhD, of the University of Maryland Medical System; Tom Emerick of Wal-Mart; Tom Elkin of Western Health Advantage; and David Jackson, PhD, Bruce Marsden, and Michael Millenson of William M. Mercer.

I would especially like to acknowledge the many substantive contributions to my learning of those who happily crossed the line from colleague to friend: David Perkins of Amgen; Kelli Back, JD, attorney and lobbyist; Mauri Okamoto-Kearney of Genentech; Carrie Walton of Healthway; Shannon Burke, Sarah Loughran, Kevin Metz, JD, Betsy Mirachi, and John McGready, formerly of HCIA; Marcos Monheit of Integrated Health Services; Chris Bartel of J.H. Whitney; Robin Platts of the Knott Foundation; Carolyn Luther of Montgomery Securities; Alexander Ford of Pfizer; Kevin Carnell, JD, of RCM&D; Bobbie Becker of the health products division of W.L. Gore & Associates; and Sandy Faust of United Behavioral Health Care.

I would like to thank the many reporters and editors I have worked with over the years, especially Thomas Donlan of *Barron's*; Keith Hammonds of *Business Week*; Gloria Lau of *Forbes*; Donald Metz and Andrea Zuercher of *Health Affairs*; Sylvia Fubini, PhD, of *Health Care Trends Report*; Scott Gottlieb, MD, of *JAMA*; Tim Troy and Tracey Walker of *Managed Healthcare*; Lisa Scott of *Modern Healthcare*; Milton Freudenheim of the *New York Times*; George Anders, Thomas Burton, Helene Cooper, Laura Johannes, Laurie McGinley, Allen Murray, Barbara Phillips, and Ron Winslow of the *Wall Street Journal*; and David Hilzenrath of the *Washington Post.* The surgical precision of your editing—or ruthlessness of your questions—has exorcised more false assumptions and sloppy thinking than I care to admit.

I would also like to acknowledge the tremendous contributions—unbeknownst to them until it came time for me to seek permission to use their work—of Paul Starr and Michael Porter. Starr's Pulitzer Prize–winning *The Social Transformation of American Medicine*, which I cite throughout this book, is a masterful history of the complex power struggles that coalesced into the modern U.S. health care system; it is detailed, profound, occasionally wry, ruthlessly nonpartisan, and always insightful; it is required reading for anyone interested in why the health care system is so complicated, paradoxical, and unyielding to easy fixes. Porter's *Competitive Strategy* and *Competitive Advantage* are groundbreaking, definitive works on corporate strategic analysis, industry structure, and the dynamic interplay of competing firms. Unlike almost all business books, Porter's are *not* of the moment: they are expansive, penetrating, crystalline, brilliantly rendered, and universally applicable to all companies in all industries in the modern era; they have stood the test of time and will continue to do so for the duration of human commerce; they are required reading for anyone involved in corporate management. Starr's and Porter's work comprises the twin pillars of my own. Without their efforts, mine would be a shambles.

I would also like to thank Mark Decker and Pam Williams, PhD, of the Johns Hopkins University for helping me craft the rudiments of this book into an acceptable graduate research project. They were both incredulous at my ambition from the outset and, I believe, are even more incredulous at its outcome.

I would like to thank Mike Brown, Jennifer Barnes-Eliot, Sandy Cannon, Kalen Conerly, Denise Coursey, Cynthia Lefton, and all the other talented people at Aspen Publishers for bringing my book to life so quickly and with such great care.

Special thanks to Suzan Westervelt, who introduced me to my first health care clients when I was still a toddler of a business writer and consultant; to Donalda King, for her strength, humor, and encouragement in those early, difficult, necessary years, and good wishes since; and to my parents, who taught me a fierce love for the power and grace of the language—a love that has proven essential to my professional successes and personal joys.

I wish to thank my tremendous friends in the physician community for keeping me honest about the realities and limitations of my theories: Joshua Blum, MD; Karen Chacko, MD; George Thomas Grace, MD; Meg Lemon, MD; Erik Mont, MD; Steven O'Brien, MD; Mara Rabin, MD; Kevin Shilling, MD; and Michelle Thomas, MD. To their ranks I would add a friend I have yet to meet: Marc Flitter, MD. I discovered his memoir, *Judith's Pavilion*, while struggling with the second rewrite of *Bleeding Edge*. Flitter's confessional is a moving, lyrical, and passionate journey through the inner dramas and sorrows of medical practice; I stumbled upon it—perhaps not accidentally—as a reminder of all the weary hearts beating just beyond the bleeding edge.

Finally, I would like to acknowledge those who personally sustained me through the struggles of this book, my work at HCIA, completion of a graduate degree, and a major personal challenge, all within a tumultuous two-year period: Sachi Morishige, for believing in this book before I did and never letting me back off from it; Brian Buchanan, Craig Havighurst, Donna Williams, Sally Armbruster, Dan Heneghan, and Kathy Goodman, for making me laugh when I was not able; Christine Yang, MD, my soulmate, playmate, and daily inspiration; and my brother Steve and sisters Betsy and Mara, for giving me the strength, scolding, and love to carry on.

INDEX

ABOUT THE AUTHOR

J.D. Kleinke is a health care executive, medical economist, and author. As a member of the editorial board of *Health Affairs* and frequent contributor to the *Wall Street Journal*, he has been a provocative voice in the most important debate in the history of the U.S. health care system: the promises and pitfalls of market-driven reform. His work has also appeared in *JAMA, Barron's, Modern Healthcare, Business & Health, Managed Healthcare, Health Affairs*, and *Compensation & Benefits Management*.

Between 1992 and 1998, Kleinke was a principal architect in the transformation of HCIA from a niche health care data analysis firm to a publicly traded provider of information systems and products to health care systems, managed care organizations, and pharmaceutical companies across the United States and Europe. During his tenure with HCIA, Kleinke spearheaded its product and market development efforts; established the company's pharmaceutical research business; and created codevelopment and marketing alliances with corporate business partners. He also directed HCIA's analyses of the impact of changing clinical practices on the U.S. health care economy.

Prior to joining HCIA, Kleinke was director of corporate programs at Sheppard Pratt Health System, the largest private psychiatric hospital in the United States. While at Sheppard Pratt, Kleinke developed and managed the nation's first provider-based, managed behavioral health care delivery system.

Kleinke holds an MSB in finance from Johns Hopkins University and a BS in economics from the University of Maryland. He lives in Denver, Colorado, and can be reached at http://www.hs-net.com.